AF675781

Atlas of Genital Dermoscopy

Series in Dermatological Treatment

About the Series
Published in association with the *Journal of Dermatological Treatment*, the *Series in Dermatological Treatment* keeps readers up to date with the latest clinical therapies to improve problems with the skin, hair, and nails. Each volume in the series is prepared separately and typically focuses on a topical theme. Volumes are published on an occasional basis, depending on the emergence of new developments.

Atlas of Genital Dermoscopy
Edited by: Giuseppe Micali and Francesco Lacarrubba

Dermatology and Solid Organ Transplantation
Edited by: Nathalie C. Zeitouni and Faramarz H. Samie

Techniques in the Evaluation and Management of Hair Disease
Edited by: Rubina Alves and Juan Grimalt

Retinoids in Dermatology
Edited by: Ayse Serap Karadag, Berna Aksoy, and Lawrence Charles Parish

Facial Skin Disorders
Edited by: Ronald Marks

Dermatologic Reactions to Cancer Therapies
Edited by: Gabriella Fabbrocini, Mario E. Lacouture, and Antonella Tosti

Acne Scars: Classification and Treatment, Second Edition
Edited by: Antonella Tosti, Maria Pia De Padova, Gabriella Fabbrocini, and Kenneth Beer

Phototherapy Treatment Protocols, Third Edition
Edited by: Steven R. Feldman and Michael D. Zanolli

Dermatoscopy in Clinical Practice: Beyond Pigmented Lesions, Second Edition
Edited by: Giuseppe Micali and Francesco Lacarrubba

Nail Surgery
Edited by: Bertrand Richert, Niton Di Chiacchio, and Eckart Haneke

For more information about this series please visit: *https://www.crcpress.com/Series-in-Dermatological-Treatment/book-series/CRCSERDERTRE*

Atlas of Genital Dermoscopy

Edited by

Giuseppe Micali, MD

Dermatology Clinic

University of Catania

Catania, Italy

Francesco Lacarrubba, MD

Dermatology Clinic

University of Catania

Catania, Italy

CRC Press
Taylor & Francis Group
Boca Raton London New York

CRC Press is an imprint of the
Taylor & Francis Group, an **informa** business

First edition published 2022
by CRC Press
6000 Broken Sound Parkway NW, Suite 300, Boca Raton, FL 33487-2742
and by CRC Press

2 Park Square, Milton Park, Abingdon, Oxon, OX14 4RN

© 2022 Taylor & Francis Group, LLC
CRC Press is an imprint of Taylor & Francis Group, LLC

This book contains information obtained from authentic and highly regarded sources. While all reasonable efforts have been made to publish reliable data and information, neither the author[s] nor the publisher can accept any legal responsibility or liability for any errors or omissions that may be made. The publishers wish to make clear that any views or opinions expressed in this book by individual editors, authors or contributors are personal to them and do not necessarily reflect the views/opinions of the publishers. The information or guidance contained in this book is intended for use by medical, scientific or health-care professionals and is provided strictly as a supplement to the medical or other professional's own judgement, their knowledge of the patient's medical history, relevant manufacturer's instructions and the appropriate best practice guidelines. Because of the rapid advances in medical science, any information or advice on dosages, procedures or diagnoses should be independently verified. The reader is strongly urged to consult the relevant national drug formulary and the drug companies' and device or material manufacturers' printed instructions, and their websites, before administering or utilizing any of the drugs, devices or materials mentioned in this book. This book does not indicate whether a particular treatment is appropriate or suitable for a particular individual. Ultimately it is the sole responsibility of the medical professional to make his or her own professional judgements, so as to advise and treat patients appropriately. The authors and publishers have also attempted to trace the copyright holders of all material reproduced in this publication and apologize to copyright holders if permission to publish in this form has not been obtained. If any copyright material has not been acknowledged please write and let us know so we may rectify in any future reprint.

Except as permitted under U.S. Copyright Law, no part of this book may be reprinted, reproduced, transmitted, or utilized in any form by any electronic, mechanical, or other means, now known or hereafter invented, including photocopying, microfilming, and recording, or in any information storage or retrieval system, without written permission from the publishers.

For permission to photocopy or use material electronically from this work, access www.copyright.com or contact the Copyright Clearance Center, Inc. (CCC), 222 Rosewood Drive, Danvers, MA 01923, 978-750-8400. For works that are not available on CCC please contact mpkbookspermissions@tandf.co.uk

Trademark notice: Product or corporate names may be trademarks or registered trademarks and are used only for identification and explanation without intent to infringe.

Library of Congress Cataloging-in-Publication Data

Names: Micali, Giuseppe, editor. | Lacarrubba, Francesco, editor.
Title: Atlas of genital dermoscopy / edited by Giuseppe Micali, Francesco Lacarrubba.
Other titles: Series in dermatological treatment
Description: First edition. | Boca Raton, FL : CRC Press, 2021. | Series: Series in dermatological treatment | Includes bibliographical references and index. | Summary: "Dermatologists, family physicians, and those involved in Sexual Health medicine will all benefit from this atlas showing the applications of dermoscopy in several external genital disorders both in males and females with large high-resolution color photographs throughout"–Provided by publisher.
Identifiers: LCCN 2021031159 (print) | LCCN 2021031160 (ebook) | ISBN 9780367440275 (hardback) | ISBN 9781032081519 (paperback) | ISBN 9781003007166 (ebook)
Subjects: MESH: Dermoscopy | Genital Diseases, Male–diagnosis | Genital Diseases, Female–diagnosis | Skin Diseases–diagnosis | Diagnosis, Differential | Atlas
Classification: LCC RC875 (print) | LCC RC875 (ebook) | NLM WJ 17 | DDC 616.6/5075–dc23
LC record available at https://lccn.loc.gov/2021031159
LC ebook record available at https://lccn.loc.gov/2021031160

ISBN: 978-0-367-44027-5 (hbk)
ISBN: 978-1-032-08151-9 (pbk)
ISBN: 978-1-003-00716-6 (ebk)

DOI: 10.1201/9781003007166

Typeset in Times LT Std
by KnowledgeWorks Global Ltd.

Contents

Preface

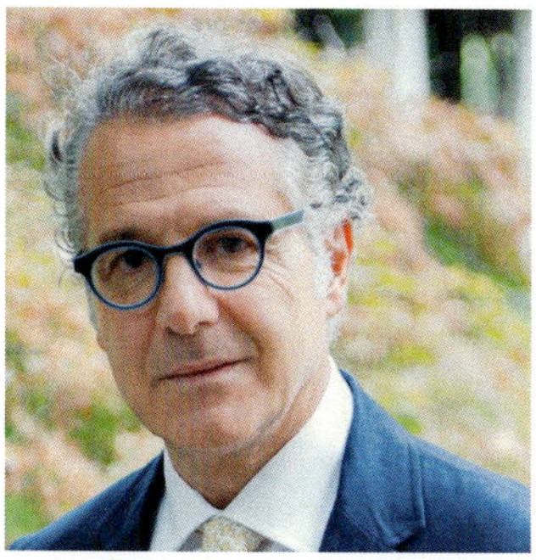

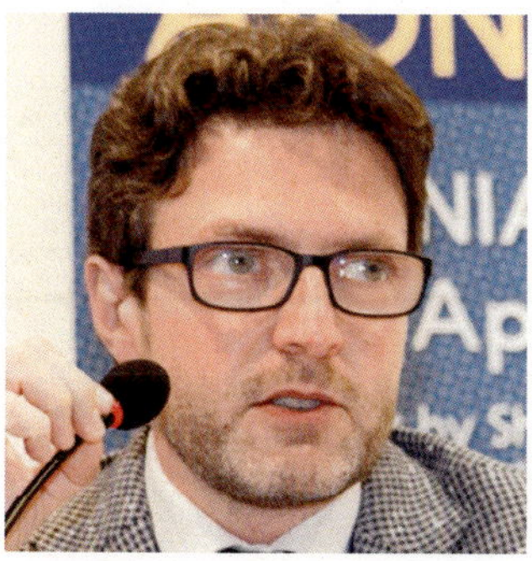

We are pleased to introduce this *Atlas of Genital Dermoscopy*, which deals with a non-invasive technique able to enhance clinical diagnosis. The male and female external genital regions are anatomical areas in which various types of skin disorders may occur. Although most of these conditions can be diagnosed by clinical examination and an accurate medical history review, in most cases further invasive procedures, such as skin biopsy are needed in order to reach a correct diagnosis.

Dermoscopy represents a modern non-invasive tool able to improve the diagnosis of pigmented and non-pigmented skin tumors along with various inflammatory and infectious skin and appendage disorders. It should be considered during clinical inspection of the genital area, especially in the presence of doubtful lesions. It is also useful for prognostic assessment and treatment monitoring. Dermoscopy may also help to rule out those conditions that may clinically appear similar but show a different dermoscopy pattern, thus narrowing down the differential diagnoses and avoiding unnecessary invasive procedures.

This Atlas, the first of its kind, provides an overview on the use of dermoscopy in genital disorders based on the authors' personal experience along with a discussion of the existing published data. It features plenty of detailed clinical and dermoscopic images with histopathological correlations. We hope that readers will find this Atlas useful for their practice, that it may serve as inspiration for further use and indications for dermoscopy of the genital area, and that it will represent an important yet relatively simple addition to the dermatologist's daily office practice.

Giuseppe Micali and Francesco Lacarrubba

Contributors

Marzia Ballesio
Dermatology Clinic
University of Catania
Catania, Italy

Alessandro Borghi
Section of Dermatology and Infectious Diseases
Department of Medical Sciences
University of Ferrara
Ferrara, Italy

Giuseppe Broggi
Department "G.F. Ingrassia" Section of Anatomic Pathology
University of Catania
Catania, Italy

Rosario Caltabiano
Department "G.F. Ingrassia" Section of Anatomic Pathology
University of Catania
Catania, Italy

Elisa Cinotti
Department of Medical, Surgical and Neurological Science
Dermatology Section
University of Siena
S. Maria alle Scotte Hospital
Siena, Italy

Monica Corazza
Section of Dermatology and Infectious Diseases
Department of Medical Sciences
University of Ferrara
Ferrara, Italy

Federica Dall'Oglio
Dermatology Clinic
University of Catania
Catania, Italy

Angelo Di Natale
Dermatology Clinic
University of Catania
Catania, Italy

Enzo Errichetti
Department of Experimental and Clinical Medicine
Institute of Dermatology
University of Udine
Udine, Italy

Roberta Gafà
Section of Anatomic Pathology
Department of Morphology, Surgery and Experimental Medicine
University of Ferrara
Ferrara, Italy

Francesco Lacarrubba
Dermatology Clinic
University of Catania
Catania, Italy

Aimilios Lallas
First Department of Dermatology
Aristotle University
Thessaloniki, Greece

Livia Liguori
Dermatology Clinic
University of Catania
Catania, Italy

Flavio Giulio Liso
Department of Medical, Surgical and Neurological Science
Dermatology Section
University of Siena
S. Maria alle Scotte Hospital
Siena, Italy

Giuseppe Micali
Dermatology Clinic
University of Catania
Catania, Italy

Alberto Monti
Section of Dermatology and Infectious Diseases
Department of Medical Sciences
University of Ferrara
Ferrara, Italy

Maria Letizia Musumeci
Dermatology Clinic
University of Catania
Catania, Italy

Maria Rita Nasca
Dermatology Clinic
University of Catania
Catania, Italy

Giulia Odorici
Section of Dermatology and Infectious Diseases
Department of Medical Sciences
University of Ferrara
Ferrara, Italy

Lucrezia Pacetti
Section of Dermatology and Infectious Diseases
Department of Medical Sciences
University of Ferrara
Ferrara, Italy

Enrico Panebianco
Dermatology Clinic
University of Catania
Catania, Italy

Jean-Luc Perrot
Department of Dermatology
Department of Pathology
University Hospital of Saint-Etienne
Saint-Etienne, France

Davide Francesco Puglisi
Dermatology Clinic
University of Catania
Catania, Italy

Nella Pulvirenti
Dermatology Clinic
University of Catania
Catania, Italy

Pietro Rubegni
Department of Medical, Surgical and Neurological Science
Dermatology Section
University of Siena
S. Maria alle Scotte Hospital
Siena, Italy

Natale Schettini
Section of Dermatology and Infectious Diseases
Department of Medical Sciences
University of Ferrara
Ferrara, Italy

Alice Sgrò
Dermatology Clinic
University of Catania
Catania, Italy

Francesca Sorci
Dermatology Clinic
University of Catania
Catania, Italy

Giuseppe Stinco
Department of Experimental and Clinical Medicine
Institute of Dermatology
University of Udine
Udine, Italy

Aurora Tedeschi
Dermatology Clinic
University of Catania
Catania, Italy

Giulia Toni
Section of Dermatology and Infectious Diseases
Department of Medical Sciences
University of Ferrara
Ferrara, Italy

Anna Elisa Verzì
Dermatology Clinic
University of Catania
Catania, Italy

Pierantonia Zedde
Section of Dermatology and Infectious Diseases
Department of Medical Sciences
University of Ferrara
Ferrara, Italy

CHAPTER 1

Fordyce's Spots

Anna Elisa Verzì MD and Giuseppe Micali MD

DEFINITION

Fordyce's spots (FS) are ectopic visible sebaceous glands that may be located either on the genitalia, the lips or the oral mucosa (1).

EPIDEMIOLOGY

Incidence of FS increases with age, being higher in adults than in children. They are present in about one-third of adult men. The prevalence in females is unknown.

ETIOLOGY

They are considered as a normal anatomic variant of the skin/mucosa surface.

CLINICAL FEATURES

FS clinically appear as painless, yellowish papules 1–2 mm in diameter that are more easily visible when the skin is stretched [Figures 1.1(a), 1.2(a) and 1.3(a)]. They usually involve the penile shaft (especially the ventral surface), the prepuce and/or the scrotum in males, the labia minora in females (2). The onset is typically after puberty and they may be a matter of concern for patients, especially when multiple lesions are present.

DIFFERENTIAL DIAGNOSIS

Differential diagnosis of FS mainly includes molluscum contagiosum, genital warts, milia and syringoma (3).

DIAGNOSIS

It is generally clinical, although sometimes it may not be easy.

DOI: 10.1201/9781003007166-1

DERMOSCOPY

FS appear at dermoscopy as yellowish lobules surrounded by a fine vascular network. Sometimes, a typical vascular garland-like aspect, whose bows (fine vessels) seem to wind around yellowish bunch-like lobules without crossing them, is evident [Figures 1.1(b), 1.2(b) and 1.3(b)] (4, 5). Other authors have described FS as swallow's nests or bottle-like formations containing a milky-white ovoid material and surrounded by non-arborizing vessels (4, 6).

HISTOPATHOLOGICAL CORRELATION

The yellowish lobules seen at dermoscopy histopathologically correlate with the sebaceous lobules located in the dermis and/or hypodermis (2).

REFERENCES

1. Massmanian A, Sorni Valls G, Vera Sempere FJ. Fordyce spots on the glans penis. Br J Dermatol 1995;133(3):498–500.
2. Lacarrubba F, Borghi A, Verzì AE, et al. Dermoscopy of genital diseases: a review. J Eur Acad Dermatol 2020;34(10):2198–207.
3. Radhakrishnan S, Agarwal DC. Fordyce spots masquerading as penile warts. Med J Armed Forces India 2016;72(4):384–5.
4. Micali G, Lacarrubba F. Augmented diagnostic capability using videodermatoscopy on selected infectious and non-infectious penile growths. Int J Dermatol 2011;50(12):1501–5.
5. Paolino G, Muscardin LM, Panetta C, et al. Linear ectopic sebaceous hyperplasia of the penis: the last memory of Tyson's glands. G Ital Dermatol Venereol 2018;153(3):429–31.
6. Ena P, Origa D, Massarelli G. Sebaceous gland hyperplasia of the foreskin. Clin Exp Dermatol 2009;34(3):372–4.

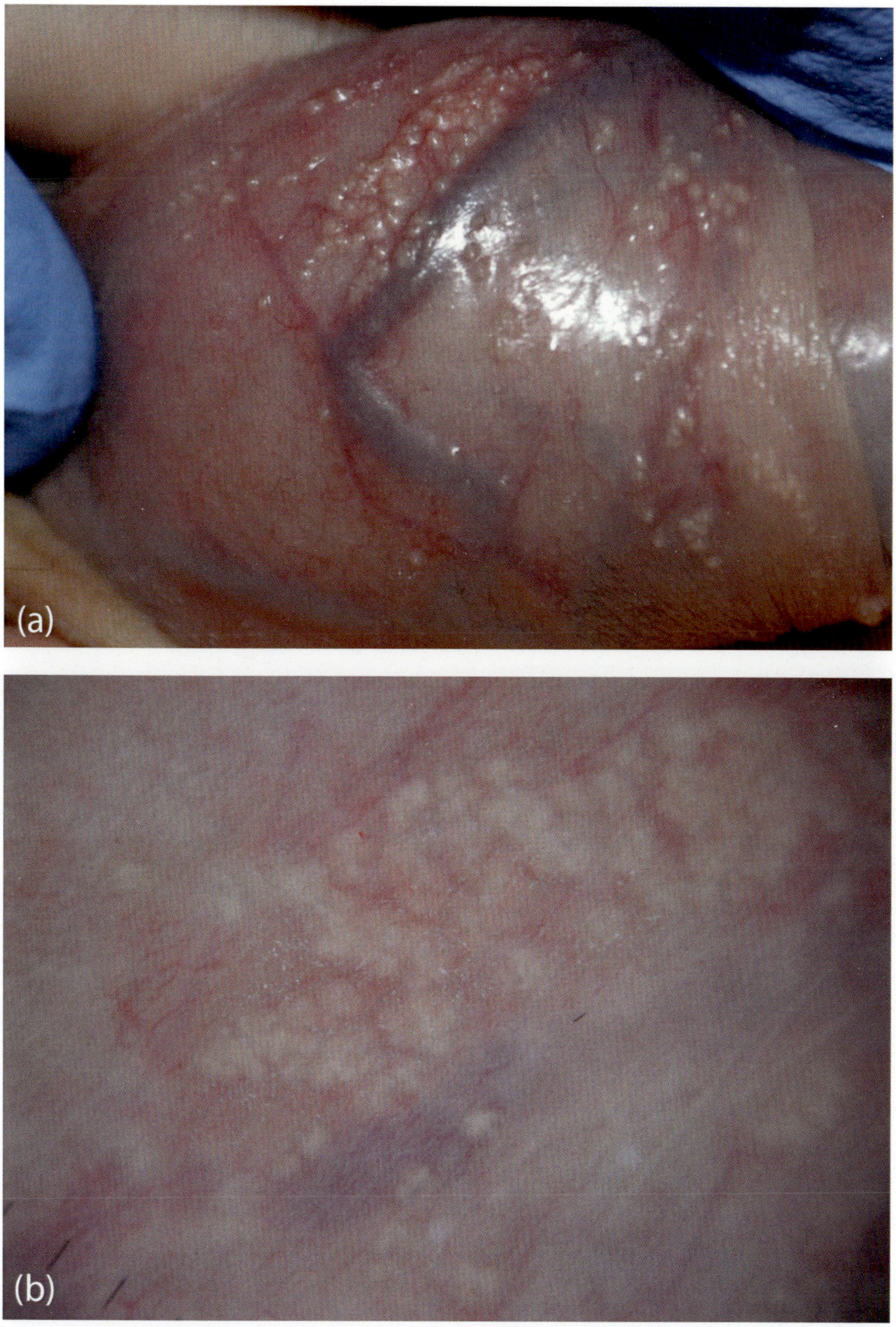

Figure 1.1 (a) Fordyce's spots. Multiple, small, yellowish papules of the prepuce in a 27-year-old man. The lesions represented an important matter of concern for the patient. (b) Dermoscopy (×10) showing typical yellowish lobules surrounded by a fine vascular network.

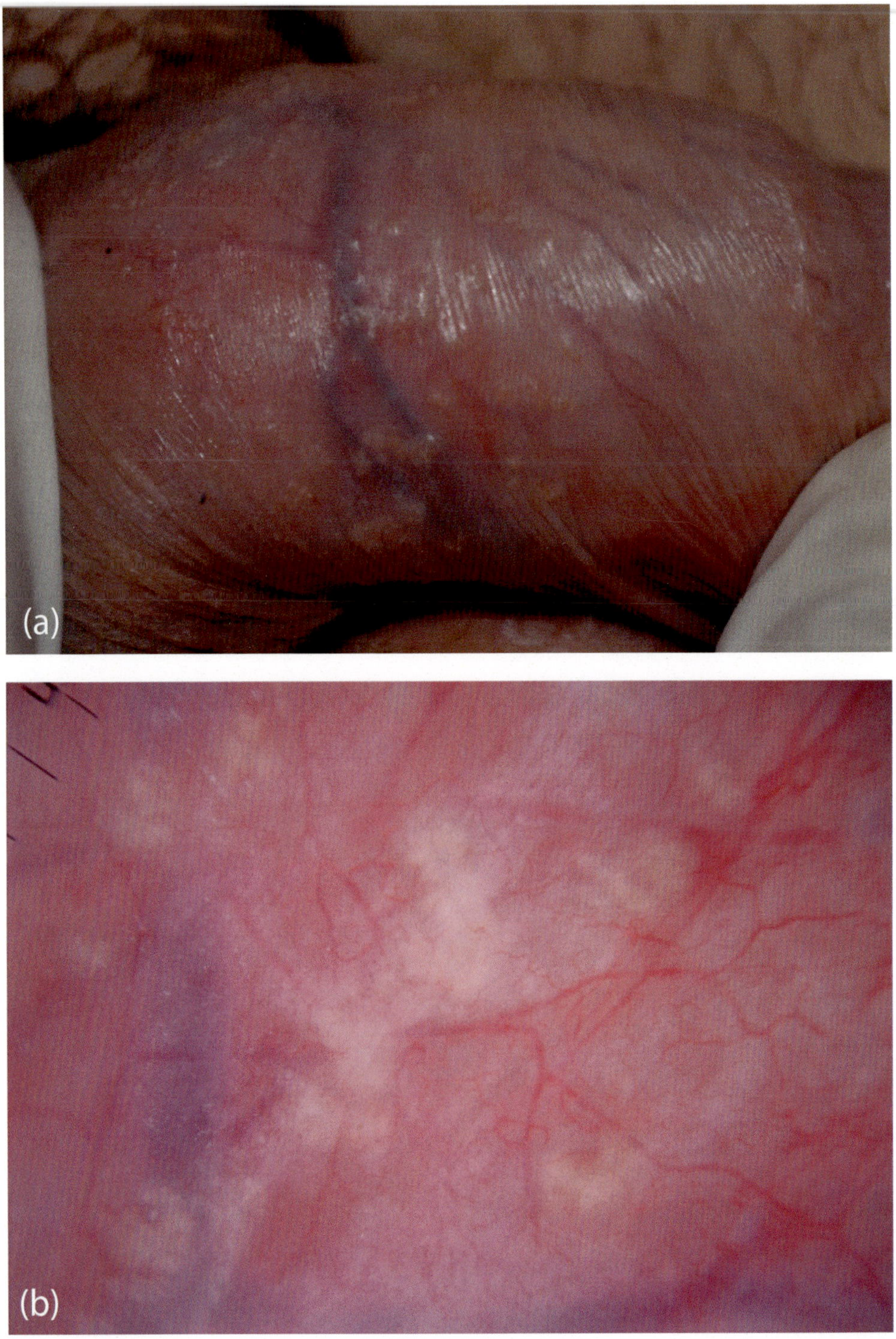

Figure 1.2 (a) Fordyce's spots. Discrete, yellowish papules of the penile shaft in a 32-year-old man. The lesions were previously misdiagnosed and treated as molluscum contagiosum. (b) Dermoscopy (×10) showing typical yellowish bunch-like lobules. The prominent vascular network in this case was unrelated to Fordyce's spots.

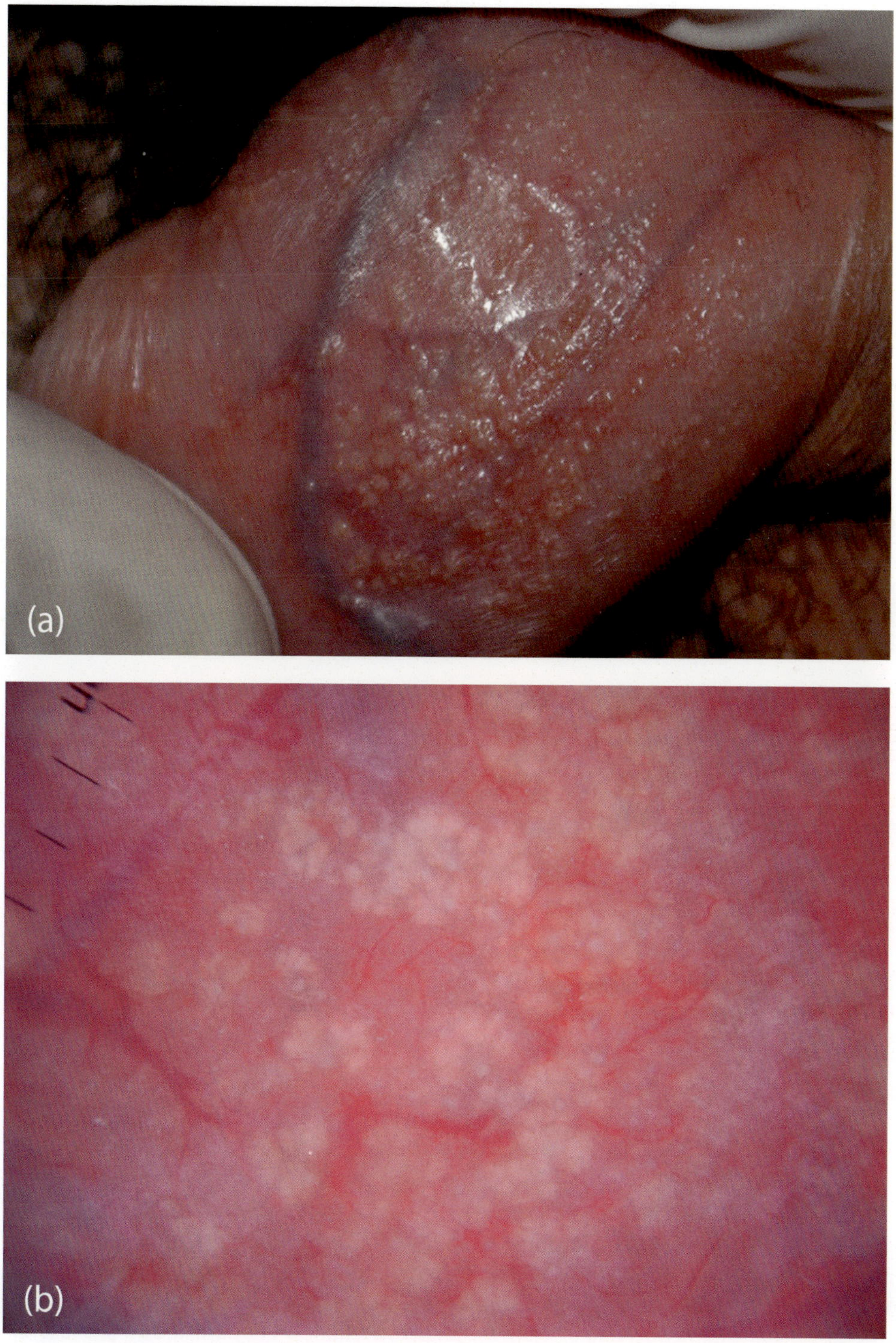

Figure 1.3 (a) Fordyce's spots. Multiple, small, yellowish papules of the penile shaft, confluent in some areas, in a 42-year-old man. (b) Dermoscopy (×10) showing the typical vascular garland-like aspect, whose bows (fine vessels) wind around yellowish bunch-like lobules without crossing them.

CHAPTER 2

Pearly Penile Papules and Vestibular Papillae

Anna Elisa Verzì MD, Davide Francesco Puglisi MD, and Francesco Lacarrubba MD

DEFINITION

Pearly penile papules (PPP) (also known as Tyson glands, hirsutoid papillomas, and hirsutis papillary corona of the penis) and vestibular papillae (VP) (also known as hirsutoid papillomas of vulvae, vulvar squamous papillomatosis, and micropapillomatosis labialis) are common, benign lesions of the male and female genitalia, respectively (1).

EPIDEMIOLOGY

PPP are present in 14–48% of males and are more common in African American and uncircumcised men (2). VP show a prevalence rate between 1% and 33% (3). Both lesions occur more frequently in the second and third decades.

ETIOLOGY

They are both common anatomical variants of the normal epithelium of the glans and the vestibular mucosa, respectively (1, 4). A causal association with *human papillomavirus* (HPV) infection has been excluded (5).

CLINICAL FEATURES

Both PPP and VP appear as multiple, 1–2 mm, soft, flesh-colored to pearly, smooth, or dome-shaped papules arranged in a single or double row. They are usually uniform in size and shape and are symmetrically distributed. PPP are located circumferentially around the corona and sulcus of the glans penis [Figures 2.1(a), 2.2(a), and 2.3(a)]. VP may be symmetrical or linear, involving the labia minora and the introitus vaginae [Figures 2.4(a) and 2.5(a)]. Although generally asymptomatic, they may be associated with itching and/or pain, especially in females. They are known to cause significant distress because of their resemblance to sexually transmitted infections (1, 2).

DOI: 10.1201/9781003007166-2

DIFFERENTIAL DIAGNOSIS

PPP and VP are quite often interpreted as genital warts, causing, on many occasions, incorrect or unnecessary treatments (4). Other misdiagnoses include molluscum contagiosum and angiokeratoma.

DIAGNOSIS

Generally, the diagnosis of both entities is clinical. A skin biopsy should be considered if the clinical presentation is doubtful (2).

DERMOSCOPY

PPP and VP show similar features at dermoscopy, namely characteristic regular, uniformly sized, whitish-pink small projections, which have separate bases [Figures 2.1(b), 2.2(b), 2.3(b), and 2.4(b)]. Delicate vascular structures may be visible within the projections. A cobblestone or grape-like aggregation may also be observed [Figure 2.5(b)] (6–12).

HISTOPATHOLOGICAL CORRELATION

Histopathologically, the whitish-pink small projections observed at dermoscopy correspond to connective tissue papillomatous structures including slight dilated and elongated vessels. The epidermis is normal or acanthotic, with no aspects of HPV infection (2, 4).

REFERENCES

1. Aldahan AS, Brah TK, Nouri K. Diagnosis and management of pearly penile papules. Am J Mens Health 2018;12(3):624–7.
2. Leung AK, Barankin B. Pearly penile papules. J Pediatr 2014;165(2):409.
3. Kakkar S, Sharma PK. Benign vulvar vestibular papillomatosis: an underreported condition in Indian dermatological literature. Indian Dermatol Online J 2017;8(1):63–5.
4. Prieto MA, Gutiérrez JV, Sambucety PS. Vestibular papillae of the vulva. Int J Dermatol 2004;43(2):143–4.
5. Moyal-Barracco M, Leibowitch M, Orth G. Vestibular papillae of the vulva. Lack of evidence for human papillomavirus etiology. Arch Dermatol 1990;126(12):1594–8.
6. Ozeki M, Saito R, Tanaka M. Dermoscopic features of pearly penile papules. Dermatology 2008; 217(1):21–2.
7. Kim SH, Seo SH, Ko HC, et al. The use of dermatoscopy to differentiate vestibular papillae, a normal variant of the female external genitalia, from condyloma acuminata. J Am Acad Dermatol 2009;60(2):353–5.
8. Watanabe T, Yoshida Y, Yamamoto O. Differential diagnosis of pearly penile papules and penile condyloma acuminatum by dermoscopy. Eur J Dermatol 2010;20(3):414–5.
9. Micali G, Lacarrubba F. Augmented diagnostic capability using videodermatoscopy on selected infectious and non-infectious penile growths. Int J Dermatol 2011;50(12):1501–5.
10. Ozkur E, Falay T, Turgut Erdemir AV, et al. Vestibular papillomatosis: an important differential diagnosis of vulvar papillomas. Dermatol Online J 2016;22(3):13030/qt7933q377.
11. Lacarrubba F, Borghi A, Verzì AE, et al. Dermoscopy of genital diseases: a review. J Eur Acad Dermatol 2020;34(10):2198–207.
12. Giuffrida G, Lacarrubba F, Boscaglia S, et al. A noninvasive aid for office-based gynecologists for the diagnosis of common external genital disorders. Obstet Gynecol Int 2019;2019:1830245.

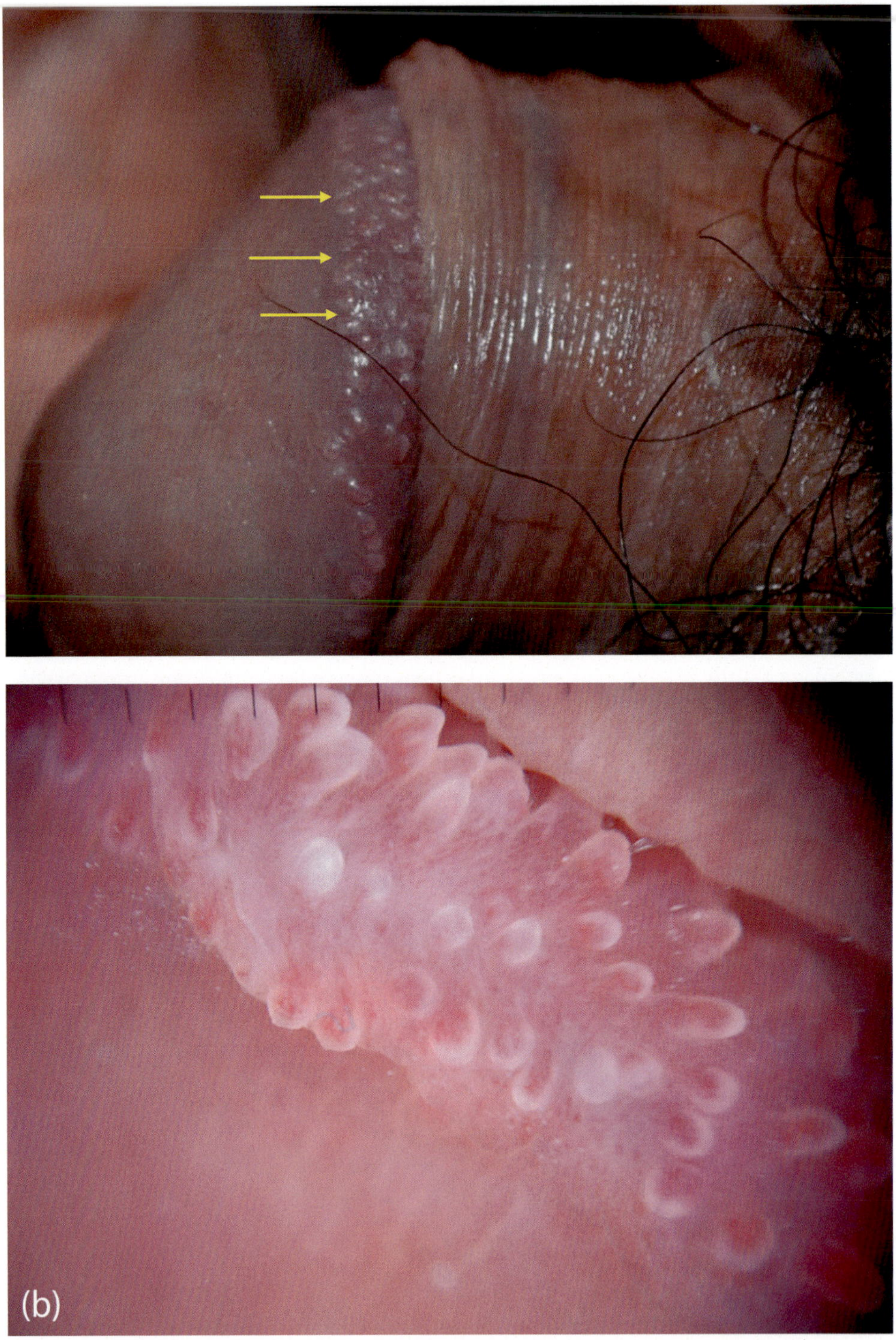

Figure 2.1 (a) Pearly penile papules. Multiple, small, flesh-colored, symmetrical papules located circumferentially around the corona glans (arrows) in a 21-year-old man. (b) Dermoscopy (×10) showing multiple rows of regular, uniformly sized, pinkish, small projections presenting delicate vascular structures and separate bases.

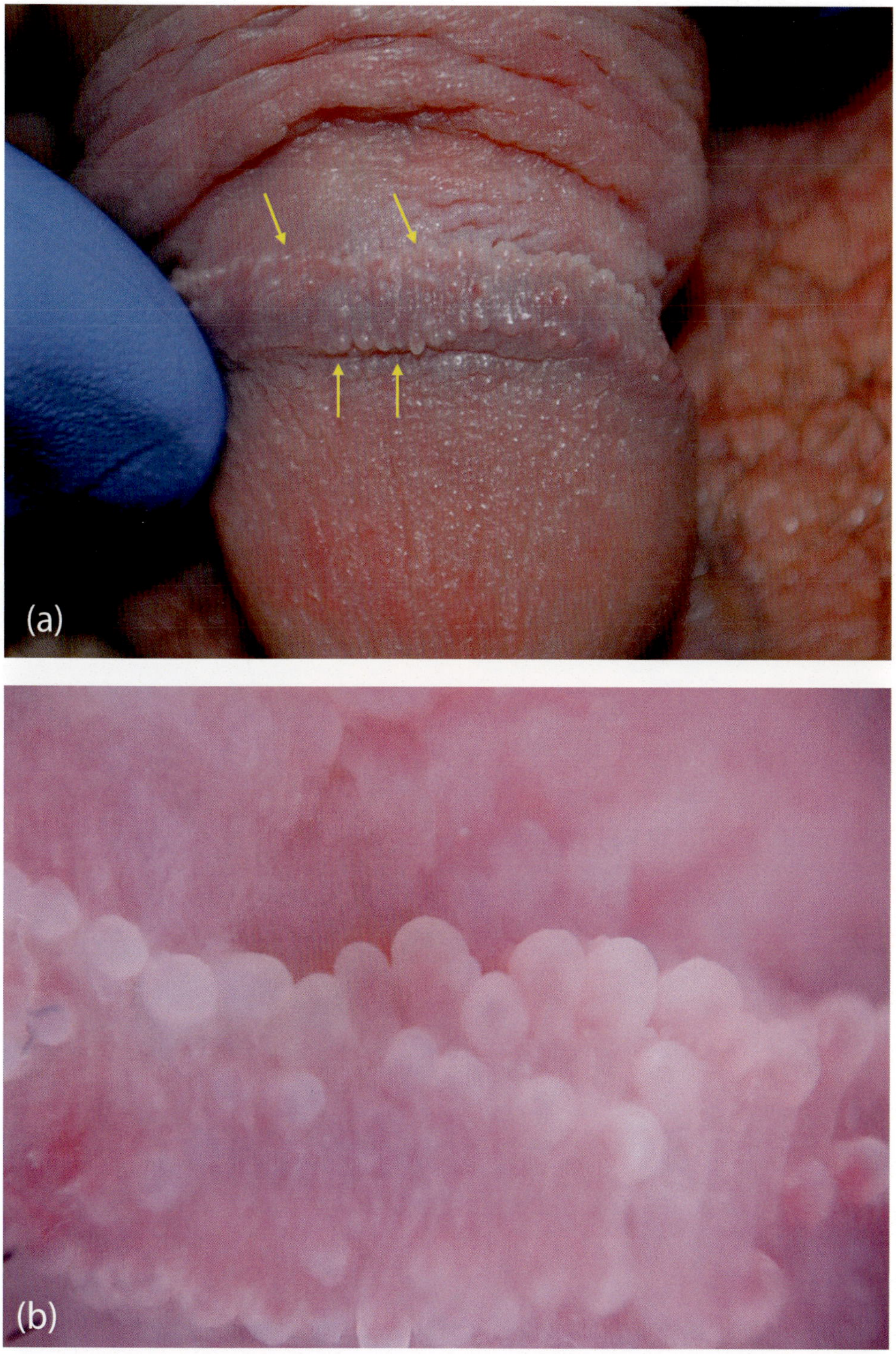

Figure 2.2 (a) Pearly penile papules. Multiple, small, flesh-colored, papules of the corona glans (arrows) in a 23-year-old man. Similar lesions in the same patients were previously treated as genital warts with laser-therapy. (b) Dermoscopy (×10) showing regular, uniformly sized, whitish-pink small projections presenting separate bases.

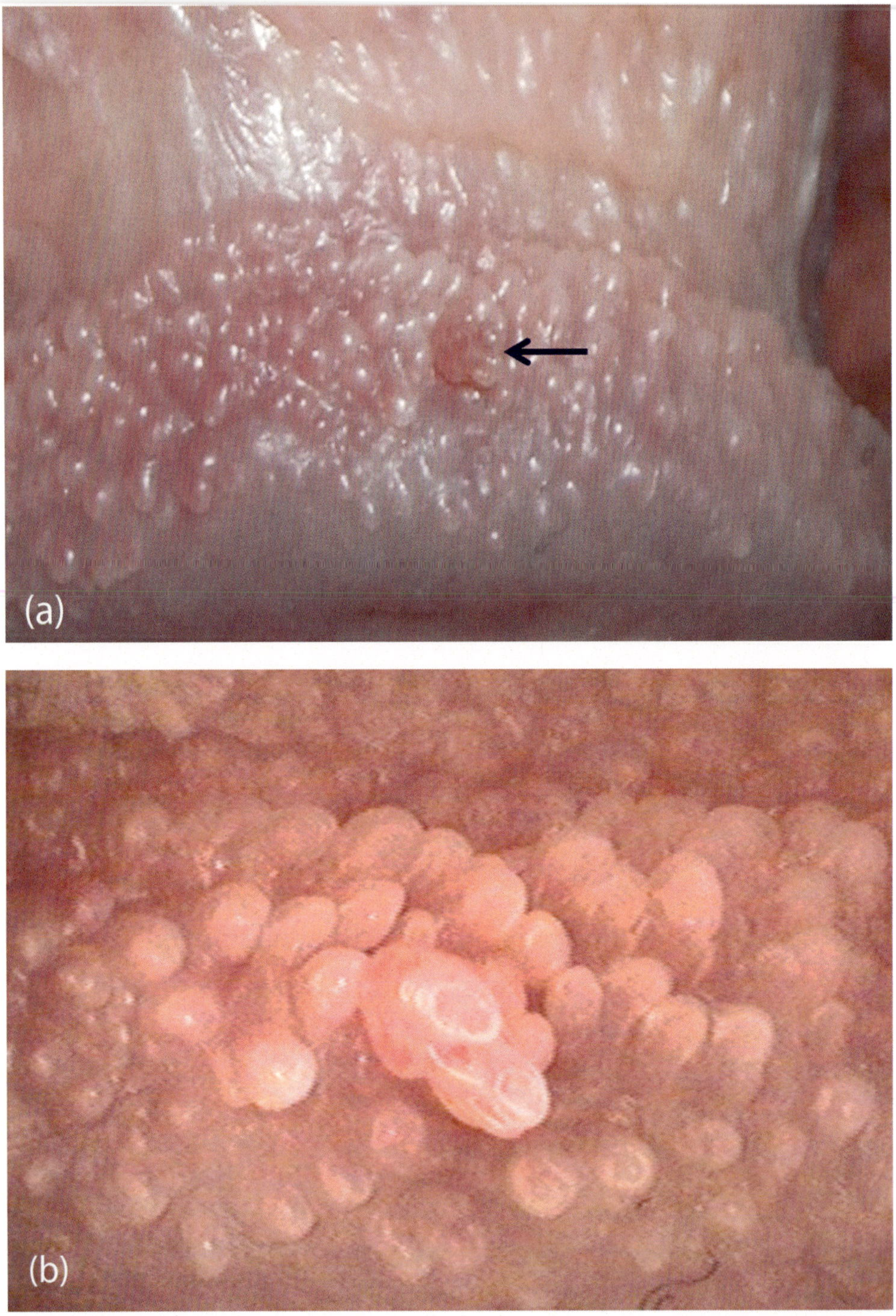

Figure 2.3 (a) Pearly penile papules. Multiple, pinkish, symmetrical papules on the corona glans in a young boy. One lesion (arrow) appears different from the others. (b) Dermoscopy (×20) showing multiple, regular, uniformly sized, pinkish, small projections. The lesion in the center is characterized by bigger projections arising from a common base and containing an elongated vessel, all features typical of genital warts (see Chapter 3).

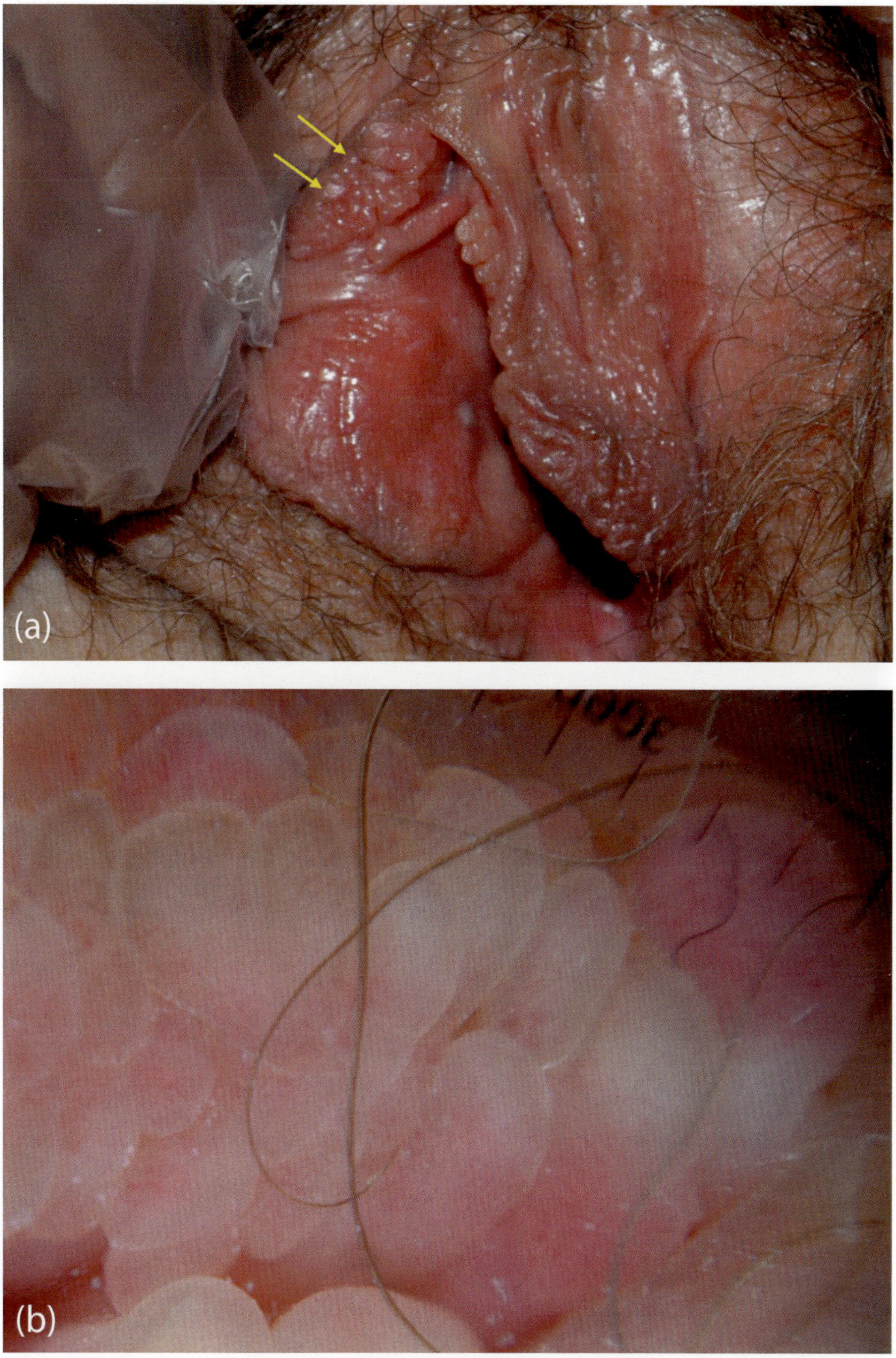

Figure 2.4 (a) Vestibular papillae. Small, smooth, flesh-colored papules of the vulva (arrows) in a 26-year-old woman. (b) Dermoscopy (×10) showing regular pinkish projections presenting separate bases.

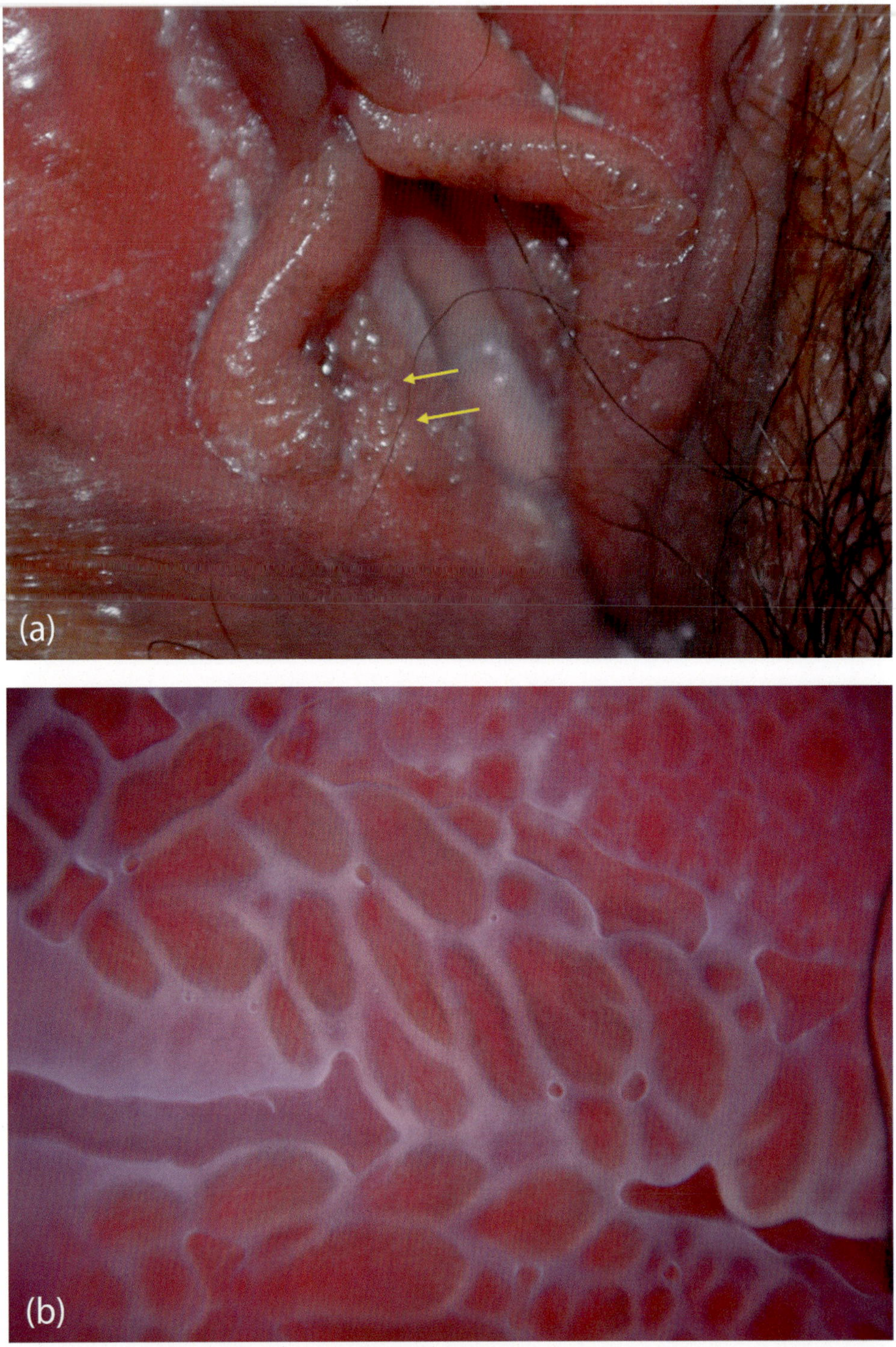

Figure 2.5 (a) Vestibular papillae. Small, smooth, flesh-colored papules of the vestibulum (arrows) in a 34-year-old woman. The lesions were previously treated as genital warts with imiquimod 5% cream. (b) Dermoscopy (×10) showing regular pinkish projections with fine vascular axis, configuring a cobblestone appearance.

CHAPTER 3

Genital Warts

Federica Dall'Oglio MD PhD, Rosario Caltabiano MD, Enrico Panebianco MD, and Giuseppe Micali MD

DEFINITION

Genital warts (GWs), also known as condylomata acuminata, represent a common, highly contagious transmissible infection of the genital and perigenital areas, more often observed in young and sexually active individuals, that are caused by *human papillomavirus* (HPV).

EPIDEMIOLOGY

GWs represent one of the most frequent sexually transmissible diseases, with a worldwide prevalence rate variable from 2% to 44% (1). In Italian women, the prevalence is 3.8 cases/1000 and incidence is 3 cases/1000 in a year (2). In the United States, every year infection occurs in 500,000–1 million residents (3). They are more commonly seen in the adult population than in children (4).

ETIOLOGY

HPVs are non-enveloped, double-stranded DNA viruses with more than 170 different subtypes (5). They can be subdivided according to their oncogenic potential into high-risk (HR) and low-risk (LR) types. LR-HPV types 6 and 11 are responsible for more than 90% of the GWs (2, 6). HR types such as HPV 16 and 18 can lead to squamous cell carcinoma, causing cervix, anal, penis, or oropharynx cancer and earlier stages thereof.

CLINICAL FEATURES

The clinical presentation of GWs is heterogeneous: they may appear as flesh-colored or brownish, broad-based, exophytic or pedunculated, papules, sometimes proliferating as papillomatous lesions or cauliflower-like plaques [Figures 3.1(a), 3.2(a), 3.3(a), 3.4(a) and 3.5(a)] (5). In men, the coronal sulcus of the penis as well as the prepuce are among the most affected areas, while in women the lesions mainly appear on the labia minora et majora and the introitus vaginae (5).

DOI: 10.1201/9781003007166-3

DIFFERENTIAL DIAGNOSIS

The main differential diagnoses of GWs include molluscum contagiosum, pearly penile papules or vestibular papillomatosis, Fordyce's spots, angiokeratoma, lymphangioma, lichen nitidus and epidermoid cyst.

DIAGNOSIS

The diagnosis of GWs is usually simple and based on the typical clinical appearance. However, early detection of minimal lesions may sometimes be challenging as they may go unnoticed or mimic other dermatologic conditions (7, 8). Histopathological examination may sometimes be necessary when dermoscopy is also doubtful.

DERMOSCOPY

Dermoscopy of GWs, extensively described in both sexes, varies depending on the clinical presentation (9–18). Small, papular lesions usually show the so-called *mosaic* pattern, consisting of a whitish reticular network circumscribing dotted vessel [Figures 3.1(b) and 3.2(b)] (8). The papillomatous, cauliflower-like GWs reveal multiple, irregular projections of different sizes, shapes and colors, from light pink to gray-whitish to brownish, arising from a common basis and comprising elongated and dilated vessels outlined by a whitish halo (*finger-like* pattern) [Figures 3.3(b), 3.4(b) and 3.5(b)]. Hemorrhagic splits can be observed inside the lesions (10, 12). Other described dermoscopic patterns include *knob-like*, *brain-like* and unspecific, which in many cases can be combined (9).

HISTOPATHOLOGICAL CORRELATION

Histopathologically, GWs are characterized by a compact stratum corneum, acanthosis and different degree of papillomatosis with increased vascularization. Scattered vacuolated keratinocytes may be observed (Figure 3.6). The whitish reticular network and the glomerular vessels that dermoscopically characterize papular GWs are related to acanthosis and tortuous/dilated capillaries in the papillary dermis, respectively. The whitish projections of the cauliflower-like GWs correspond to marked papillomatosis, acanthosis and hyperkeratosis (10).

REFERENCES

1. Suligoi B, Vittori G, Salfa MC, et al. Prevalence and incidence of external genital warts in a sample of Italian general female population. Genital Warts 2 (GW2) Working Group. BMC Infect Dis 2017;17(1):126.
2. Steben M, Garland SM. Genital warts. Best Pract Res Clin Obstet Gynaecol 2014;28(7):1063–73.
3. Cates W Jr. Estimates of the incidence and prevalence of sexually transmitted diseases in the United States. American Social Health Association Panel. Sex Transm Dis 1999;26(Suppl 4):S2–7.
4. Myhre AK, Dalen A, Berntzen K, Bratlid D. Anogenital human papillomavirus in non-abused preschool children. Acta Paediatr 2003;92:1445–52.
5. Clanner-Engelshofen BM, Marsela E, Engelsberger N, et al. Condylomata acuminata: a retrospective analysis on clinical characteristics and treatment options. Heliyon 2020;6(3):e03547.
6. Bussen S, Sutterlin M, Schmidt U, Bussen D. Anogenital warts in childhood—always a marker for sexual abuse? Geburtshilfe Frauenheilkd 2012;72(1):43–8.
7. Micali G, Lacarrubba F. Augmented diagnostic capability using videodermatoscopy on selected infectious and non-infectious penile growths. Int J Dermatol 2011;50(12):1501–5.

8. Giuffrida G, Lacarrubba F, Boscaglia S, et al. A noninvasive aid for office-based gynecologists for the diagnosis of common external genital disorders. Obstet Gynecol Int 2019;2019:1830245.
9. Dong H, Shu D, Campbell TM, et al. Dermatoscopy of genital warts. J Am Acad Dermatol 2011;64(5):859–64.
10. Lacarrubba F, Dinotta F, Nasca MR, Micali G. Enhanced diagnosis of genital warts with videodermatoscopy: histopatologic correlation. G Ital Dermatol Venereol 2012;147(2):215–6.
11. Jiang S, Zhang Y, Zou X. Condyloma acuminata at urethral orifice complicated with hemophilia A. An Bras Dermatol 2017;92(2):289–90.
12. Ozdemir F, Kilinc-Karaarslan I, Akalin T. A pigmented, hemorrhagic genital wart: clinical, dermoscopic, and histopathologic features. Arch Dermatol 2008;144(8):1072–3.
13. Watanabe T, Yoshida Y, Yamamoto O. Differential diagnosis of pearly penile papules and penile condyloma acuminatum by dermoscopy. Eur J Dermatol 2010;20(3):414–5.
14. Veasey JV, Framil VM, Nadal SR, et al. Genital warts: comparing clinical findings to dermatoscopic aspects, in vivo reflectance confocal features and histopathologic exam. An Bras Dermatol 2014;89(1):137–40.
15. Campos MA, Sousa A, Lage G, et al. Blue-gray plaque of the penis. JAAD Case Rep 2018;4(6):531–3.
16. Chuh A, Zawar V, Ooi C, Lee A. A case-control study in primary care settings on the roles of dermatoscopy in infectious diseases affecting the skin. Part 1: viral and bacterial infections. Skin Med 2018;16(4):247–54.
17. Zhang Y, Jiang S, Lin H, et al. Application of dermoscopy image analysis technique in diagnosing urethral condylomata acuminata. An Bras Dermatol 2018;93:67–71.
18. Lacarrubba F, Borghi A, Verzì AE, et al. Dermoscopy of genital diseases: a review. J Eur Acad Dermatol 2020;34(10):2198–207.

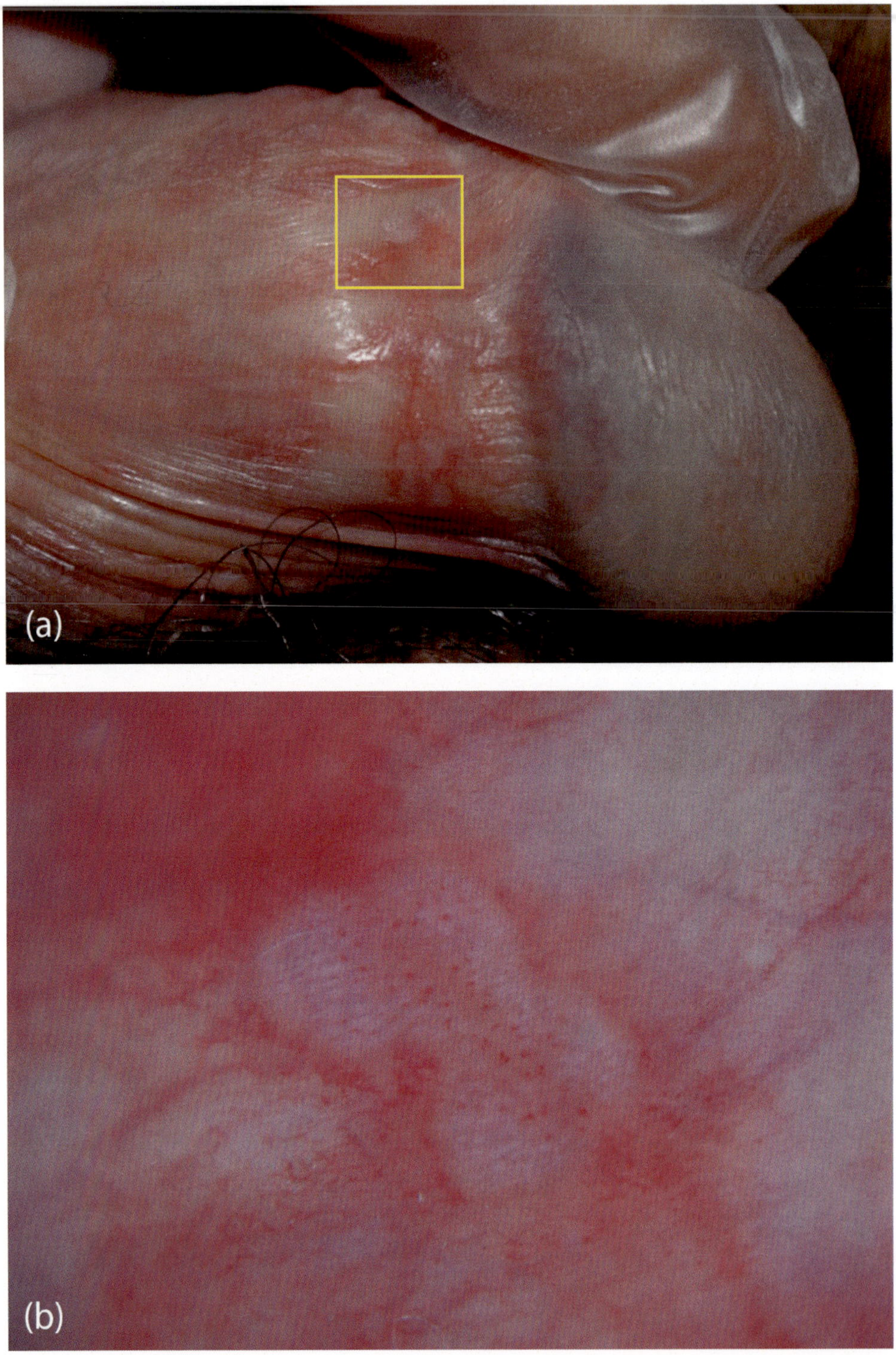

Figure 3.1 (a) Genital wart. Single, small and pinkish papule of the prepuce (square) in a 19-year-old boy. (b) Dermoscopy (×10) showing a whitish network circumscribing dotted vessels ("mosaic pattern").

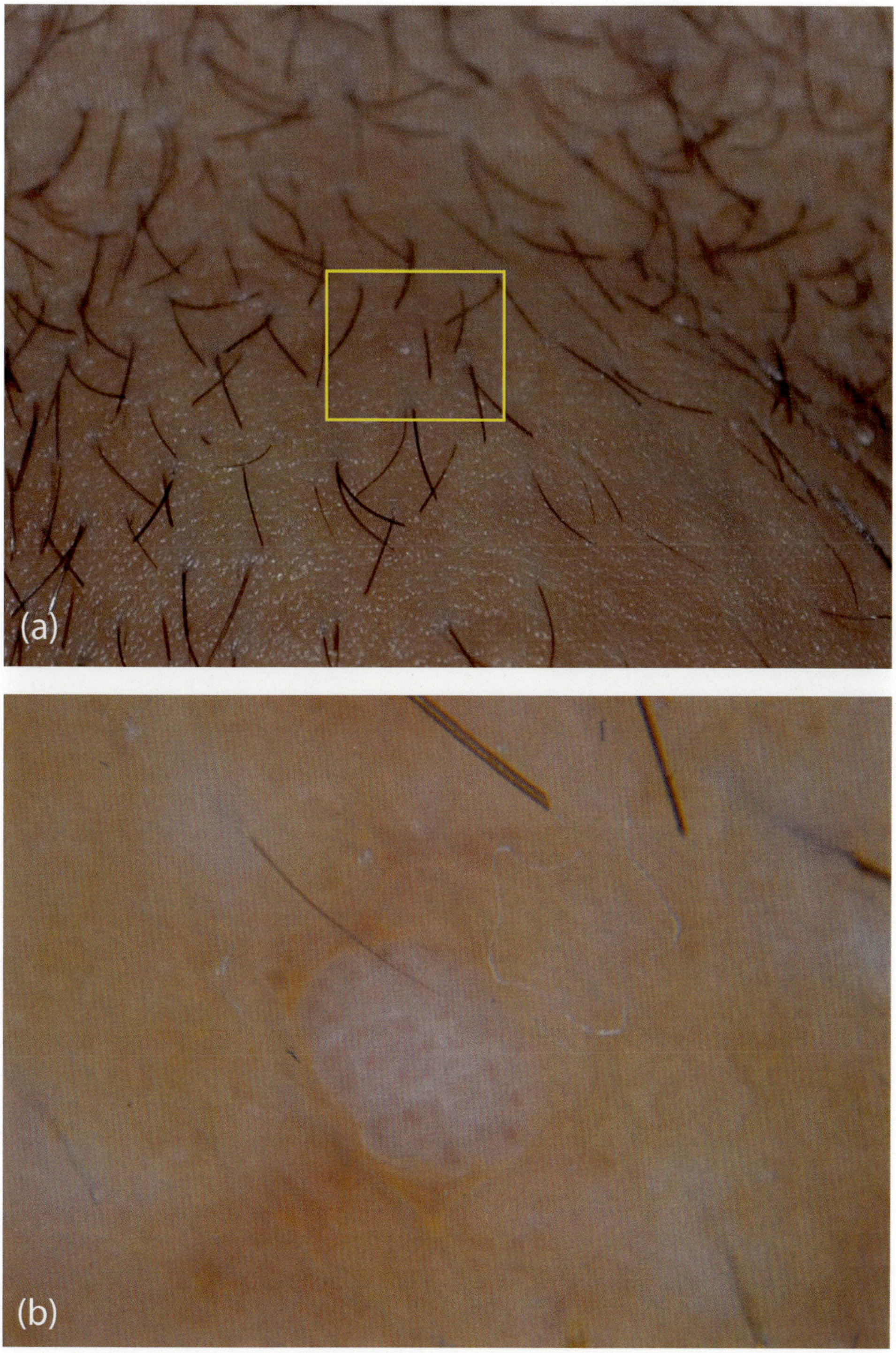

Figure 3.2 (a) Genital wart. Very small and skin-colored papule of the pubis (square) in a 25-year-old man. The patient noticed the lesion after epilation. (b) Dermoscopy (×10) showing a whitish network circumscribing dotted vessels ("mosaic pattern").

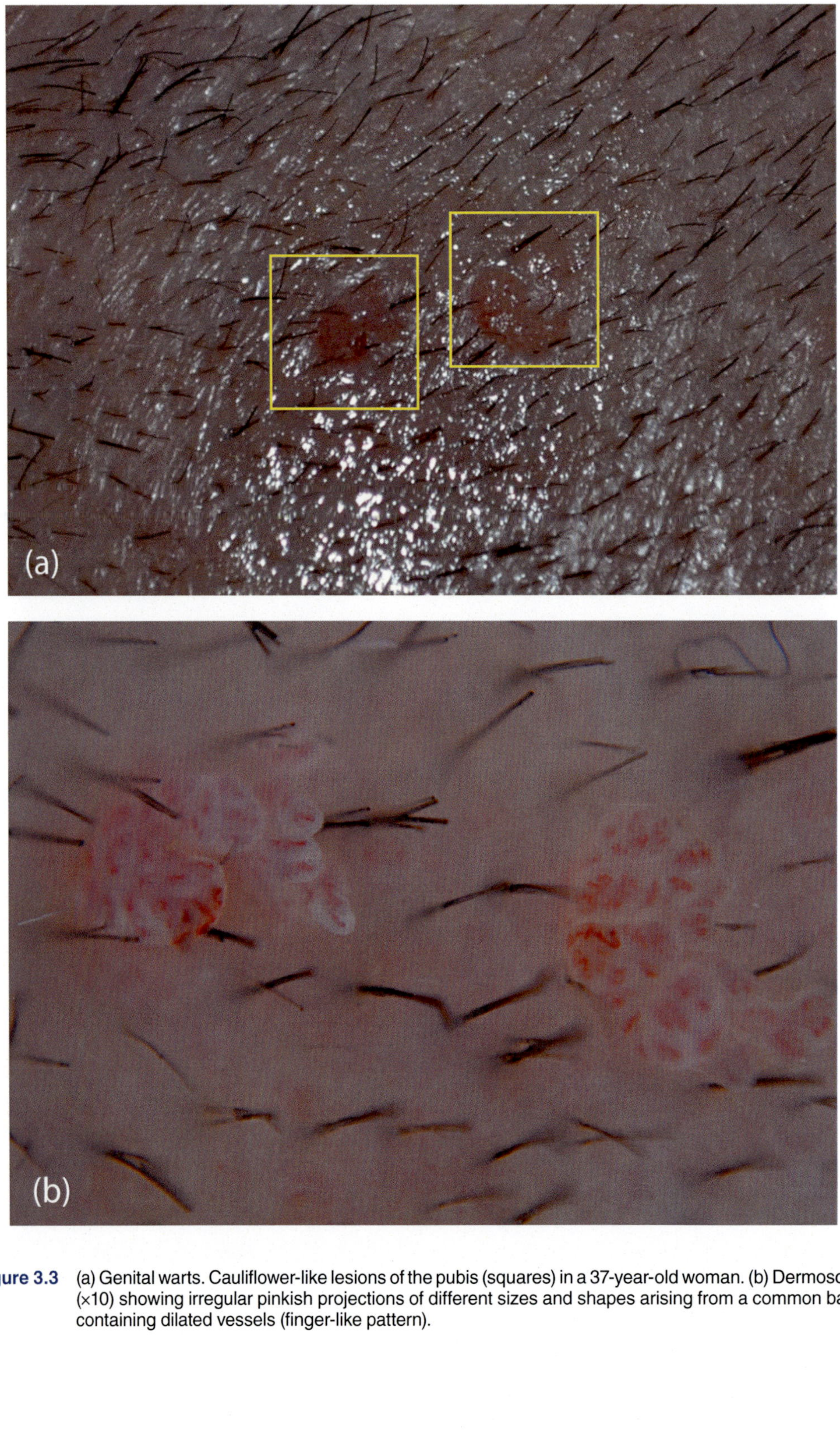

Figure 3.3 (a) Genital warts. Cauliflower-like lesions of the pubis (squares) in a 37-year-old woman. (b) Dermoscopy (×10) showing irregular pinkish projections of different sizes and shapes arising from a common basis, containing dilated vessels (finger-like pattern).

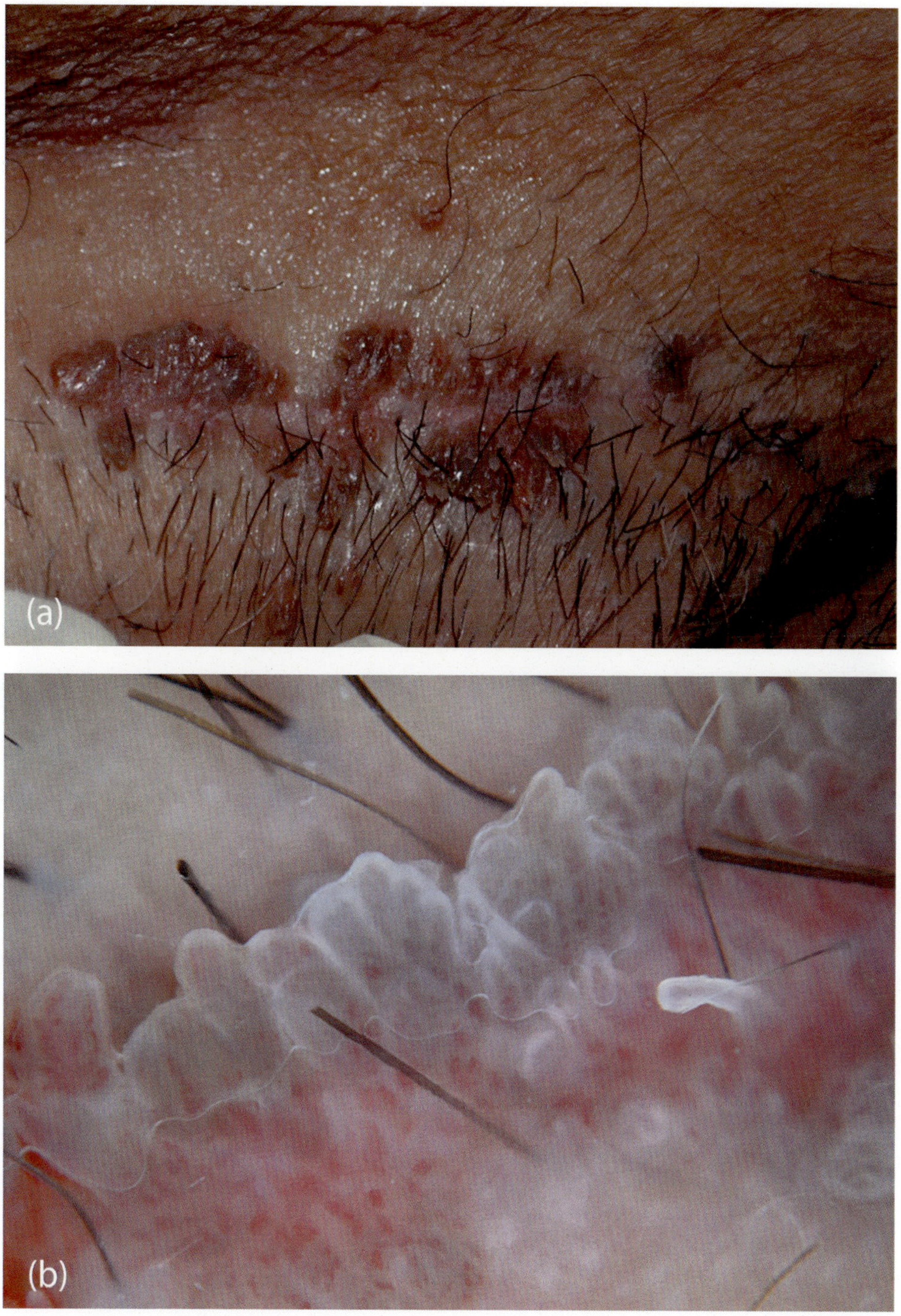

Figure 3.4 (a) Genital warts. Multiple, confluent, reddish and cauliflower-like lesions of the peri-genital area in a 31-year-old woman. (b) Dermoscopy (×10) showing irregular whitish projections of different sizes arising from a common basis, containing dilated vessels (finger-like pattern).

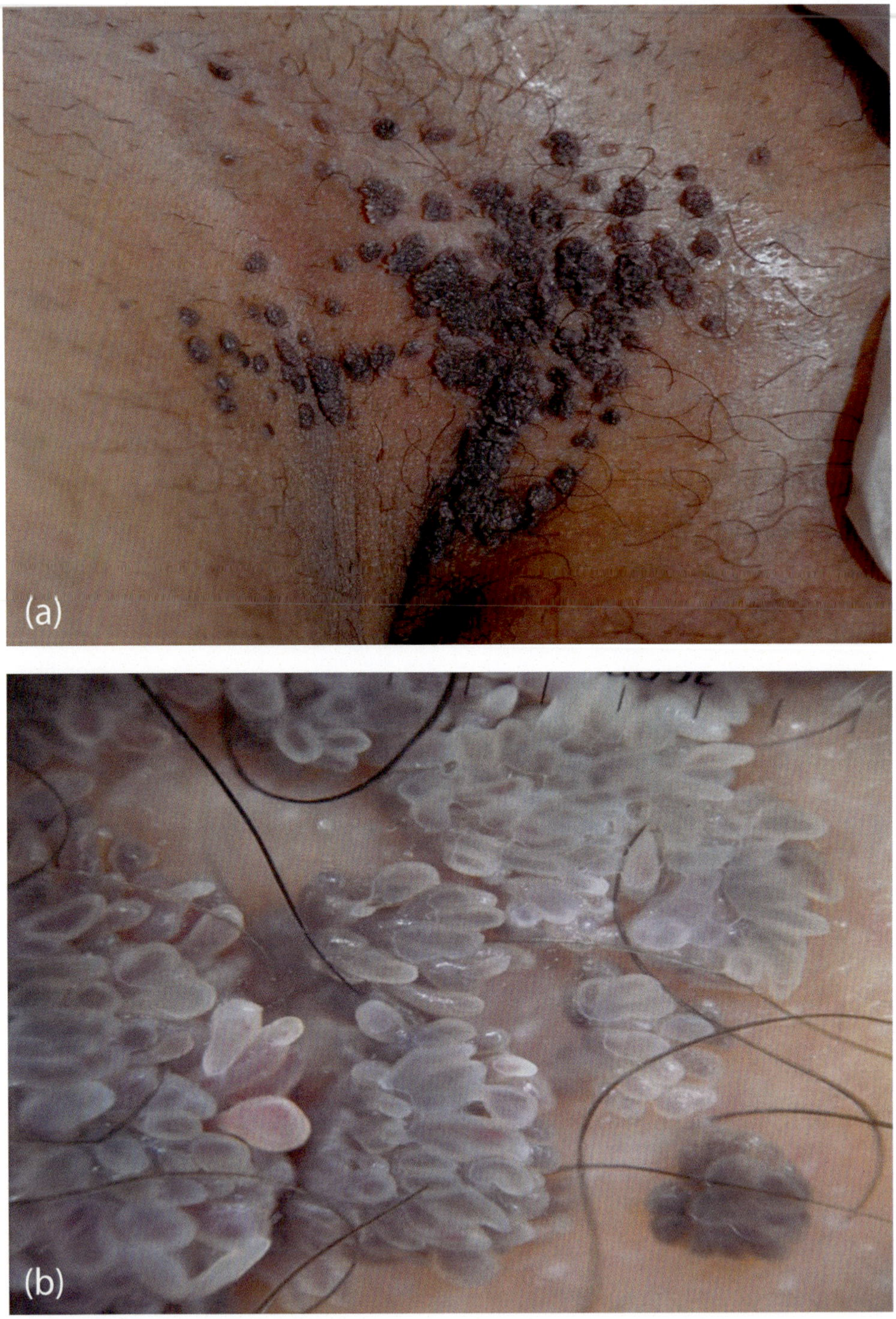

Figure 3.5 (a) Genital warts. Brownish and cauliflower-like lesions of the peri-genital area in a 37-year-old man. (b) Dermoscopy (×10) showing irregular grayish projections arising from a common basis, containing dilated vessels (finger-like pattern).

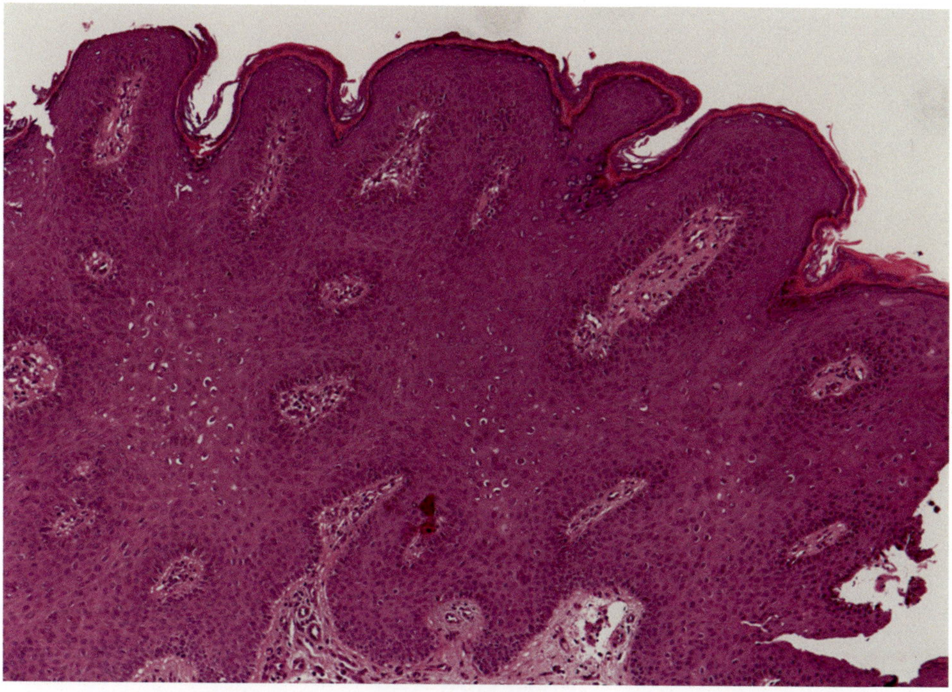

Figure 3.6 Histopathology of genital wart showing marked acanthosis, papillomatosis and a broad exophytic growth. The surface of the lesion is hyperkeratotic and parakeratotic and the deep margin is sharp and regular (H&E, ×100).

CHAPTER 4

Molluscum Contagiosum

Anna Elisa Verzì MD, Giuseppe Broggi MD, Marzia Ballesio MD, and Francesco Lacarrubba MD

DEFINITION

Molluscum contagiosum (MC) is a common viral infection, frequent in the paediatric population, sexually active adults, and immunocompromised individuals (1).

EPIDEMIOLOGY

The worldwide incidence of MC is estimated to be between 2% and 8% (1). Although the infection is more frequent among children (between 2 and 5 years old), with a prevalence estimated between 5.1% and 11.5% (2), over past decades its incidence in adults has been increasing, mainly as a sexually transmitted disease, and/or as a result of concurrent human immunodeficiency virus (HIV) infection (1).

ETIOLOGY

MC is caused by the *Molluscum contagiosum virus* (MCV) a double-stand DNA, epidermotropic virus which belongs to the Poxviridae family. There are four main subtypes of MCV: MCV1, MCV2, MCV3, and MC4. MCV1 is the most common genotype (75–96%) and it is more frequent in children, while MCV2 is more frequent among adults (3). The virus is transmitted through direct sexual or non-sexual skin contact with an infected individual, or by autoinoculation. It can also be transmitted by fomites such as bath towels or sponges and tattoo instruments. The average incubation time is between 2 and 7 weeks with a range extending to 6 months (4).

CLINICAL FEATURES

MC is clinically characterized by asymptomatic, small, skin-colored, and translucent papules with a typical, central, whitish depression or umbilication [Figures 4.1(a), 4.2(a), 4.3(a), and 4.4]. Lesions may vary in size from 1 to 10 mm, although occasionally giant lesions may be seen, especially in immunocompromised individuals. They may be single or, more frequently, multiple or clustered. Sometimes they may be linearly arranged due to scratching (pseudo-Koebner). In some cases, the lesions may have an erythematous halo or may be pedunculated. The genital and perigenital area are usually affected in young adults as a result of a sexual transmission (5). MC is mostly localized on the penile shaft and the pubis

DOI: 10.1201/9781003007166-4

in males, on vulvar skin, pubis, and perineum in females. In immunocompetent patients, lesions may be self-limiting, lasting from 6 to 9 months although in some cases they can persist for more than 3–4 years.

DIFFERENTIAL DIAGNOSIS

Differential diagnosis of genital MC includes several dermatological conditions such as viral warts, melanocytic nevi, Fordyce's spots, syringoma, lymphangioma, angiokeratoma, and pyogenic granuloma. Giant MC may be confused with a squamous cell carcinoma or a keratoacanthoma.

DIAGNOSIS

The diagnosis of MC is generally clinical, based on the recognition of the typical aspect. However, sometimes the lesions have a different morphology or unusual body location, and the diagnosis may be more difficult. Histopathological examination is rarely indicated. Besides dermoscopy, reflectance confocal microscopy, which reveals microscopic details closely related to histopathology, may represent an adjunctive non-invasive diagnostic option for difficult cases (6).

DERMOSCOPY

The main dermoscopic feature of MC consists of the presence of single or multiple, white-yellowish, roundish structures ("pores" or "orifices"), generally in the center of the lesion. Sometimes, a "four-leaved clover-like" structure may be observed; in other cases several "pores" may be clustered forming a polylobular structure [Figures 4.1(b), 4.2(b), 4.3(b), and 4.4] (6–10). Vessels are usually visible at the periphery of the lesions with different arrangements, namely crown, radial, and/or dotted patterns (11). In some cases, the pores, the polylobular structures, or the vascular component may be absent, making the dermoscopic diagnosis more difficult (9).

HISTOPATHOLOGICAL CORRELATION

Histopathologically, MC is characterized by a well-circumscribed, endophytic, lobulated, epidermal hyperplasia composed of enlarged keratinocytes containing typical eosinophilic cytoplasmic inclusion bodies (Henderson-Paterson bodies) (Figure 4.5). The roundish or polylobular white-yellowish structures ("pores") seen at dermoscopy, histopathologically correspond to the areas of epidermal invagination, while the peripheral vascular pattern correlates to dilatated vessels in the dermis (4).

REFERENCES

1. Hanson D, Diven DG. Molluscum contagiosum. Dermatol Online J 2003;9(2):2.
2. Olsen JR, Gallacher J, Piguet V, Francis NA. Epidemiology of molluscum contagiosum in children: a systematic review. Fam Pract 2014;31(2):130–6.
3. Meza-Romero R, Navarrete-Dechent C, Downey C. Molluscum contagiosum: an update and review of new perspectives in etiology, diagnosis, and treatment. Clin Cosmet Investig Dermatol 2019;12:373–81.

4. Lacarrubba F, Verzì AE, Dinotta F, et al. Dermatoscopy in inflammatory and infectious skin disorders. G Ital Dermatol Venereol 2015;150(5):521–31.
5. Lacarrubba F, Borghi A, Verzì AE, et al. Dermoscopy of genital diseases: a review. J Eur Acad Dermatol 2020;34(10):2198–207.
6. Lacarrubba F, Verzì AE, Ardigò M, Micali G. Handheld reflectance confocal microscopy for the diagnosis of molluscum contagiosum: histopathology and dermoscopy correlation. Australas J Dermatol 2017;58(3):e123–5.
7. Micali G, Lacarrubba F. Augmented diagnostic capability using videodermatoscopy on selected infectious and non-infectious penile growths. Int J Dermatol 2011;50(12):1501–5.
8. Ku SH, Cho EB, Park EJ, et al. Dermoscopic features of molluscum contagiosum based on white structures and their correlation with histopathological findings. Clin Exp Dermatol 2015;40(2):208–10.
9. Zhuang K, Ran Y, Xu F, Lama J. Atypical infantile genital molluscum contagiosum. An Bras Dermatol 2015;90:403–5.
10. Chuh A, Zawar V, Ooi C, Lee A. A case-control study in primary care settings on the roles of dermatoscopy in infectious diseases affecting the skin, Part 1: viral and bacterial infections. Skinmed 2018;16(4):247–54.
11. Ianhez M, CestariSda C, Enokihara MY, Seize MB. Dermoscopic patterns of molluscum contagiosum: a study of 211 lesions confirmed by histopathology. An Bras Dermatol 2011;86(1):74–9.

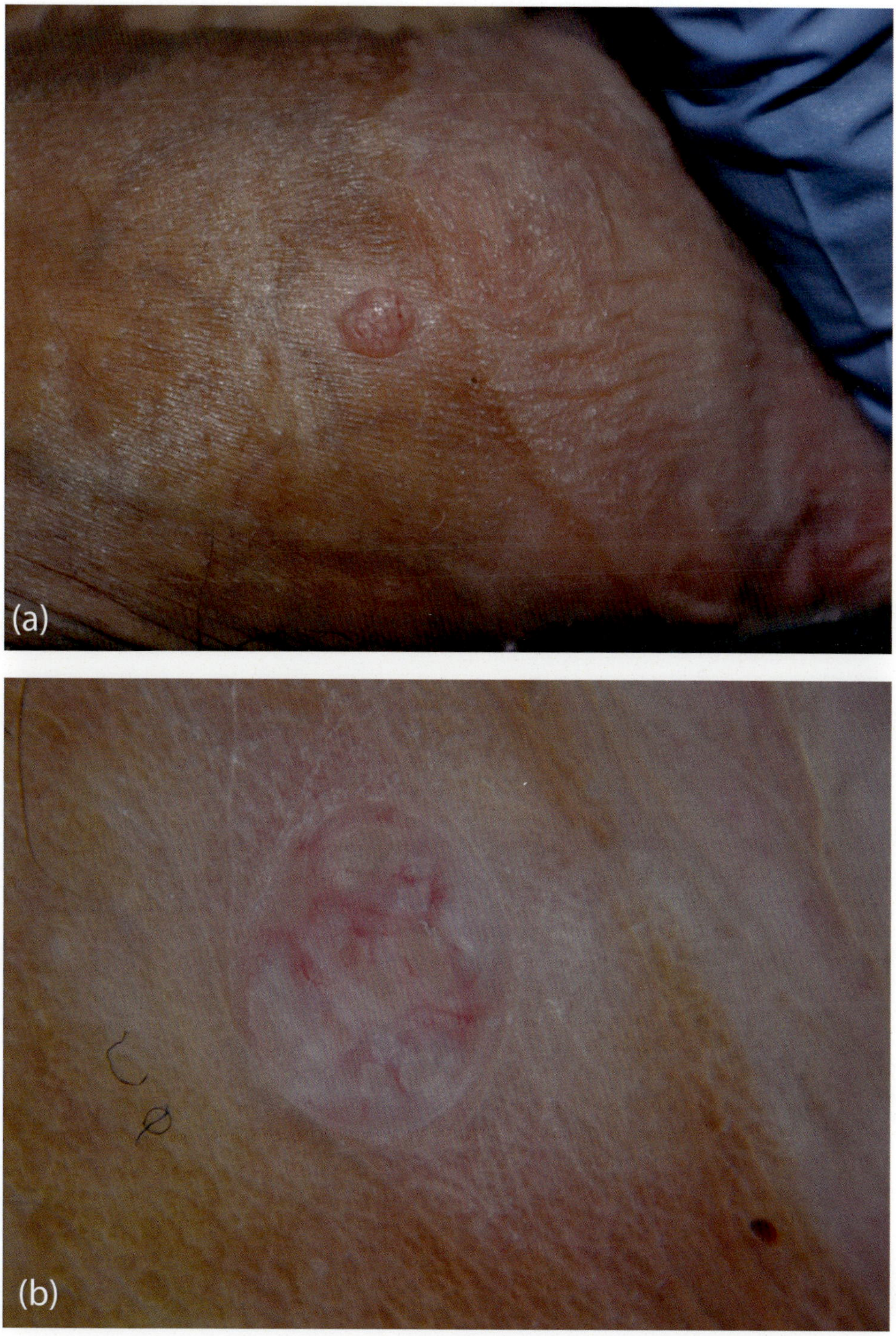

Figure 4.1 (a) Molluscum contagiosum. Single, dome-shaped, and pinkish papule of the penile shaft in a 45-year-old man. (b) Dermoscopy (×10) showing multiple, roundish, and yellowish structures ("pores") surrounded by irregular vessels.

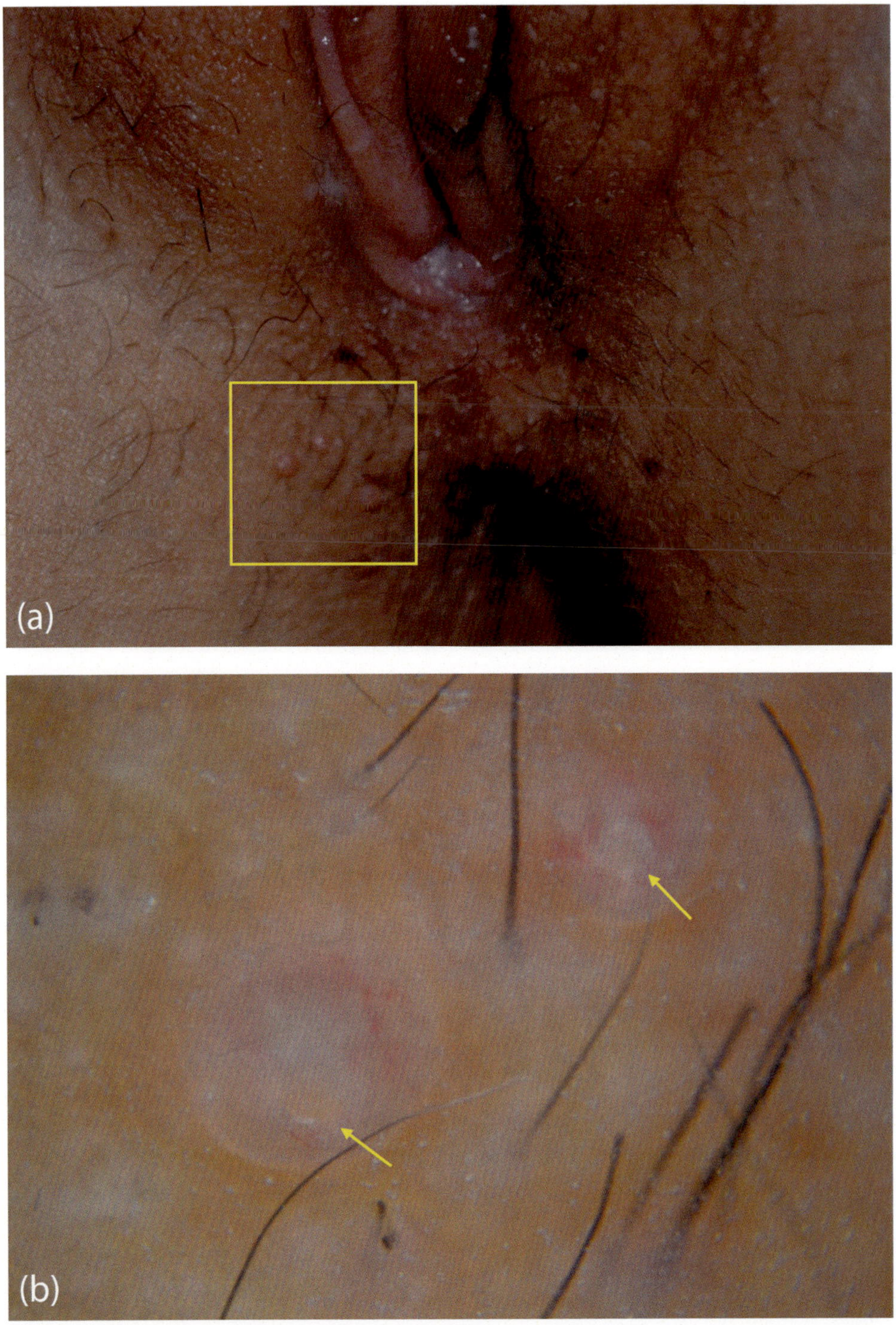

Figure 4.2 (a) Molluscum contagiosum. Multiple, small, and skin-colored papules of the perineum (square) in a 33-year-old woman. (b) Dermoscopy (×10) of two lesions showing central, roundish, and yellowish "pores" (arrows) surrounded by fine vessels.

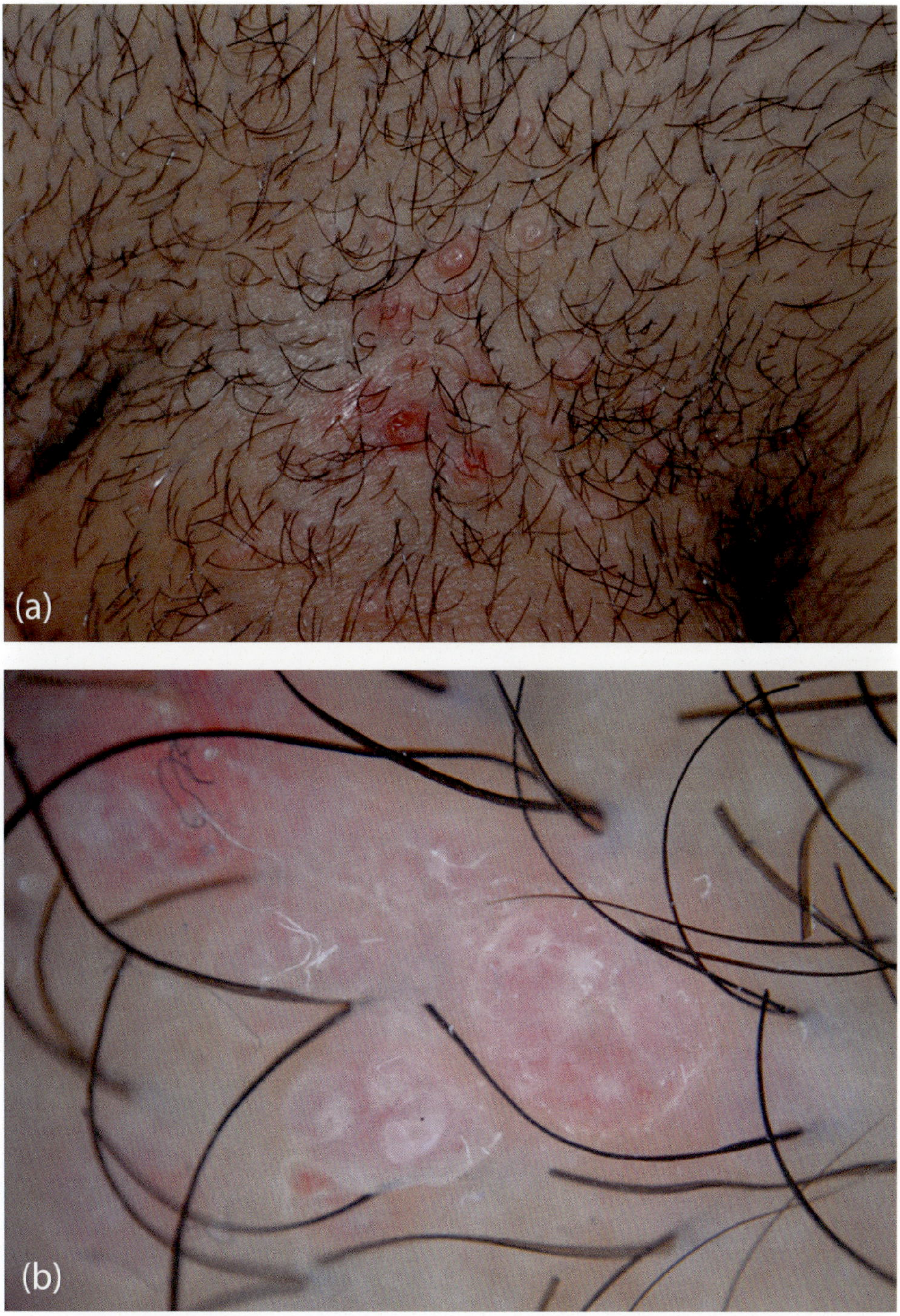

Figure 4.3 (a) Molluscum contagiosum. Multiple, confluent, and pinkish papules of the pubis in a 22-year-old man, some of them showing the typical umbilication. (b) Dermoscopy (×10) showing polylobular, yellowish structures, and irregular vessels.

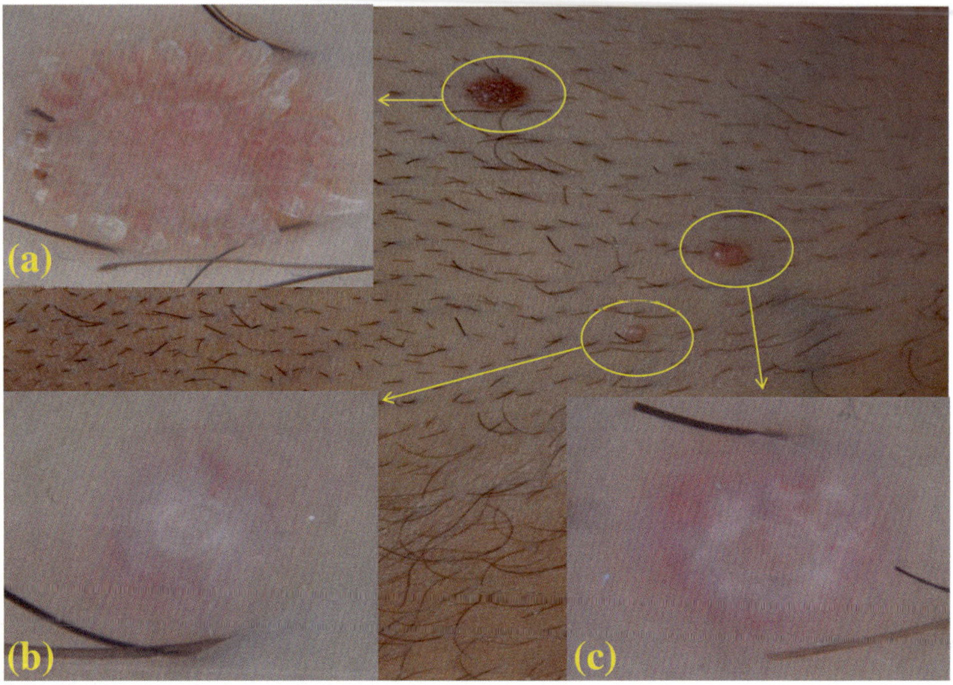

Figure 4.4 A 28-year-old man showing molluscum contagiosum and genital warts on the pubic area. (a) Dermoscopy (×10) of a wart showing irregular whitish projections of different sizes containing dilated vessels (see Chapter 3). (b, c) Dermoscopy (×10) of molluscum contagiosum showing central, roundish, and yellowish "pores" surrounded by fine vessels.

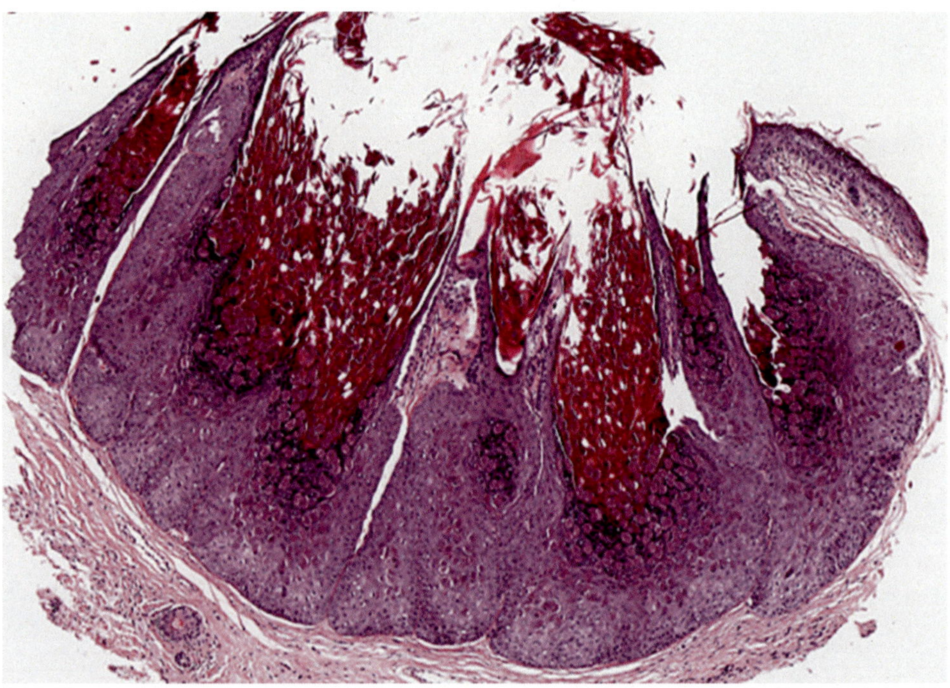

Figure 4.5 Histopathology of molluscum contagiosum showing a cup-shaped, invaginated, and lobulated epidermal hyperplasia composed of enlarged keratinocytes (H&E, ×100).

CHAPTER 5

Scabies

Anna Elisa Verzì MD, Angelo Di Natale MD, and Giuseppe Micali MD

DEFINITION

Scabies is a highly contagious ectoparasitosis caused by *Sarcoptes scabiei* var. *hominis* and characterized by diffuse and intense pruritus (1).

EPIDEMIOLOGY

Scabies is estimated to affect around 150–200 million people globally (1, 2). The prevalence is highest in low- and middle-income tropical countries, where scabies is an endemic disease (1, 2). In industrialized countries, outbreaks are common in institutions and communities such as hospitals, schools, nursing homes, prisons, retirement homes, and long-term care facilities. Genital lesions are reported to occur in up to 10–30% of males with scabies (2).

ETIOLOGY

S. scabiei var. *hominis* is a human-specific ectoparasite of approximately 0.4 mm in size that is not visible to the naked eye. Scabies infestation begins when a fertilized female mite burrows into the patient's epidermis. Following primary infestation, individuals are usually asymptomatic for the incubation period of 4–6 weeks. Itch is common and is related to a cutaneous hypersensitivity reaction to the mite and its products (3). *S. scabiei* can survive outside of the host for up to 24–36 hours (4). The risk of transmission is related to the frequency, duration, and surface area of skin contacts.

CLINICAL FEATURES

The pathognomonic lesion of scabies is the burrow, a slightly raised, silvery-gray, whitish or light brown, linear or sinuous tract measuring about 3–7 mm in length and approximately 0.4 mm in width (2). Other scabies lesions consist of small, raised, erythematous papules due to hypersensitivity. Both burrows and papules are typically located on interdigital spaces, creases of the palms and soles, volar aspects of the wrists, and ankles. The genital region [Figures 5.1(a) and 5.2(a)], breasts, buttocks, and axillae are often involved (2, 5). Larger, nodular lesions may occur and persist for several weeks, even after mites are successfully eradicated. Papules or larger

DOI: 10.1201/9781003007166-5

nodules found on the penis (shaft, corona, glans, and prepuce) and/or scrotum are highly specific for scabies.

Itch is typically described as more severe at night and can induce sleep disruption. Excoriations, scratching marks, and secondary bacterial infections (mainly due to *Staphylococcus aureus* and *Streptococcus pyogenes*) are related to itching (2).

DIFFERENTIAL DIAGNOSIS

The differential diagnosis includes all cutaneous disorders characterized by diffuse pruritus such as arthropod bites, papular urticaria, body and pubic lice, atopic dermatitis, prurigo nodularis, dermatitis herpetiformis, mycosis fungoides, and delusionary parasitosis.

DIAGNOSIS

The diagnosis of scabies can be clinically suspected when typical skin lesions with characteristic distribution are present in patient with diffuse pruritus. However, microscopic and/or instrumental identification of the scabies mite or its products (eggs or fecal pellets) is recommended to confirm the diagnosis. According to the 2020 International Alliance for the Control of Scabies (IACS) Consensus Criteria for the Diagnosis of Scabies (2), "clinical scabies" needs at least one of the following: 1) scabies burrows; 2) typical lesions affecting male genitalia; 3) typical lesions in a typical distribution and two history features. On the other hand, "confirmed scabies" should include at least one of the following: 1) mites, eggs, or feces on light microscopy of skin samples; 2) mites, eggs, or feces visualized on individual using high-powered imaging device (videodermatoscopy, reflectance confocal microscopy, or optical coherence tomography); 3) mite visualized on individual using dermoscopy.

DERMOSCOPY

Since 1992, the use of epiluminescence microscopy has been suggested in diagnosing scabies (6). Nowadays, dermoscopy is a common diagnostic practice for scabies in many dermatologic centers. At low magnification (×10), the typical feature of scabies consists of a small dark brown triangular structure located at the end of a subtle linear segment, resembling a delta wing jet with contrail [Figures 5.1(b) and 5.2(b)]. Of note, splinter hemorrhages due to scratching may mimic the dark brown triangular structure (Figure 5.3). Higher magnifications (>×100) allow a clear visualization of the oval, translucent body of the mite and its legs, rostrum, eggs, and feces (Figure 5.4) (1, 2, 7–9). Compared to skin scraping, dermoscopy is more sensitive, fast, and well accepted by patients (5, 9, 10).

Although a limitation of the use of high-quality devices may be their high cost, recently low-cost videomicroscopes, allowing magnification up to ×1000 (cost is about $30) and available for nonmedical use, have been reported to enable adequate and optimal visualization of the typical signs of scabies, similar to that observed by standard videodermatoscopes (8).

HISTOPATHOLOGICAL CORRELATION

The "delta wing jet" and the "contrail" histopathologically correspond to the pigmented anterior part of the mite and the burrow, respectively.

REFERENCES

1. Thomas C, Coates SJ, Engelman D, et al. Ectoparasites: scabies. J Am Acad Dermatol 2020;82(3):533–48.
2. Engelman D, Yoshizumi J, Hay RJ, et al. The 2020 IACS consensus criteria for the diagnosis of scabies. Br J Dermatol 2020;183(5):808–20.
3. Bhat SA, Mounsey KE, Liu X, Walton SF. Host immune responses to the itch mite, *Sarcoptes scabiei*, in humans. Parasit Vectors 2017;10:385.
4. Arlian LG, Morgan MS. A review of *Sarcoptes scabiei*: past, present and future. Parasit Vectors 2017;10(1):297.
5. Lacarrubba F, Borghi A, Verzì AE, et al. Dermoscopy of genital diseases: a review. J Eur Acad Dermatol 2020;34(10):2198–207.
6. Kreusch J. Incident light microscopy: reflection on microscopy of the living skin. Int J Dermatol 1992;31:618–20.
7. Lacarrubba F, Micali G. Videodermatoscopy and scabies. J Pediatr 2013;163(4):1227–1227.e1.
8. Micali G, Lacarrubba F, Verzì AE, Nasca MR. Low-cost equipment for diagnosis and management of endemic scabies outbreaks in underserved populations. Clin Infect Dis 2015;60(2):327–9.
9. Micali G, Lacarrubba F, Verzì AE, et al. Scabies: advances in noninvasive diagnosis. PLOS Negl Trop Dis 2016;10(6):e0004691.
10. Suh KS, Han SH, Lee KH, et al. Mites and burrows are frequently found in nodular scabies by dermoscopy and histopathology. J Am Acad Dermatol 2014;71(5):1022–3.

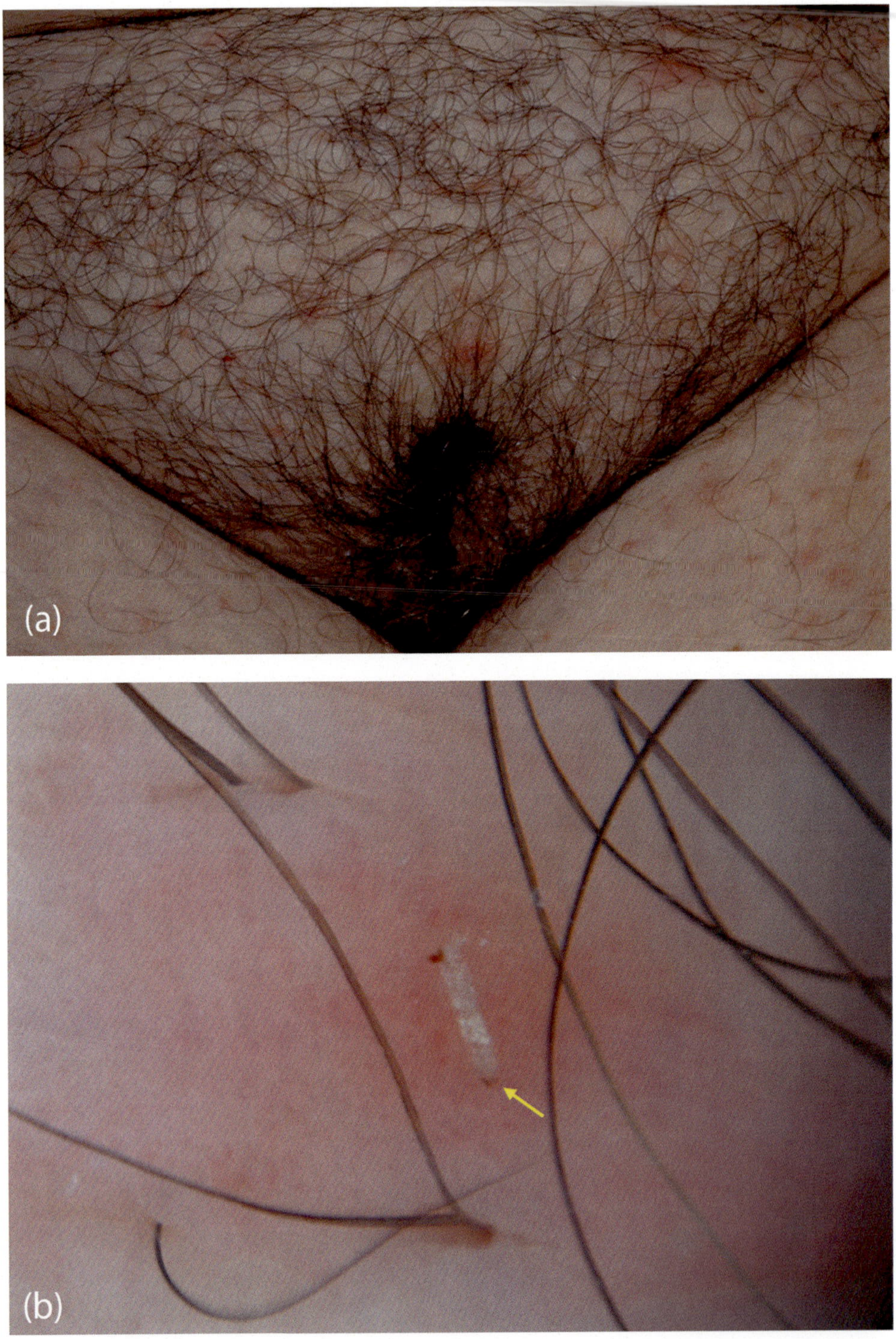

Figure 5.1 (a) Scabies. Multiple erythematous papules and scratching marks on the pubic area of a 42-year-old woman. Similar, itchy lesions were observed on the breasts and wrists. (b) Dermoscopy (×10) showing a burrow with the typical "jet with contrail" shape: the brownish triangular structure located at the lower extremity (arrow) corresponds to the anterior structures of *Sarcoptes scabiei*.

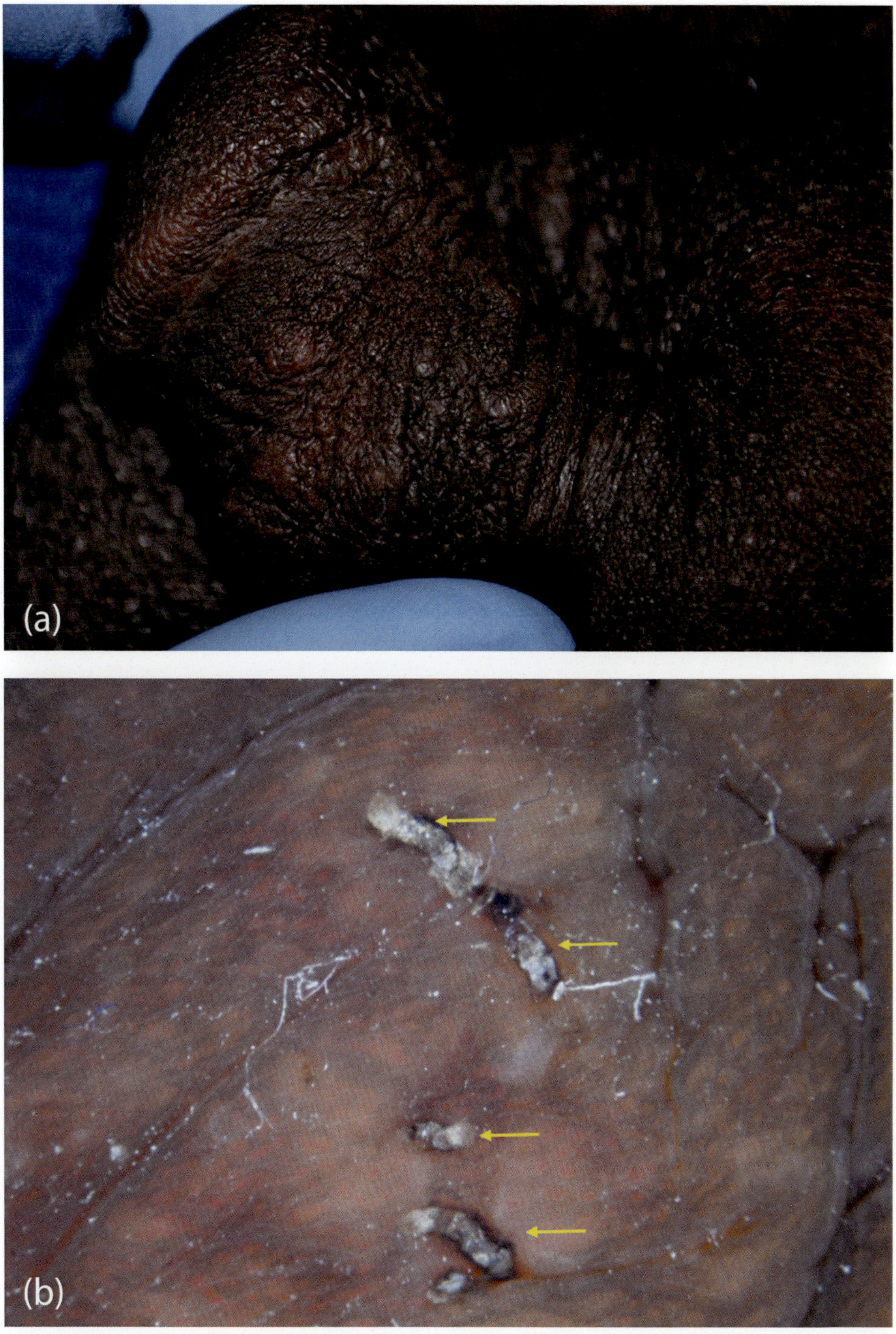

Figure 5.2 (a) Scabies. Multiple skin-colored papules of the penile shaft in a 24-year-old black patient. The patient had been previously treated with topical steroids. (b) Dermoscopy (×10) showing multiple burrows (arrows).

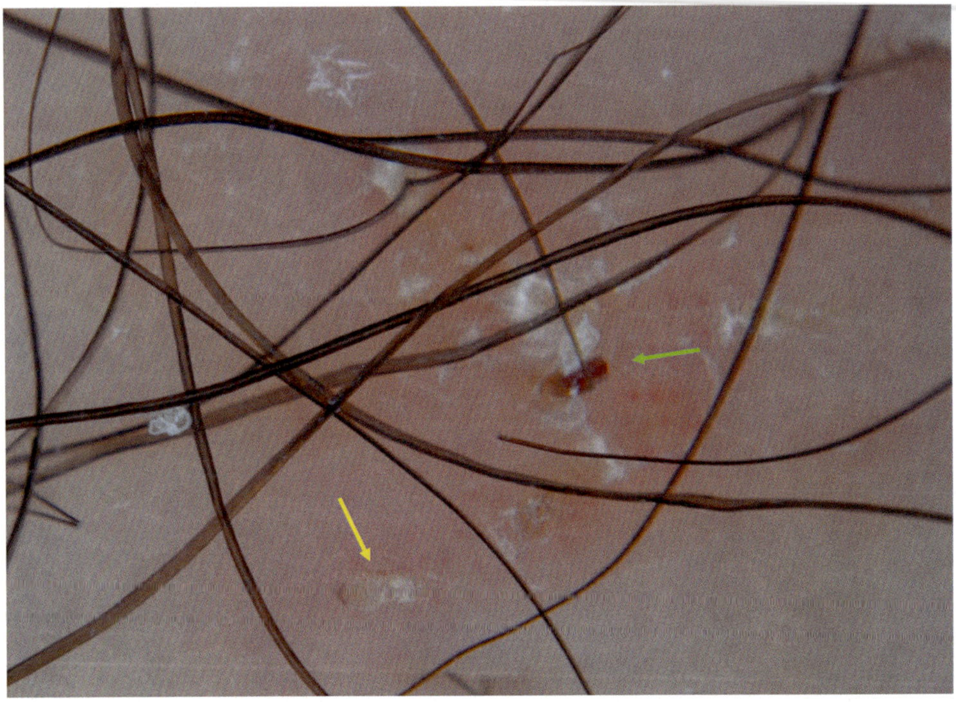

Figure 5.3 Dermoscopy (×10) showing a burrow with the typical "jet with contrail" shape (yellow arrow). Note the splinter hemorrhage in the center of the image (green arrow) resembling the mite.

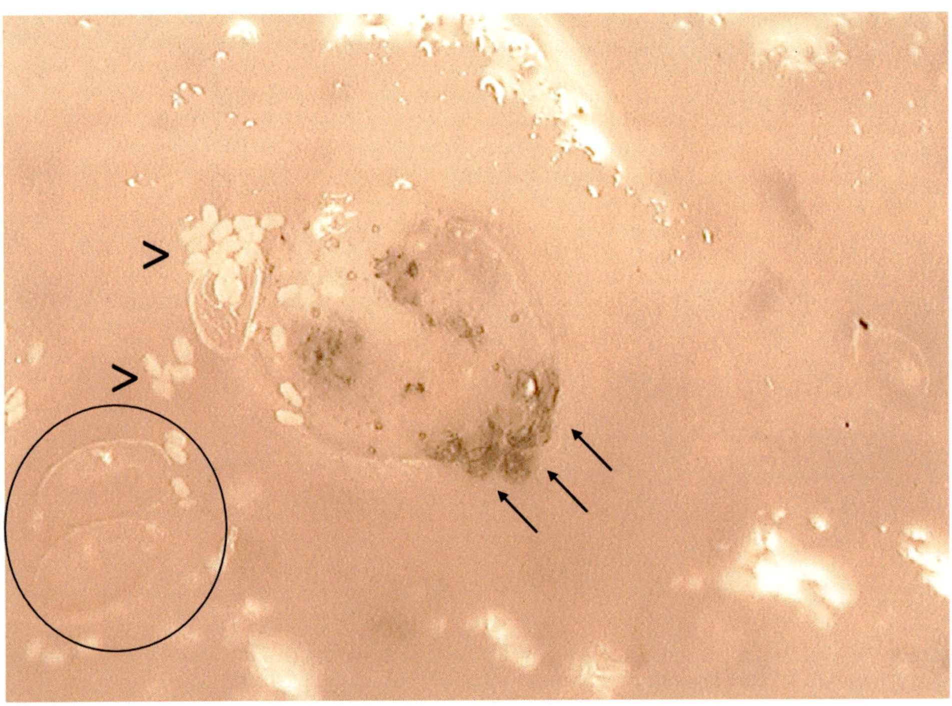

Figure 5.4 High-magnification dermoscopy (×500) of *Sarcoptes scabiei* on the skin showing the roundish body with a pigmented area (arrows) corresponding to the mouth parts and the two anterior pairs of legs. Two eggs (circle) and small feces (arrowheads) are also visible.

CHAPTER 6

Pediculosis Pubis

Maria Rita Nasca MD PhD, Francesca Sorci MD, and Francesco Lacarrubba MD

DEFINITION

Pediculosis pubis (PP) is an ectoparasitosis caused by *Phthirus pubis* (also known as crab louse) and typically transmitted by sexual or intimate contact.

EPIDEMIOLOGY

Accurate epidemiologic data are difficult to collect because PP cases are not rigorously registered. However, the infestation occurs worldwide and affects both genders (1) being particularly prevalent in groups that live in crowded spaces with poor sanitary conditions. It seems slightly more prevalent in men aged from 15 to 40 years (2).

ETIOLOGY

P. pubis is a blood-sucking insect and obligate human parasite (3). Lice have a light brown body, crab shape, measuring about 0.8–1.2 mm in length with three pairs of legs. *P. pubis* lives on average 15 days, the female lays 25 eggs, the incubation of the nits lasts 7 days, and the nymphs mature in 14 days (4). The infection is usually transmitted through physical or sexual contact or by fomites (underwear, bedding material).

CLINICAL FEATURES

Pruritus, due to lice bites and saliva's hypersensitivity, is the main symptom of PP. Clinical signs mainly include erythematous papules, scratching lesions, and bluish macules ("maculae ceruleae") at the site of crab bites, especially on the lower abdomen and thighs. An associated locoregional lymphadenopathy due to secondary infections may be sometimes observed. The infestation typically involves the pubis and genital area [Figures 6.1(a) and 6.2(a)], but other hairy regions may also be interested, such as axillae, chest, limbs, eyebrows, and eyelashes (phthiriasis palpebrarum) (3). PP may be associated with other sexually transmitted diseases that are present in about 30% of infested individuals; thus, screening for other infections is strongly recommended (5, 6).

DOI: 10.1201/9781003007166-6

DIFFERENTIAL DIAGNOSIS

Different pruritic dermatosis may simulate PP of the genital area, such as scabies, tinea cruris, trichomycosis, contact dermatitis, and seborrheic dermatitis.

DIAGNOSIS

The diagnosis of PP is usually clinical, based on the identification of the crab lice, nymphs, or nits at close inspection, possibly with the aid of a magnifying glass. Nits appear as small, gray-brownish granules attached to the hair. When present, maculae ceruleae are a characteristic finding.

DERMOSCOPY

Dermoscopy is useful to establish a quick and definitive diagnosis of PP (6). It clearly shows the presence of adult crab lice [Figures 6.1(b) and 6.2(b)] or nymphs and white-brownish nits attached to hair shafts. Viable nits appear as ovoid, brown structures characterized by a convex free ending (Figure 6.3), while empty nits appear as ovoid, translucent structures with flat free endings (Figure 6.4). This information represents an essential clue to a correct therapeutic approach (7). Dermoscopy also allows a clear differentiation from other entities that mimic nits (pseudonits), such as scales of atopic dermatitis or trichomycosis pubis (8). Moreover, it improves the monitoring of the clinical response to treatment, also allowing to establish the optimal times of application of the drugs, in order to minimize the risk of excessive treatment and the side effects (9).

HISTOPATHOLOGICAL CORRELATION

Histopathology examination is not necessary to diagnose pediculosis.

REFERENCES

1. Coates SJ, Thomas C, Chosidow O, et al. Ectoparasites: pediculosis and tungiasis. J Am Acad Dermatol 2020;82(3):551–69.
2. Wang T, Fan YM. White eggs and yellow-brown spots on the pubic-perineal hairs. BMJ 2019;367:l6559.
3. Chosidow O. Scabies and pediculosis. Lancet 2000;355(9206):819–26.
4. Shakya M, Jayraw AK, Singh M. Pubic lice infestation in man from Mhow, Madhya Pradesh. J Parasit Dis 2018;42(3):402–4.
5. Salavastru CM, Chosidow O, Janier M, Tiplica GS. European guideline for the management of pediculosis pubis. J Eur Acad Dermatol Venereol 2017;31(9):1425–28.
6. Scott GR, Chosidow O, IUSTI/WHO. European guideline for the management of pediculosis pubis, 2010. Int J STD AIDS 2011;22(6):304–5.
7. Giuffrida G, Lacarrubba F, Boscaglia S, et al. A noninvasive aid for office-based gynecologists for the diagnosis of common external genital disorders. Obstet Gynecol Int 2019;2019:1830245.
8. Lacarrubba F, Verzì AE, Micali G. Trichoscopy in the differential diagnosis of pseudonits. Skin Appendage Disord 2019;5(3):142–5.
9. Micali G, Tedeschi A, West DP, Dinotta F, Lacarrubba F. The use of videodermatoscopy to monitor treatment of scabies and pediculosis. J Dermatolog Treat 2011;22(3):133–37.

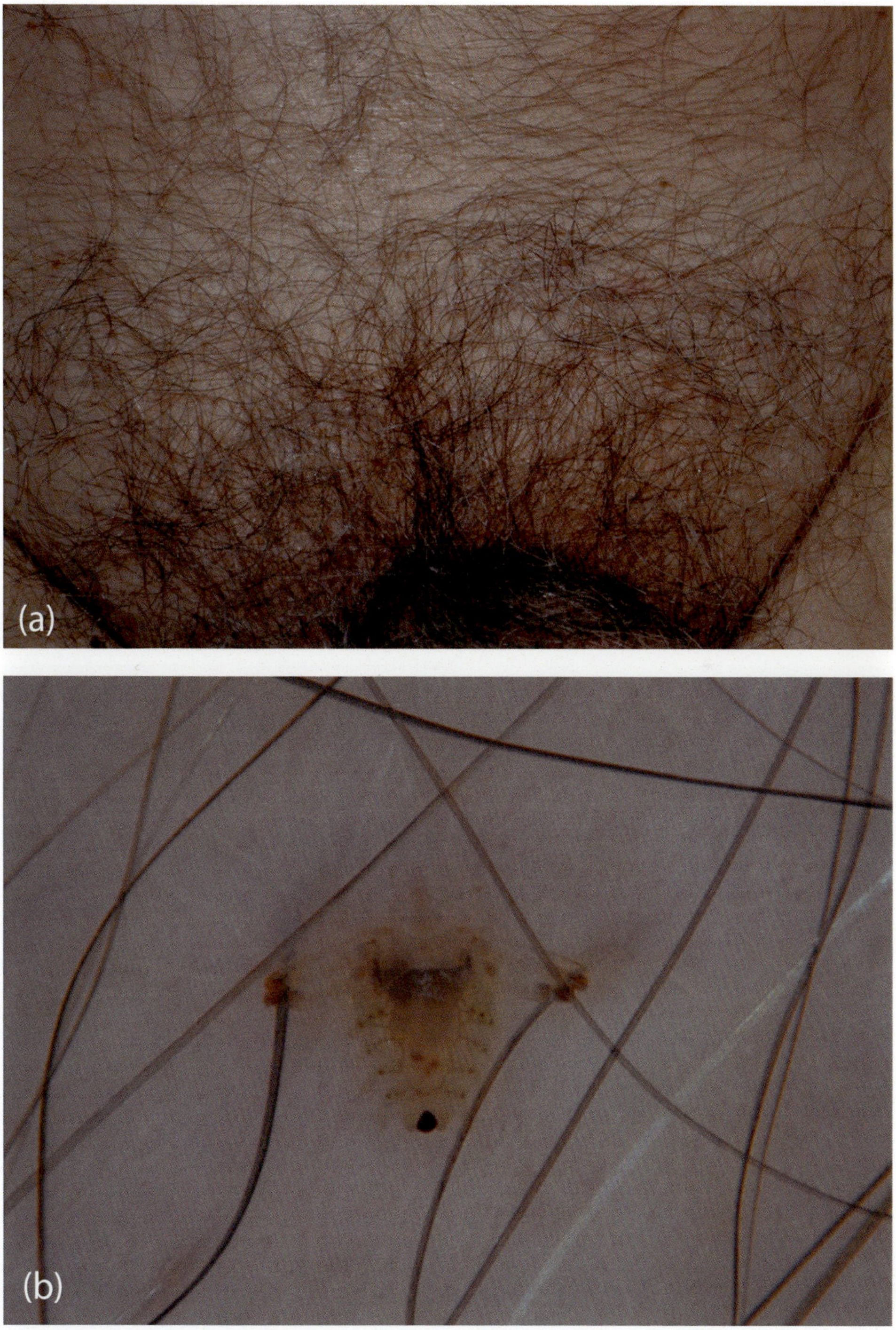

Figure 6.1 (a) Pediculosis pubis. Multiple erythematous papules of the pubis in a 56-year-old man. (b) Dermoscopy (×10) showing *Phthirus pubis* firmly attached to two adjacent hairs with the anterior legs.

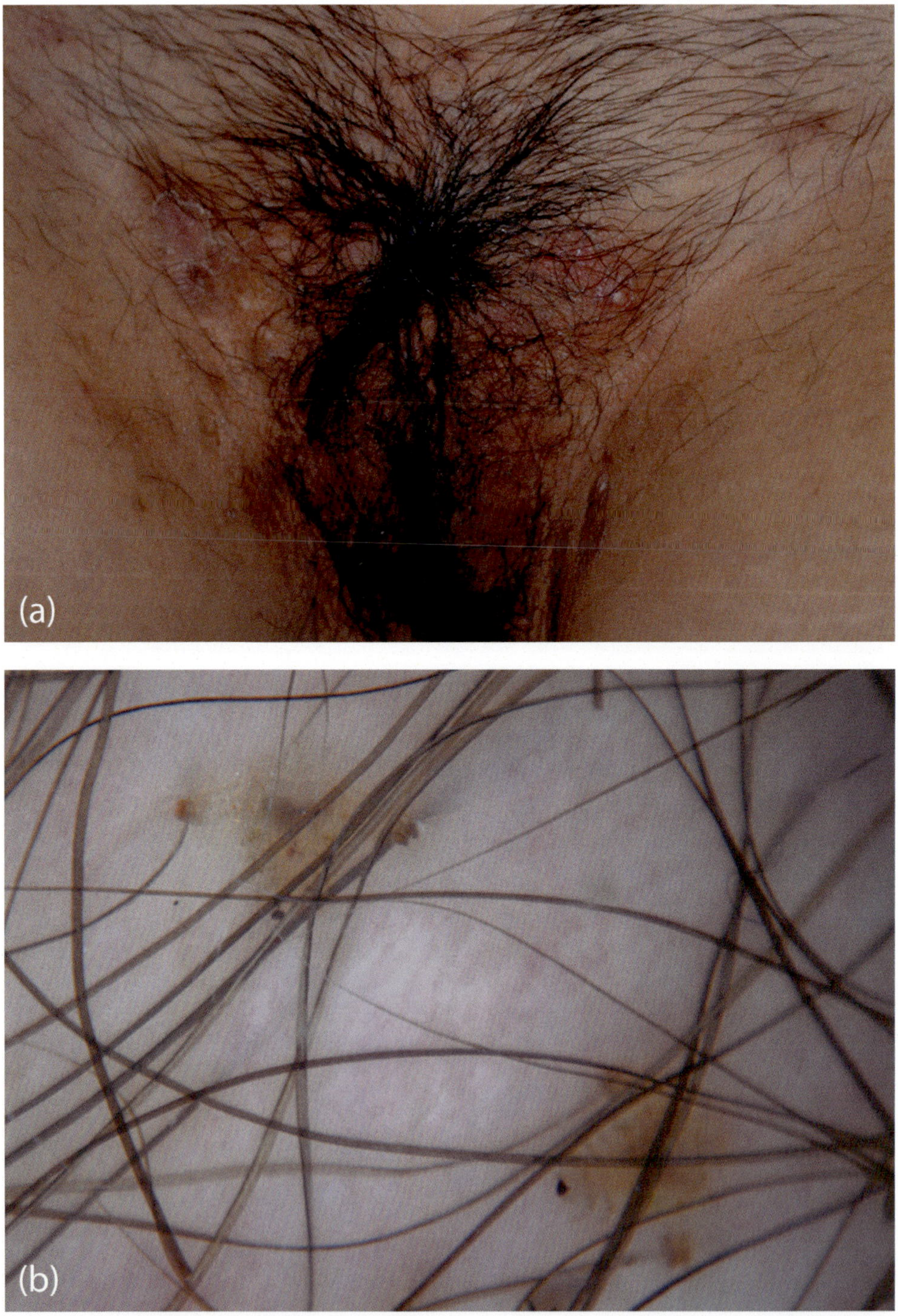

Figure 6.2 (a) Pediculosis pubis. Multiple erythematous papules and scratching marks of the genital area in a 24-year-old woman. The patient had been treated for 1 month for eczema. (b) Dermoscopy (×10) showing two crab lice firmly attached to the hairs.

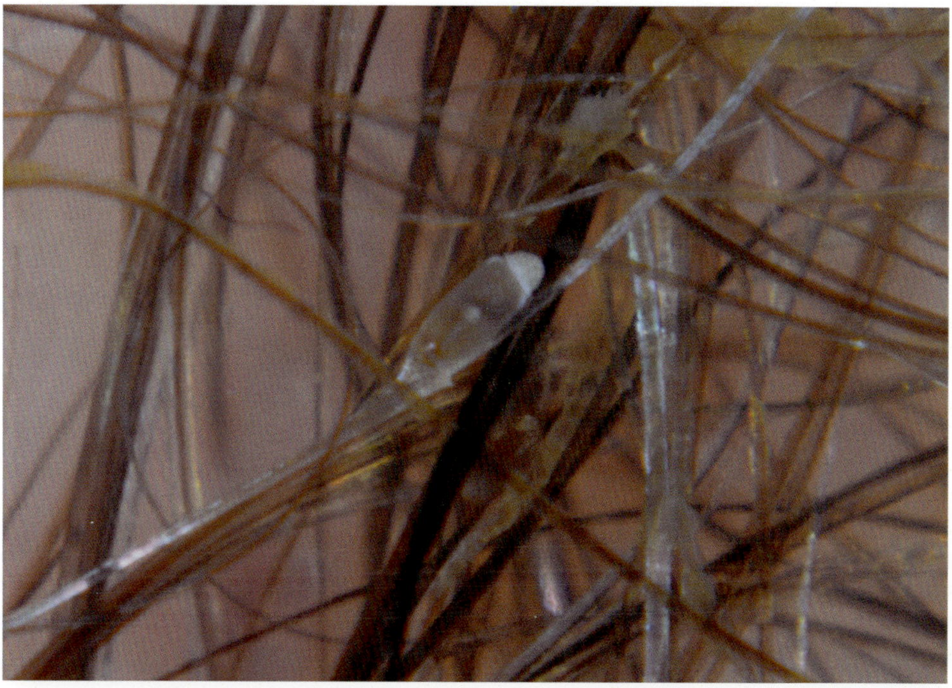

Figure 6.3 Pediculosis pubis. Dermoscopy (×10) showing a full, viable nit appearing as an ovoid, brown structure with a convex free ending and attached to the hair shaft.

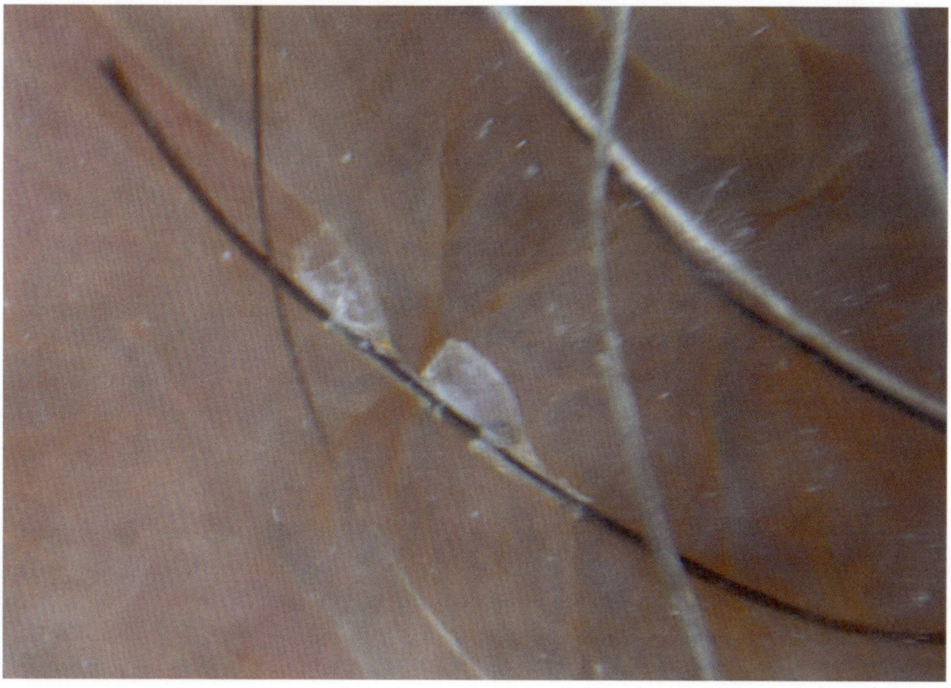

Figure 6.4 Pediculosis pubis. Dermoscopy (×10) showing two empty nits appearing as ovoid, translucent structures with flat free endings.

CHAPTER 7

Candidiasis

Enzo Errichetti MD and Giuseppe Stinco MD

DEFINITION

Cutaneous candidiasis is a superficial opportunistic infection of the skin due to yeasts of the *Candida* species (1, 2). Two main forms exist, primary (without specific underlying skin disease) and secondary (i.e., forms arising on the background of other dermatoses, such as atopic dermatitis, psoriasis or diaper dermatitis) (1, 2).

EPIDEMIOLOGY

It is a frequent disease that may potentially affect all age groups, though it is more prevalent in old age and infancy (1–4). It accounts for approximately 1% of all outpatient and 7% of all inpatient visits to dermatological clinics (3, 4).

ETIOLOGY

A variety of *Candida* species may be responsible, with *C. albicans* being the most common one (1, 2). They are part of the normal microflora of several districts (e.g., oral cavity, gastrointestinal tract, vagina, and penis) and become pathogenic only when favorable conditions arise (1, 2). Albeit all body areas may be involved, cutaneous candidiasis mainly affects skin folds and anogenital areas, as such regions are characterized by a high humidity degree, which remarkably favors *Candida* growth (1, 2). Other predisposing factors include immunosuppression, diabetes mellitus, systemic corticosteroids, and broad-spectrum antibiotic use, pregnancy, and endocrine disorders (1, 2).

CLINICAL FEATURES

The patient with candidal vulvovaginitis [Figures 7.1(a) and 7.2(a)] may present with intense itching and irritation in the vagina and vulva, a burning sensation with urination which can be mistaken for urinary tract infection, vaginal soreness or pain, a dry erythematous rash, and a thick white discharge (1, 2). On the other hand, the penis is less commonly affected and may present itchy reddish and/or whitish patches of the glands and/or foreskin [Figure 7.3(a)] (1, 2). *Candida* infection may very rarely spread from such districts to other parts of the body resulting in fevers along with other symptoms (1, 2).

DOI: 10.1201/9781003007166-7

DIFFERENTIAL DIAGNOSIS

Candidal vulvovaginitis should be differentiated from conditions characterized by inflammation, pruritus and/or whitish discharge, including bacterial vaginosis, trichomonas vaginitis, atrophic vaginitis, and psoriasis, while candidal balanitis may be mistaken for other forms of balanitis, especially Zoon's balanitis, irritative balanitis and psoriatic balanitis (1, 2, 5, 6).

DIAGNOSIS

Genital candidiasis is diagnosed according to clinical presentation and mycological assessment of vaginal or penile discharge, including microscopic examination and fungal culture; under the microscope, budding yeast is visible (1, 2).

DERMOSCOPY

Cutaneous candidiasis is dermoscopically typified by erythema and epidermal detachment presenting as large scales usually having a peripheral distribution and an outward direction of extension (1, 2, 5, 6). However, genital lesions typically lack scaling due to the higher humidity degree of such areas, whereas it is possible to appreciate vascular features (mainly in the form of sparse, blurred arborizing, dotted, or linear-irregular vessels) and, most importantly, a fragmented, multifocal, white film, also known as "cottage cheese"-like structures [Figures 7.1(b) and 7.3(b)] (1, 2, 5, 6). Finally, dermoscopy may be of aid also in highlighting peripheral (satellite) pustules [Figure 7.2(b)] (1, 2, 5, 6).

HISTOPATHOLOGICAL CORRELATION

From a dermoscopic-pathological correlation point of view, white scaling is related to hyperkeratosis and acanthosis, while vascular features and "cottage cheese"-like structures correspond to inflammation/vasodilation and the presence of fungal colonies, respectively (1, 2, 5, 6).

REFERENCES

1. R AN, Rafiq NB. Candidiasis. 2020 Nov 20. In: StatPearls [Internet]. Treasure Island, FL: StatPearls Publishing; 2021 Jan. PMID: 32809459.
2. Taudorf EH, Jemec GBE, Hay RJ, Saunte DML. Cutaneous candidiasis – an evidence-based review of topical and systemic treatments to inform clinical practice. J Eur Acad Dermatol Venereol 2019;33:1863–73.
3. Sei Y. 2011 epidemiological survey of dermatomycoses in Japan. Med Mycol J 2015;56:J129–35.
4. Penate Y, Guillermo N, Melwani P, et al. Dermatologists in hospital wards: an 8-year study of dermatology consultations. Dermatology 2009;219:225–31.
5. Errichetti E, Lallas A, Di Stefani A, et al. Accuracy of dermoscopy in distinguishing erythroplasia of Queyrat from common forms of chronic balanitis: results from a multicentric observational study. J Eur Acad Dermatol Venereol 2019;33:966–72.
6. Lekkas D, Lacarrubba F, Verzì AE, Micali G. Mycoses. In: Dermoscopy in General Dermatology (Lallas A, Errichetti E, Ioannides D, eds), 1st edn. Boca Raton, FL: CRC Press, 2018:210–20.

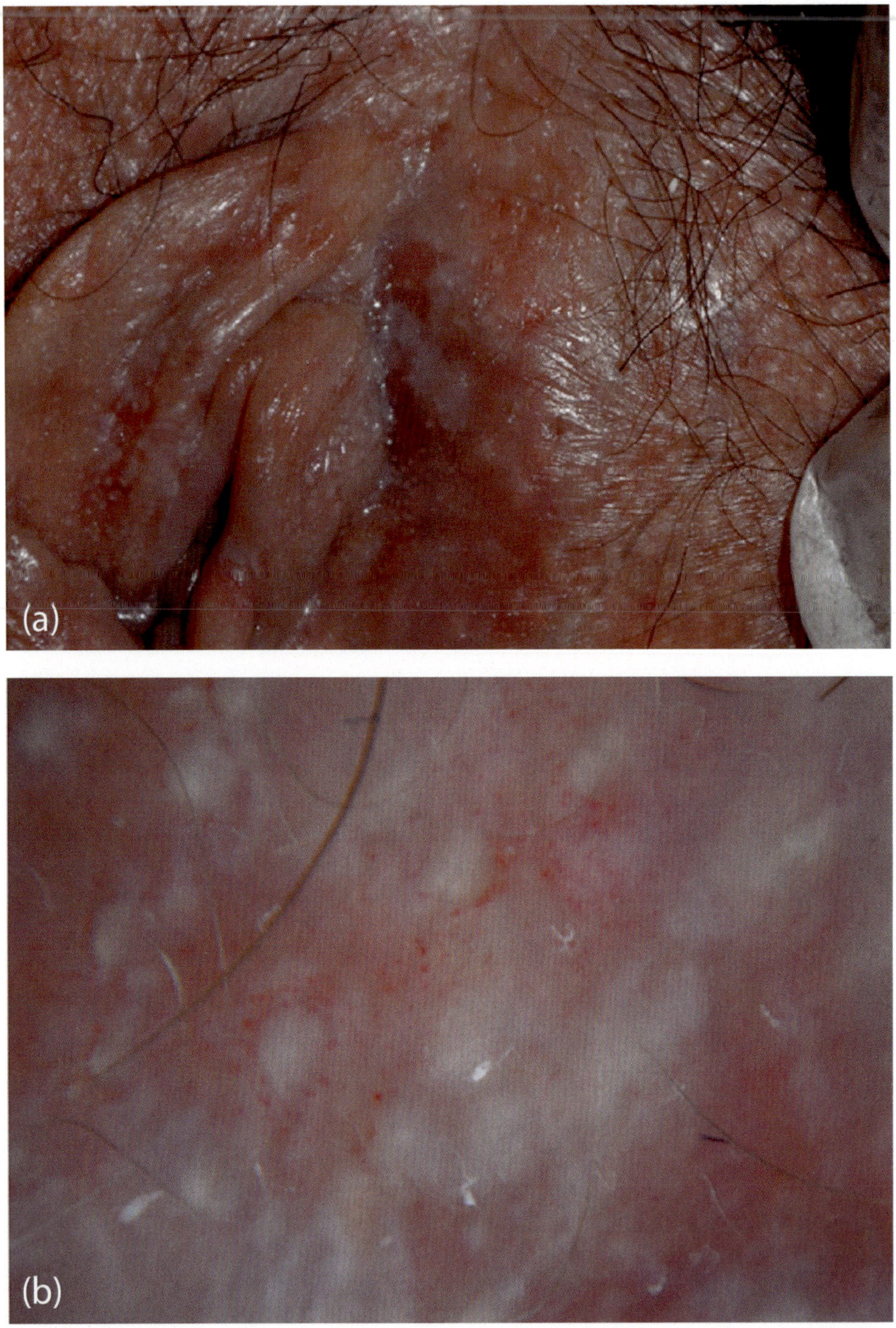

Figure 7.1 (a) Candidal vulvovaginitis. Erythema and whitish plaques involving the vulva. (b) Dermoscopy (×10) showing a multifocal white film ("cottage cheese"-like structures) along with sparse dotted vessels.

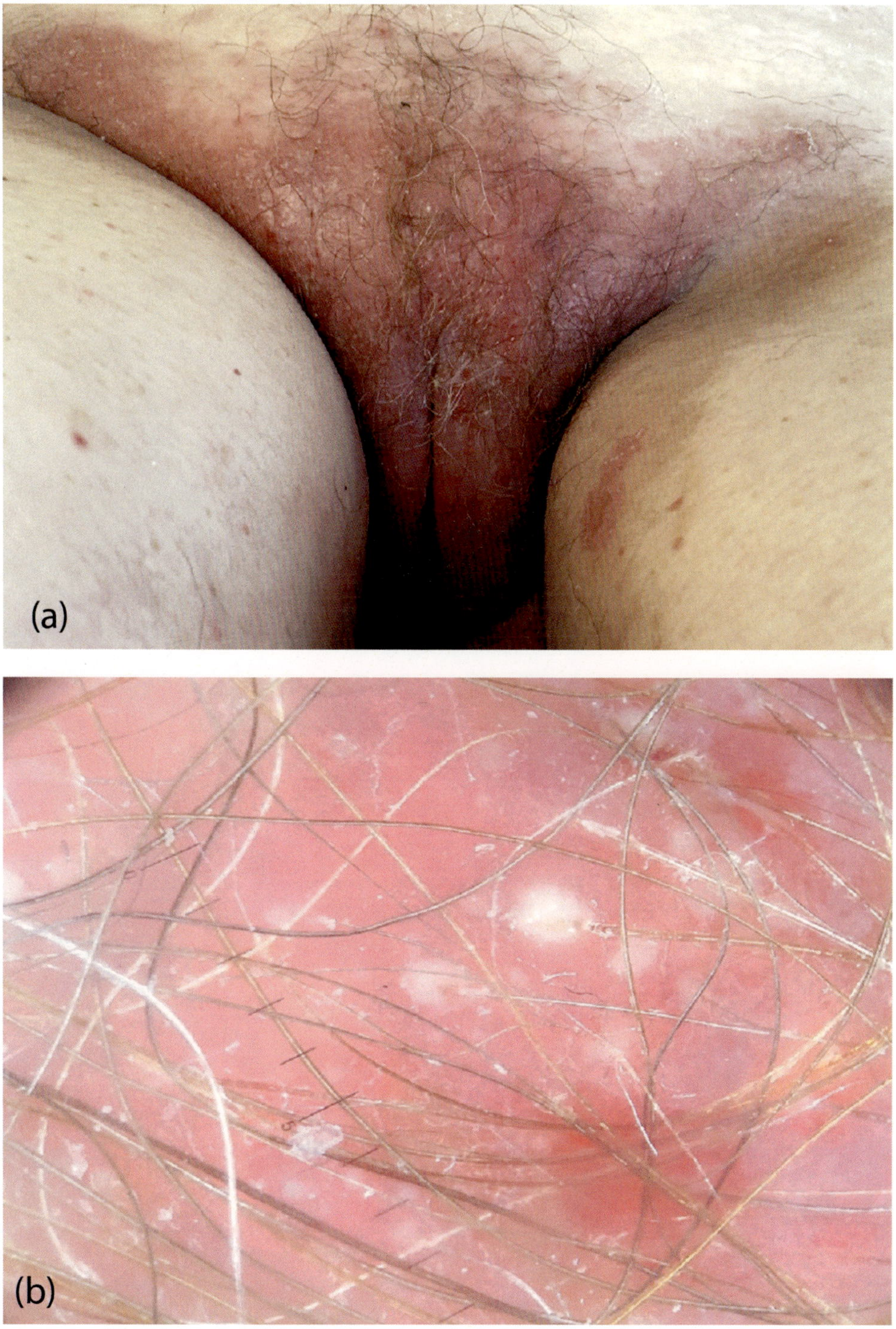

Figure 7.2 (a) Candidal vulvovaginitis. Diffuse erythema involving the perivulvar and pubic area. (b) Dermoscopy (×10) revealing an erythematous background and follicular pustules.

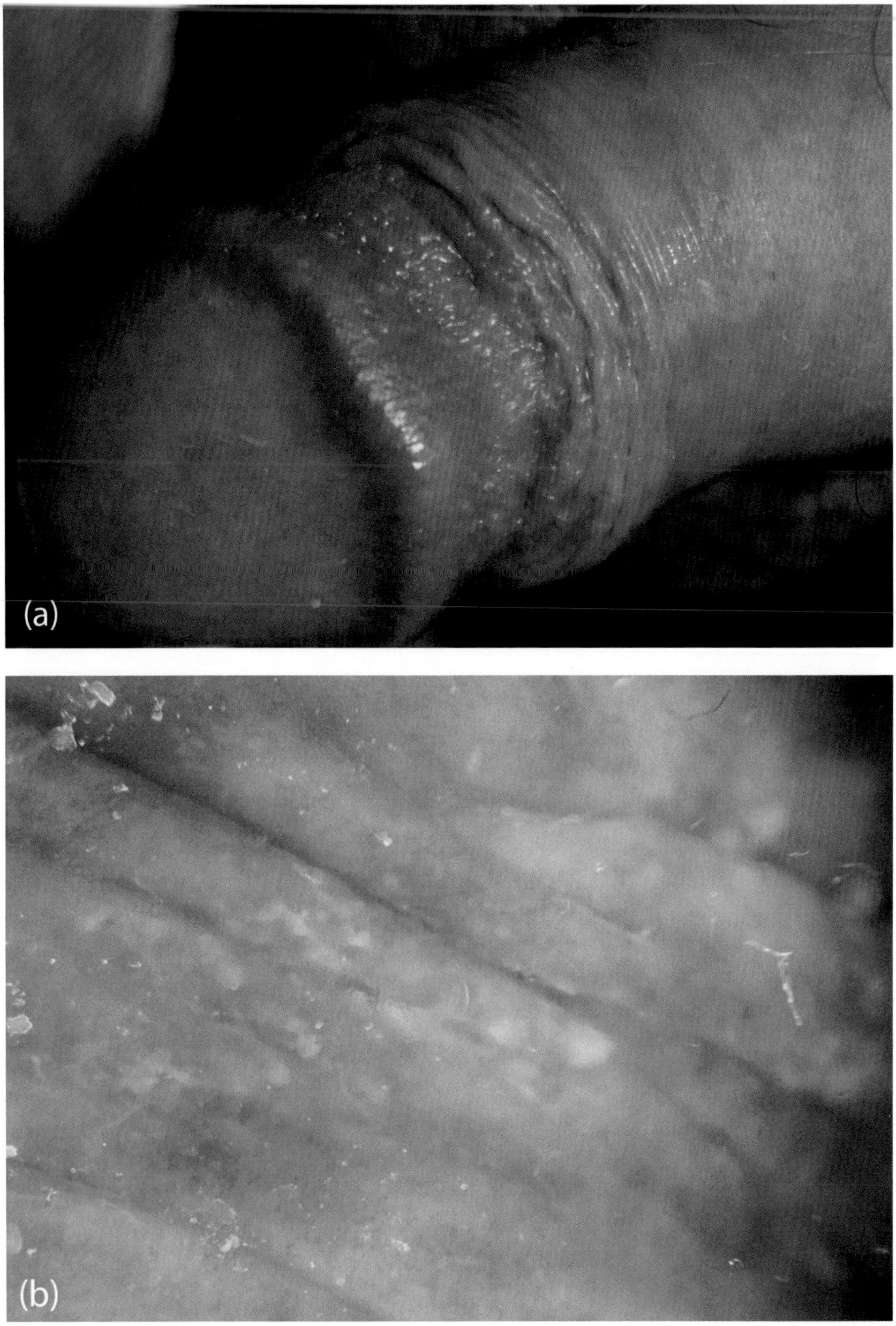

Figure 7.3 (a) Candidal balanitis. Diffuse erythema involving the glans and foreskin. (b) Dermoscopy (×10) displaying an erythematous background and a multifocal white film ("cottage cheese"-like structures).

CHAPTER 8

Lichen Planus

Alessandro Borghi MD, Giulia Toni MD, Giulia Odorici MD, Roberta Gafà MD, and Monica Corazza MD

DEFINITION

Lichen planus (LP) is a chronic, relapsing muco-cutaneous inflammatory disease with unknown etiology (1, 2).

EPIDEMIOLOGY

Genital LP (GLP) may be isolated or occur in association with either oral or skin involvement (2–5). Vulvovaginal LP (VVLP) mostly affects women in their perimenopausal and postmenopausal years but it may present at any time in adult life. A prevalence of 3.7% for VVLP on vulvar biopsies was found in the practice of a vulvar clinic (6). GLP constituted approximately 2–9% of cases of male non-venereal genital dermatoses in some reported series (7).

ETIOLOGY

LP etiology is not completely understood, but an autoimmune pathomechanism on a predisposing genetic background is hypothesized (8). LP is considered a prototypic 'interface dermatitis', in which a T cell-mediated response to unidentified either altered self-antigens or foreign antigens leads to an attack directed against basal keratinocytes (1). Various potential triggers, such as viral or bacterial antigens, metal ions, drugs, or physical factors, are supposed to initiate this autoimmune cell-mediated process, which leads to keratinocyte apoptosis (9).

CLINICAL FEATURES

In female patients, GLP involves the inner surface of the labia minora, but it may also affect the vagina. The hair-bearing areas are uncommon sites. From a clinical point of view, VVLP can present with three different variants: classic type or papulosquamous, hypertrophic, and erosive, which is the most common subtype (10). Erosive VVLP [Figures 8.1(a) and 8.2(a)] presents with a glazed erythema that may easily undergo bleeding and erosion (10). Mucous erythema is often surrounded by a lacy, white border, with or without Wickham striae (WS) in the surrounding skin. An alteration of the normal architecture may be observed. In papulosquamous VVLP, lesions may appear darkish red instead of the typical violaceous color of skin LP. The rare hypertrophic VVLP presents with

DOI: 10.1201/9781003007166-8

whitish papules/plaques with irregular borders and thickened irregular surface (7). Women with erosive VVLP can present with pain, dyspareunia, and dysuria while non-erosive forms are typically itching (2, 6, 10). A risk of malignant progression of 1–3% is reported (11).

In males, GLP typically presents with either an annular or reticular pattern [Figure 8.3(a)], with white streaks corresponding to WS, and is mainly located on glans penis. The penile shaft and coronal sulcus may be involved too. Koebernization can be seen. In papular form, penile LP (PLP) may show whitish, violaceous or reddish-brown papules, without scaling, which tend to coalesce into plaques [Figure 8.4(a)]. Other less common variants include erosive, bullous, atrophic, and hypertrophic LP (9). Itching is the most common symptom in annular and papular types; pain, burning, and sexual dysfunction occur in erosive PLP.

DIFFERENTIAL DIAGNOSIS

GLP may clinically resemble other inflammatory, infectious, or tumoral diseases such as plasma cell mucositis, lichen sclerosus, contact dermatitis, psoriasis, fixed drug reaction, erythema multiforme, autoimmune blistering disorders, genital warts, candidiasis, and genital intraepithelial neoplasia.

DIAGNOSIS

Diagnosis of GLP may be challenging, especially in the absence of cutaneous lesions, so the histopathological examination of a biopsy may be necessary (see below).

DERMOSCOPY

To date, only vulvovaginal cases of GLP have been described from a dermoscopic point of view (12). The following dermoscopic parameters, variously combined, enhance VVLP diagnostics: 1) thick linear, irregular vessels arranged diffusely throughout LP lesions; 2) peripheral WS, which can exhibit different morphological patterns; 3) an intense red background, especially in erosive subtypes [Figure 8.1(b)]. In VVLP, the vessels present different morphologies variously combined, including linear vessels, which appear as red telangiectasias of different calibre and size, and hairpin vessels. A parallel arrangement, mainly peripheral or close to WS, has been described. WS represent the dermoscopic hallmark of LP, which seem to be further highlighted by dermoscopic observation. Dermoscopy shows WS as pearly whitish structures, arranged in different patterns similar to those described in cutaneous LP, namely reticular, annular, dotted/"starry sky" and rounded/globular configuration (13–15). WS can also appear as peripheral thin projections, configuring a comb-like pattern, intermingled with parallel vessels. In some cases, WS present as structureless, blue-white, or gray-white areas, similar to a veil (12, 15). This latter one should not be confused with the white homogeneous areas observed at the sinuous, hyperkeratotic edge of the characteristic erythematous background, which correspond to the macerate border surrounding the erosive VVLP surfaces [Figure 8.2(b)]. Whereas WS are a constant dermoscopic feature in skin LP, they may be absent in a small rate of cases at a genital level. Finally, as reported in genital lichen sclerosus (16), gray-brown dots with a characteristic peppered arrangement may also be present in VVLP.

Based on our experience (unpublished cases) and sporadic reports (17), PLP with reticular configuration at dermoscopic observation shows white striae, corresponding to WS, with reticular (crossing lines) or crystalline (snow crystal-like) or leaf venation pattern, over a richly vascularized basis [Figures 8.3(b) and 8.4(b)]. Vessels are mainly dotted in shape. Black-grayish pigmentation arranged either in dots or in streaming lines can be observed on the outskirts of the waned white striae.

In summary, whitish WS with different arrangements are common dermoscopic clues in female and male GLP. A rich vascularization is mostly linear in shape at both erosive and mucosal surfaces and is predominantly dotted at the skin level. Vascular features are less evident or absent in dark-skinned patients (17). Erosive GLP presents light red background whereas in cutaneous LP a dull red color is predominant (18). Different patterns of pigmentation, namely pigmented dots, lines, globules and diffuse hyperpigmentation, the latter mainly at a cutaneous level and within mature lesions, are further dermoscopic features.

HISTOPATHOLOGICAL CORRELATION

The histological examination of GLP lesion reveals lichenoid dermatitis, with a band-like lymphohistiocytic infiltrate obscuring the dermo-epidermal junction (Figure 8.5) (7). Histological features that may be particularly useful for differentiating LP from other inflammatory disorders, mainly lichen sclerosus, include a wedge-shaped hypergranulosis, numerous cytoid bodies, and pointed rete ridges. The histological correlate of WS is a compact orthokeratosis above the zones of wedge-shaped hypergranulosis. The gray-brown dots with peppered arrangement and the globules correspond to melanophages in the dermis, as observed in cutaneous LP (13, 18). Linear vessels are the dermoscopic expression of the deeper ectatic horizontal subpapillary capillaries.

REFERENCES

1. Le Cleach L, Chosidow O. Clinical practice. Lichen planus. N Engl J Med 2012;366:723–32.
2. Fahy CMR, Torgerson RR, Davis MDP. Lichen planus affecting the female genitalia: a retrospective review of patients at Mayo Clinic. J Am Acad Dermatol 2017;77:1053–9.
3. Belfiore P, Di Fede O, Cabibi D, et al. Prevalence of vulval lichen planus in a cohort of women with oral lichen planus: an interdisciplinary study. Br J Dermatol 2006;155:994–8.
4. Kirtschig G, Wakelin SH, Wojnarowska F. Mucosal vulval lichen planus: outcome, clinical and laboratory features. J Eur Acad Dermatol Venereol 2005;19:301–7.
5. Eisen D. The clinical features, malignant potential, and systemic associations of oral lichen planus: a study of 723 patients. J Am Acad Dermatol 2002;46:207–14.
6. Micheletti L, Preti M, Bogliatto F, et al. Vulval lichen planus in the practice of a vulval clinic. Br J Dermatol 2000;143:1349–50.
7. Khurana A, Tandon S, Marfatia YS, Madnani N. Genital lichen planus: an underrecognized entity. Indian J Sex Transm Dis AIDS 2019;40:105–12.
8. Cooper SM, Ali I, Baldo M, Wojnarowska F. The association of lichen sclerosus and erosive lichen planus of the vulva with autoimmune disease: a case-control study. Arch Dermatol 2008;144:1432–5.
9. Lehman JS, Tollefson MM, Gibson LE. Lichen planus. Int J Dermatol 2009;48:682–94.
10. Lewis FM, Bogliatto F. Erosive vulval lichen planus—a diagnosis not to be missed: a clinical review. Eur J Obstet Gynecol Reprod Biol 2013;171:214–9.
11. Simpson RC, Littlewood SM, Cooper SM, et al. Real-life experience of managing vulval erosive lichen planus: a case-based review and UK multicentre case note audit. Br J Dermatol 2012;167:85–91.
12. Borghi A, Corazza M, Minghetti S, et al. Preliminary study on dermoscopic features of vulvar lichen planus: new insights for diagnosis. J Eur Acad Dermatol Venereol 2016;30:1063–5.
13. Vázquez-López F, Manjón-Haces JA, Maldonado-Seral C, et al. Dermoscopic features of plaque psoriasis and lichen planus: new observations. Dermatology 2003;207:151–6.
14. Vázquez-López F, Gómez-Díez S, Sánchez J, et al. Dermoscopy of active lichen planus. Arch Dermatol 2007;143:1092.
15. Tan C, Min ZS, Xue Y, et al. Spectrum of dermoscopic patterns in lichen planus: a case series from China. J Cutan Med Surg 2014;18:28–32.
16. Borghi A, Corazza M, Minghetti S, et al. Dermoscopic features of vulvar lichen sclerosus in the setting of a prospective cohort of patients: new observations. Dermatology 2016;232:71–7.
17. García-García B, Munguía-Calzada P, Aubán-Pariente L, et al. Dermoscopy of Lichen planus: vascular and Wickham striae variations in the skin of colour. Australas J Dermatol 2019;60:301–4.
18. Lallas A, Kyrgidis A, Tzellos TG et al. Accuracy of dermoscopic criteria for the diagnosis of psoriasis, dermatitis, lichen planus and pityriasis rosea. Br J Dermatol 2012;166:1198–205.

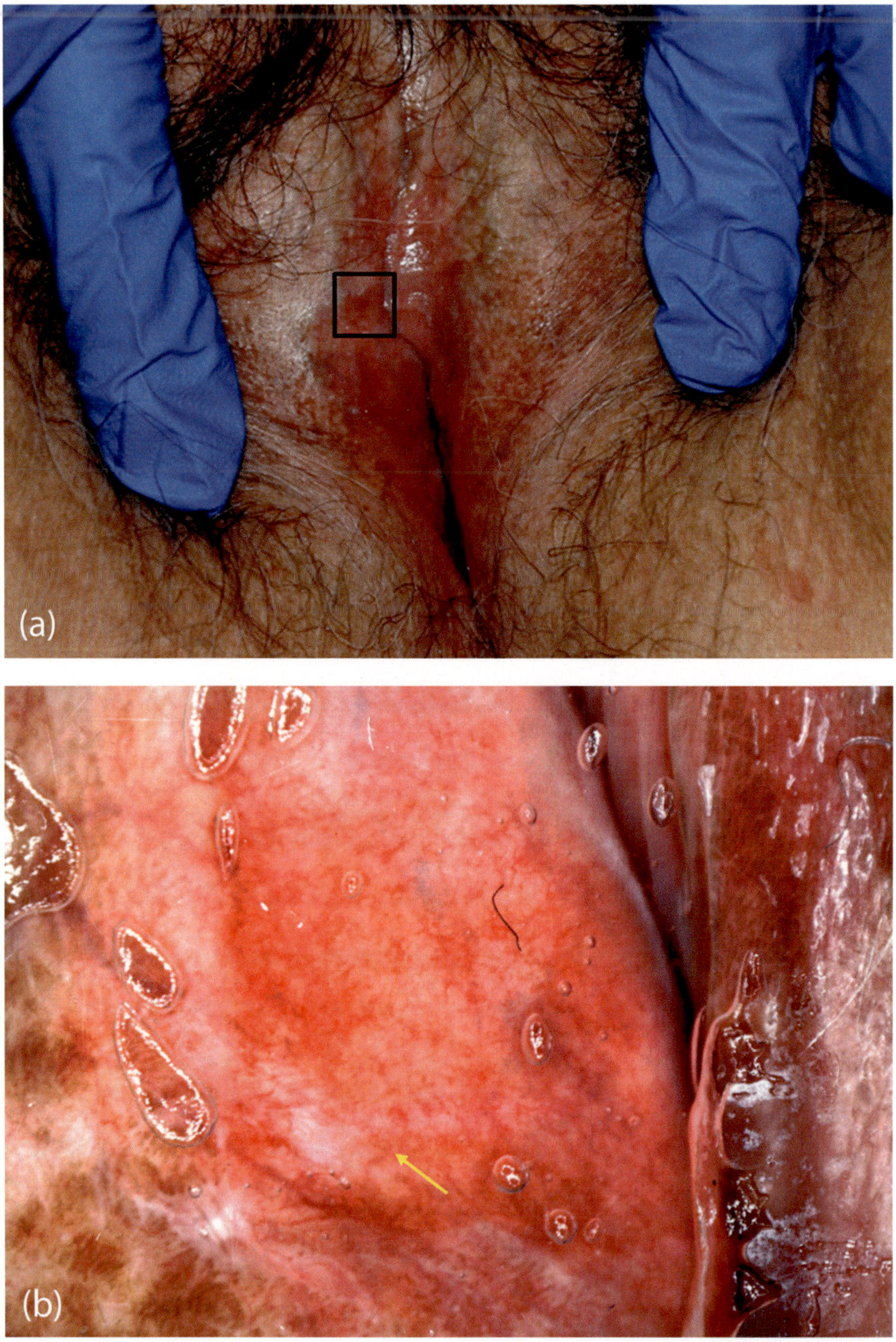

Figure 8.1 (a) Erosive vulvovaginal lichen planus. The square indicates the area where dermoscopy was performed. (b) Dermoscopy (×20) showing thick linear irregular vessels arranged diffusely over an intense red background, edged by a lacy, white-grayish border. Whitish structures arranged in a reticular pattern, corresponding to Wickham striae, are observed on the skin (arrow).

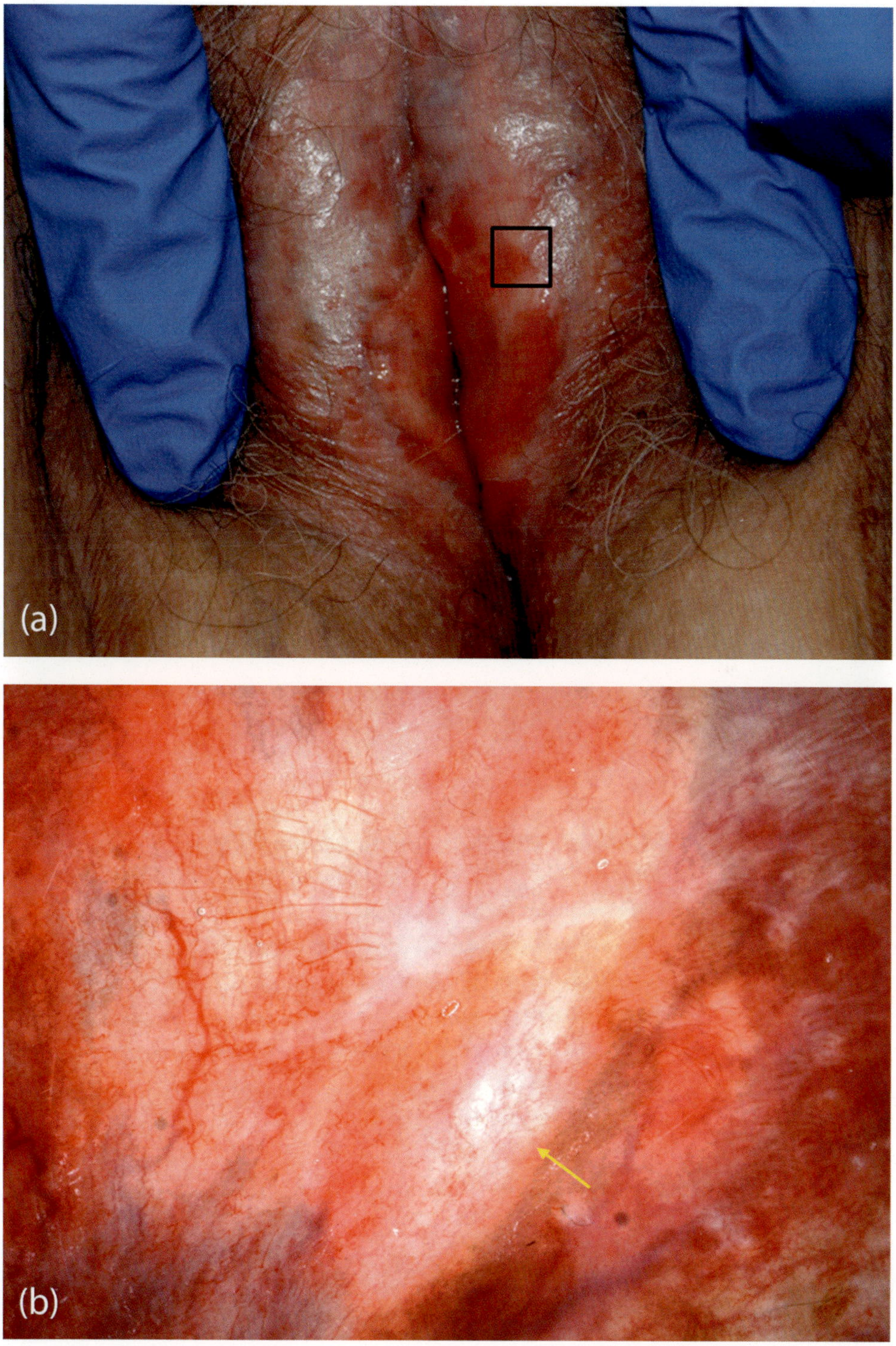

Figure 8.2 (a) Erosive vulvovaginal lichen planus. The square indicates the area where dermoscopy was performed. (b) Dermoscopy (×20) showing white homogeneous areas observed at the sinuous edge of the erythematous background (arrow), which correspond to the macerate border surrounding the erosive surfaces.

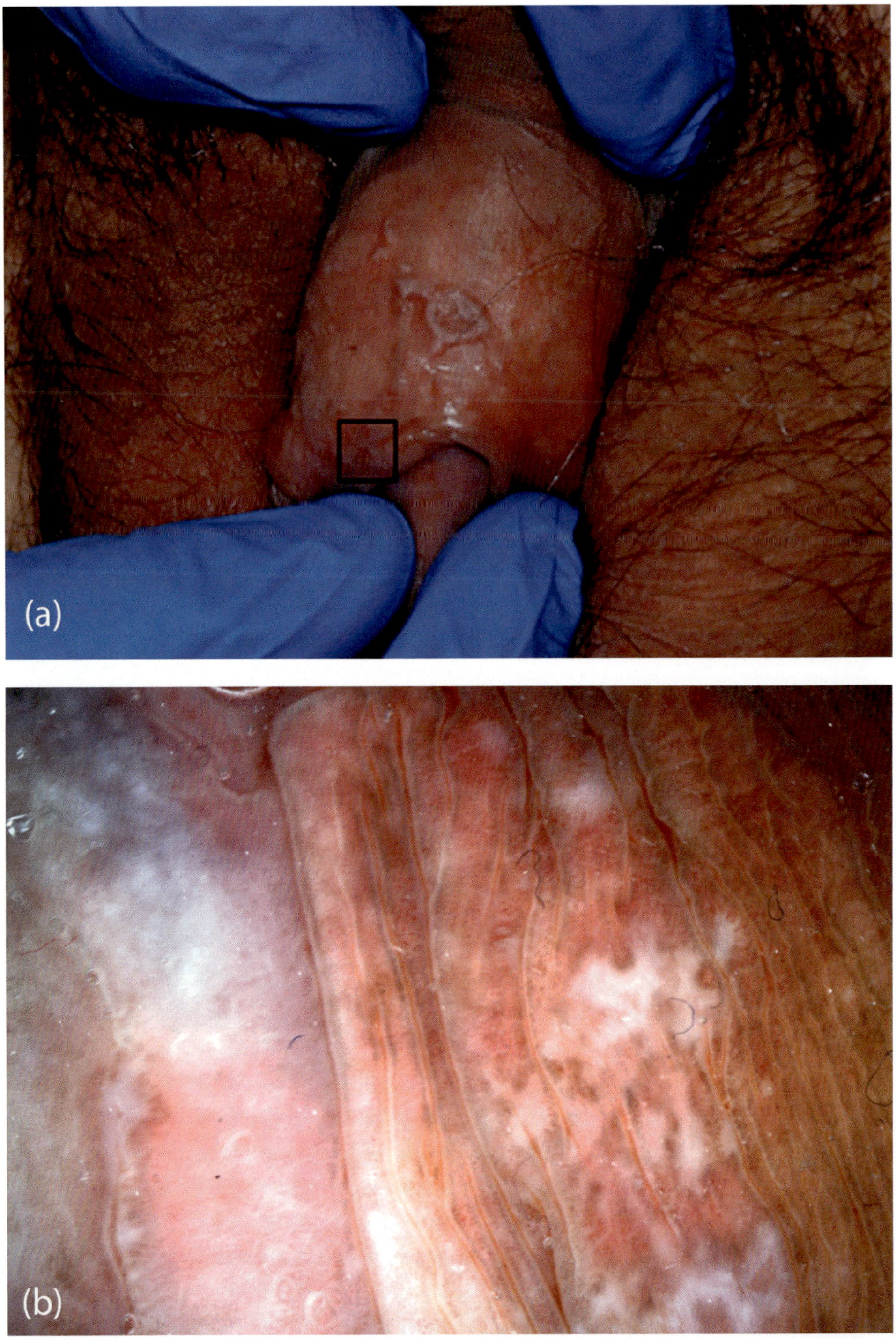

Figure 8.3 (a) Penile lichen planus. The lesions show an annular and reticular pattern. The square indicates the area where dermoscopy was performed. (b) Dermoscopy (×20) showing white streaks arranged in a snow crystal-like pattern (Wickham striae), with adjacent gray pigmentation.

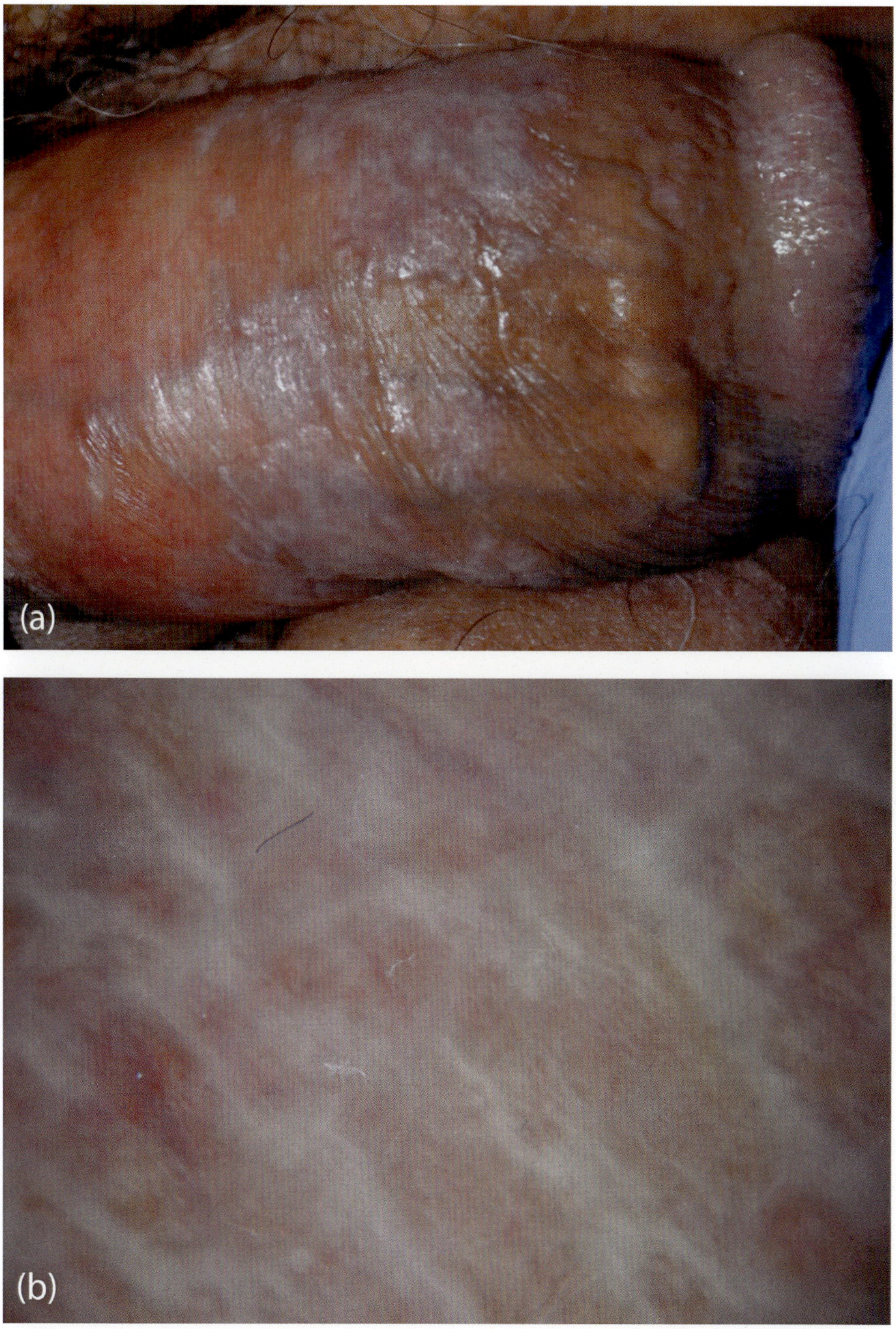

Figure 8.4 (a) Penile lichen planus. Whitish, irregular plaque involving the shaft and the prepuce. (b) Dermoscopy (×10) showing typical white streaks arranged in a reticular pattern (Wickham striae).

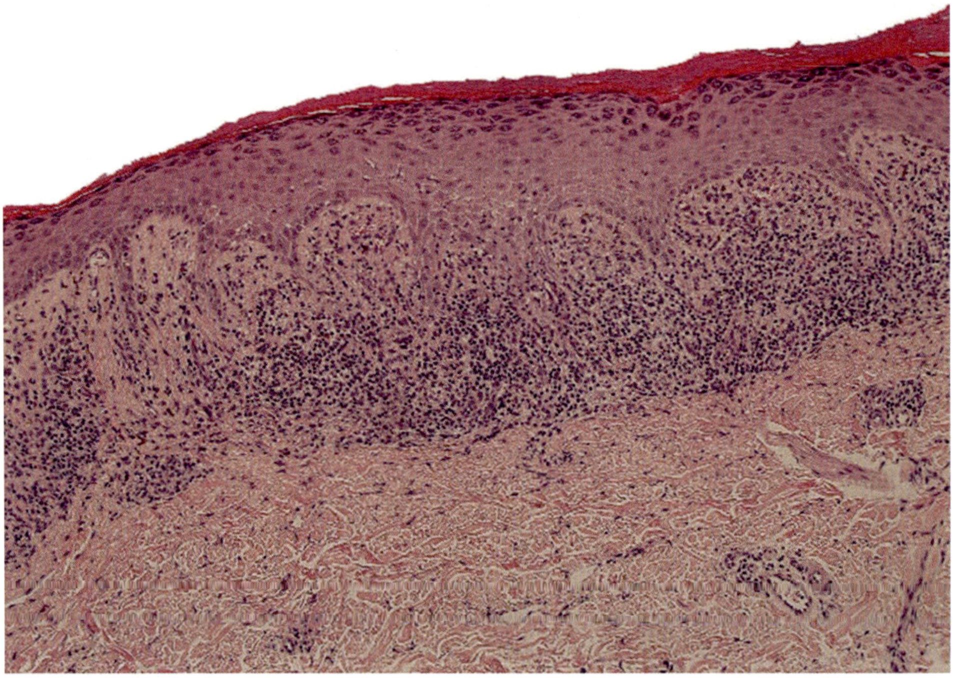

Figure 8.5 Histopathology of lichen planus showing compact hyperkeratosis of the epidermis and thickened granular layer with lichenoid infiltrate of the dermis and basal vacuolization (H&E, ×100).

CHAPTER 9

Lichen Sclerosus

Monica Corazza MD, Pierantonia Zedde MD, Roberta Gafà MD, and Alessandro Borghi MD

DEFINITION

Lichen sclerosus (LS) is a distressing, chronic inflammatory disease that affects mostly the anogenital areas (1, 2). An increased risk of genital cancer is also recognized, especially for vulvar LS (3, 4).

EPIDEMIOLOGY

The exact prevalence of LS is unknown. The ratio of women to men is approximately 3:1–10:1 (1). In females, vulvar LS onset peaks in the prepubertal and postmenopausal periods, with prevalence of about 0.1% and 3%, respectively (2). The prevalence of genital localization in male patients is estimated to be between 0.0014% and 0.07% (5).

ETIOLOGY

The etiology of LS is not well understood, but there is an association with autoimmune disorders, genetic and epigenetic factors (2, 6, 7). Immunological alterations and chronic inflammation seem to be key pathomechanisms (8). An abnormal activation of a Th1 autoimmune response, together with a reduced Treg activity, has been found in affected tissue (9). Both a cell-mediated attack against self-antigens and an upregulation of pro-inflammatory cytokines are direct consequences of this immune imbalance. Promoting fibroblast growth and activity, as well as collagen synthesis, is another key event in LS pathogenesis (8, 10). Infections, hormonal influences, trauma (Koebner phenomenon), chronic irritation and overweight have been suggested as possible triggers in predisposed individuals (1, 8, 11).

CLINICAL FEATURES

LS primary lesions are flat, ivory-colored spots, which may coalesce into pale, crinkly thin patches and plaques [Figures 9.1(a), 9.2(a), 9.3(a) and 9.4(a)]. Erythema, ecchymosis and itching-related excoriations are common, and occasionally hyperkeratosis is prominent.

DOI: 10.1201/9781003007166-9

The sites most characteristically involved by vulvar LS are the inter-labial sulci, labia minora and labia majora, clitoris and clitoral hood. LS may involve the entire vulva, with possible extension to perineum and perianus, giving rise to the characteristic “figure-of-eight” shape. The vagina is usually spared. In males, LS presents with whitish or grayish depigmentation of the glans and/or the inner surface of the prepuce. Gradual sclerosis of the prepuce, which becomes tightened, nonretractile and prone to fissuring, leads to phimosis. Perineum and perianal skin are rarely involved. Post-inflammatory progressive scarring may cause destruction of anogenital architecture. Distressing symptoms include itching and burning and affect females more than males (1, 2, 12, 13). Sexual dysfunctions are common (14).

DIFFERENTIAL DIAGNOSIS

The main differential diagnoses of genital LS are lichen planus, vitiligo, lichen simplex chronicus, immunobullous disorders and vulvar or penile intraepithelial neoplasia (2).

DIAGNOSIS

The diagnosis of genital LS is generally clinical, but a biopsy may be necessary when the clinical picture is not diagnostic.

DERMOSCOPY

Whitish background and patchy structureless areas, varying in color from white to white-yellowish to milky-pinkish, are the most prevalent and typical dermoscopic features of genital LS in both females and males [Figures 9.1(b) and 9.2(b)] (16–19). These dermoscopic clues may be observable also in the case of absence of pallor at the clinical assessment. A marked decrease in vessel concentration, which configures a sort of “vascular desertification”, within genital LS lesions when compared with surrounding unaffected surfaces is the other dermoscopic hallmark of this disease. The sparse vessels are polymorphic in shape, without any specific arrangement (20). A dermoscopic picture which combines whitish background, whitish patchy structureless areas and vascular desertification is highly suggestive of genital LS. Gray-brown dots arranged in a peppering pattern may frequently be observed in genital LS, as in other genital inflammatory diseases (19). Red to purpuric, structureless, well circumscribed dots, globules or blotches, which correspond to blood spots, are common features of genital LS. Yellow, comedo-like openings are dermoscopic findings that may be observed in some cases of genital LS [Figures 9.3(b) and 9.4(b)], whereas are quite constant in extragenital sites (21, 22). Short white shiny lines are observed in a variable proportion of cases (17, 23). White scales are occasional dermoscopic features of LS also at a genital level.

HISTOPATHOLOGICAL CORRELATION

Typical histological features of genital LS include orthohyperkeratosis, loss of rete ridges, epidermal atrophy, basal cell degeneration, dermal hyalinization with homogenized band of dense fibrosis at papillary dermis and a band-like lymphocytic infiltrate (Figure 9.5) (15).

Whitish background and patchy structureless areas are the dermoscopic expression of dermal sclerosis, homogenization of collagen fibres and hyalinization (16). The dermoscopic appearance of “vascular desertification” does not seem to have a specific histological counterpart; in fact, in LS vessels appear ectatic at histology. It can be hypothesized that the homogenization of collagen in the upper dermis may hinder the dermoscopic assessment of vessels. Gray-brown peppering corresponds to melanophages displaced in the upper dermis and at perifollicular site, as a consequence of the inflammatory process (17). The yellow comedo-like openings histopathologically correlate with dilated infundibula with follicular cornified plugging. Some dermoscopic features of vulvar LS change following corticosteroid treatment (24) mirroring the histological changes observed as a treatment effect (25).

REFERENCES

1. Kirtschig G, Becker K, Günthert A, et al. Evidence-based (S3) guideline on (anogenital) lichen sclerosus. J Eur Acad Dermatol Venereol 2015;29,e1–43.
2. Fistarol SK, Itin PH. Diagnosis and treatment of lichen sclerosus: an update. Am J Clin Dermatol 2013;14:27–47.
3. Halonen P, Jakobsson M, Heikinheimo O, et al. Lichen sclerosus and risk of cancer. Int J Cancer 2017;140:1998–2002.
4. Powell J, Robson A, Cranston D, et al. High incidence of lichen sclerosus in patients with squamous cell carcinoma of the penis. Br J Dermatol 2001;145:85–9.
5. Nelson DM, Peterson AC. Lichen sclerosus: epidemiological distribution in an equal access health care system. J Urol 2011;185:522–5.
6. Kreuter A, Kryvosheyeva Y, Terras S, et al. Association of autoimmune diseases with lichen sclerosus in 532 male and female patients. Acta Derm Venereol 2013;93:238–41.
7. Trietsch MD, Nooij LS, Gaarenstroom KN, van Poelgeest MI. Genetic and epigenetic changes in vulvar squamous cell carcinoma and its precursor lesions: a review of the current literature. Gynecol Oncol 2015;136:143–57.
8. Tran DA, Tan X, Macri CJ, et al. Lichen sclerosus: an autoimmunopathogenic and genomic enigma with emerging genetic and immune targets. Int J Biol Sci 2019;15:1429–39.
9. Farrell AM, Dean D, Millard PR, et al. Cytokine alterations in lichen sclerosus: an immunohistochemical study. Br J Dermatol 2006;155:931–40.
10. Ren L, Zhao Y, Huo X, Wu X. MiR-155–5p promotes fibroblast cell proliferation and inhibits FOXO signaling pathway in vulvar lichen sclerosis by targeting FOXO3 and CDKN1B. Gene 2018;653:43–50.
11. Virgili A, Borghi A, Cazzaniga S, et al. New insights into potential risk factors and associations in genital lichen sclerosus: data from a multicentre Italian study on 729 consecutive cases. J Eur Acad Dermatol Venereol 2017;31:699–704.
12. Virgili A, Borghi A, Toni G et al. Prospective clinical and epidemiologic study of vulvar lichen sclerosus: analysis of prevalence and severity of clinical features, together with historical and demographic associations. Dermatology 2014;228:145–51.
13. Cazzaniga S, Naldi L, Virgili A, et al. An original exploration of genital lichen sclerosus: the semantic connectivity map. J Eur Acad Dermatol Venereol 2019;33:e59–e62.
14. Corazza M, Virgili A, Minghetti S, Borghi A. Dyspareunia in vulvar lichen sclerosus: an overview of a distressing symptom. G Ital Dermatol Venereol 2020;155(3):299–305.
15. Niamh L, Naveen S, Hazel B. Diagnosis of vulval inflammatory dermatoses: a pathological study with clinical correlation. Int J Gynecol Pathol 2009;28:554–8.
16. Larre Borges A, Tiodorovic-Zivkovic D, Lallas A, et al. Clinical, dermoscopic and histopathologic features of genital and extragenital lichen sclerosus. J Eur Acad Dermatol Venereol 2013;27:1433–9.
17. Borghi A, Corazza M, Minghetti S, et al. Dermoscopic features of vulvar lichen sclerosus in the setting of a prospective cohort of patients: new observations. Dermatology 2016;232:71–7.
18. Lacarrubba F, Verzì AE, Ardigò M, Micali G. Handheld reflectance confocal microscopy, dermatoscopy and histopathological correlation of common inflammatory balanitis. Skin Res Technol 2018;24:499–503.
19. Borghi A, Virgili A, Corazza M. Dermoscopy of inflammatory genital diseases: practical insights. Dermatol Clin 2018;36:451–61.

20. Lacarrubba F, Dinotta F, Nasca MR, et al. Localized vascular lesions of the glans in patients with lichen sclerosus diagnosed by dermatoscopy. G Ital Dermatol Venereol 2012;147:510–1.
21. Horcajada-Reales C, Campos-Domínguez M, et al. Comedo-like openings in dermoscopy: an essential diagnostic clue for lichen sclerosus, even in children. J Am Acad Dermatol 2015;72:S4–S5.
22. Lacarrubba F, Pellacani G, Verzì AE, et al. Extragenital lichen sclerosus: clinical, dermoscopic, confocal microscopy and histologic correlations. J Am Acad Dermatol 2015;72:S50–2.
23. Liu J, Hao J, Liu Y, Lallas A. Dermoscopic features of lichen sclerosus in Asian patients: a prospective study. J Eur Acad Dermatol Venereol 2020;34(11):e720–1.
24. Borghi A, Corazza M, Minghetti S, et al. Clinical and dermoscopic changes of vulvar lichen sclerosus after topical corticosteroid treatment. J Dermatol 2016;43:1078–82.
25. Dalziel KL, Millard PR, Wojnarowska F. The treatment of vulval lichen sclerosus with a very potent topical steroid (clobetasol propionate 0.05%) cream. Br J Dermatol 1991;124:461–4.

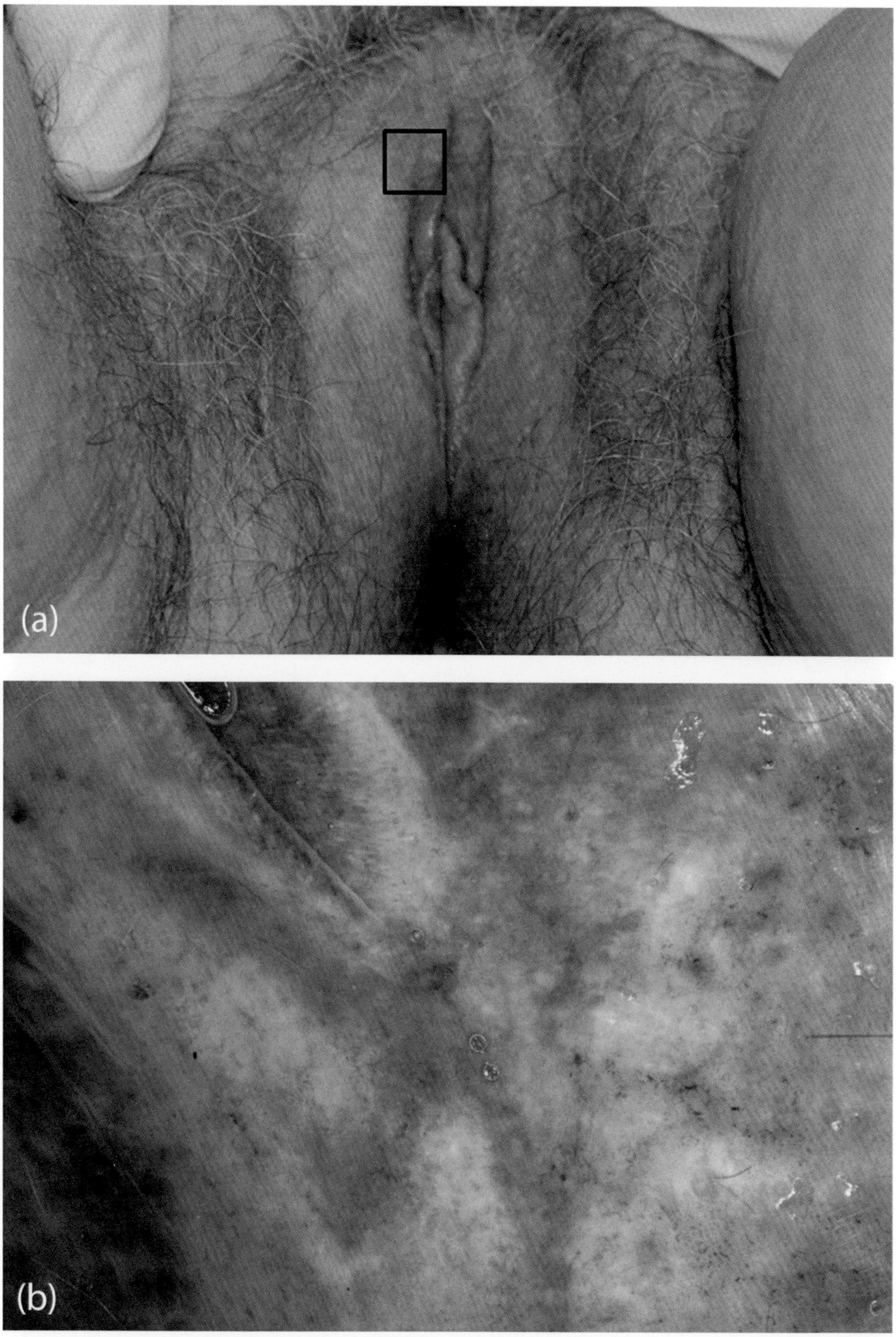

Figure 9.1 (a) Vulvar lichen sclerosus involving labia minora and majora, inter-labial sulci, fourchette and perineum. The square indicates the area where dermoscopy was performed. (b) Dermoscopy (×20) showing white and milky-pinkish structureless areas on a whitish background, with sparse vessels (vascular "desertification"). Gray/brownish dots arranged in a peppering pattern are also visible.

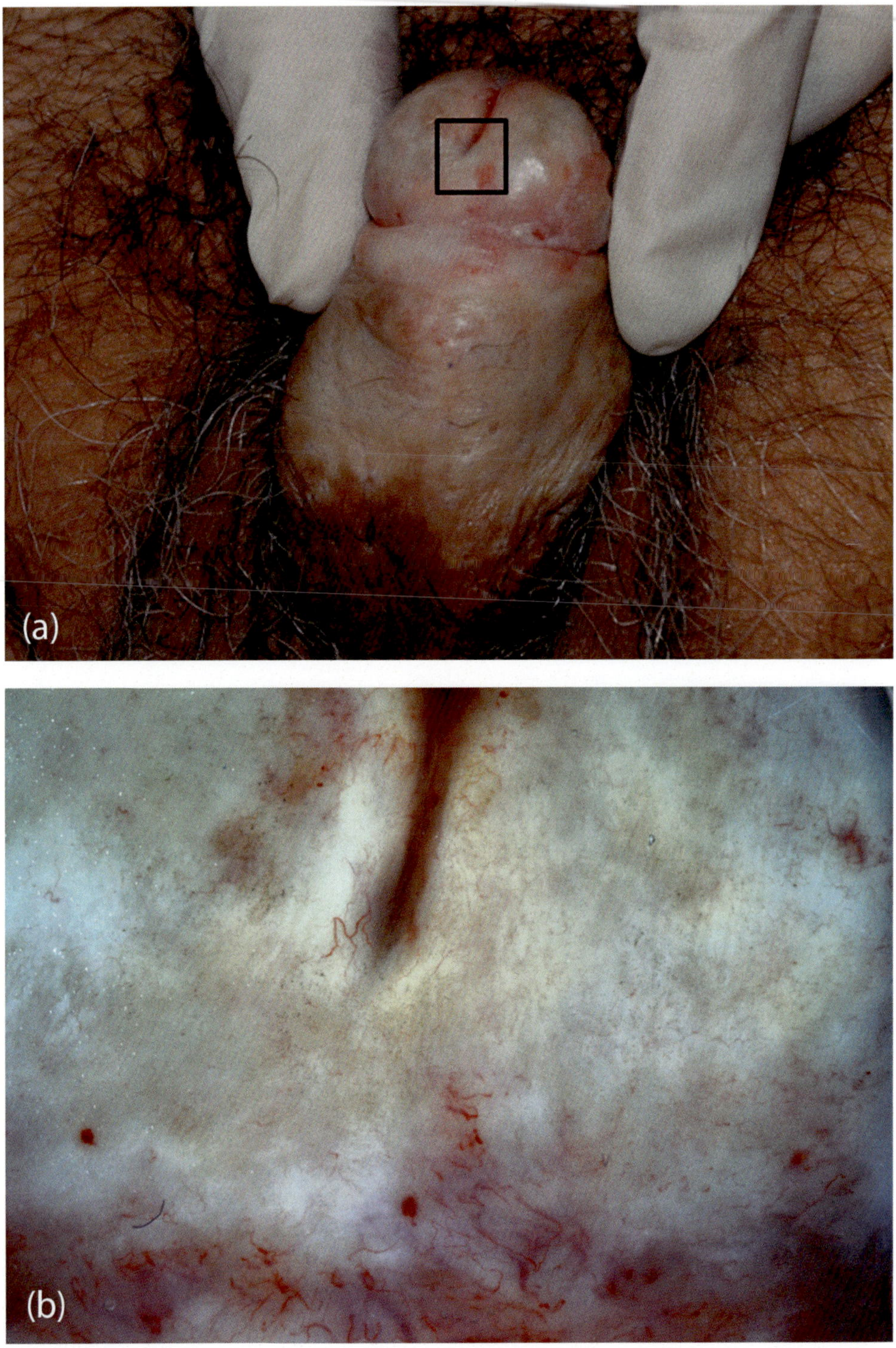

Figure 9.2 (a) Lichen sclerosus of glans, inner surface of the prepuce and penis shaft. The square indicates the area where dermoscopy was performed. (b) Dermoscopy (×30) showing white background with red globules and dots corresponding to ecchymosis. Polymorphic linear vessels, without any specific arrangement, are observed at the periphery. Sparse gray/brownish peppering is visible.

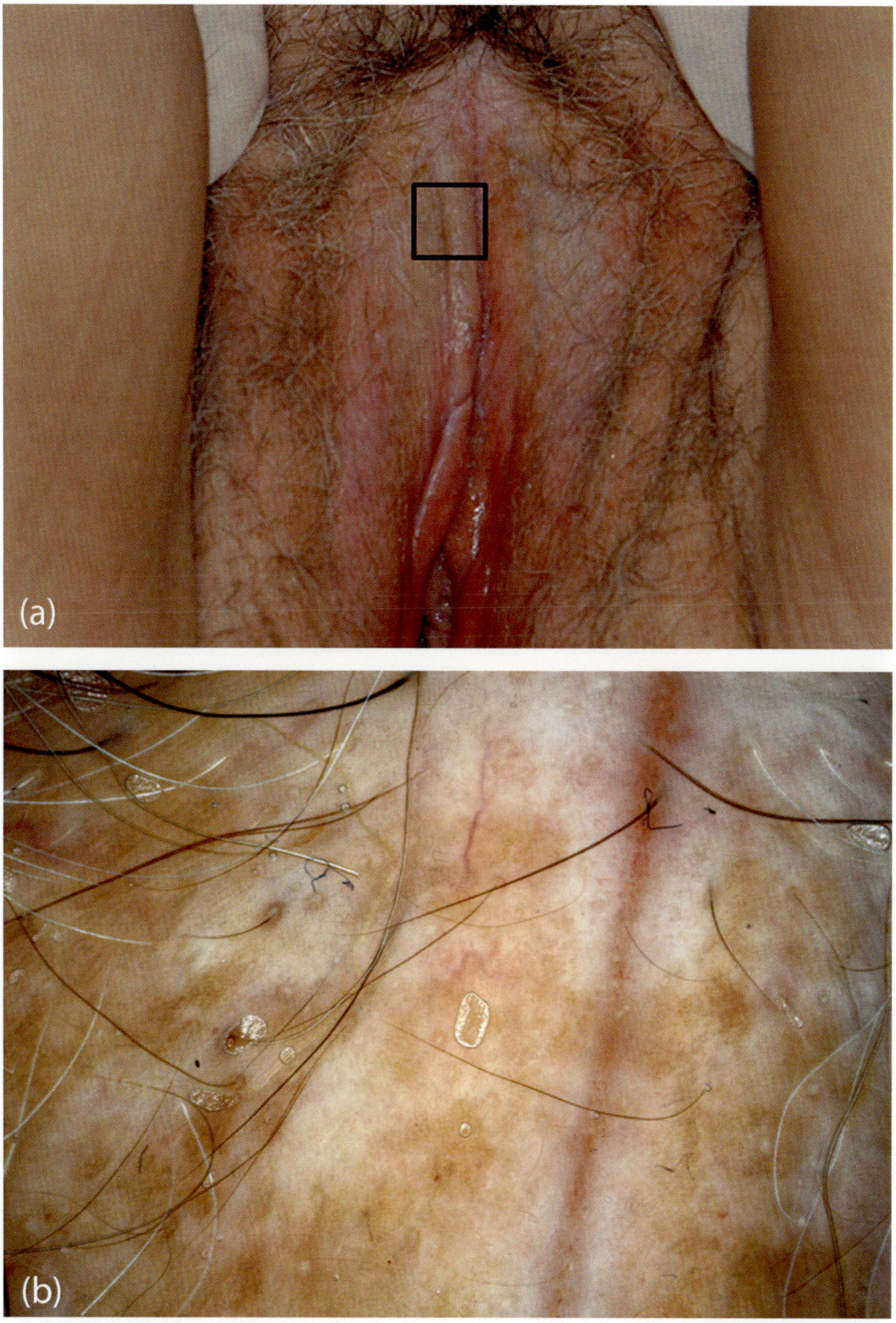

Figure 9.3 (a) Vulvar lichen sclerosus affecting labia minora and majora, inter-labial sulci and perineum. The square indicates the area where dermoscopy was performed. (b) Dermoscopy (×20) showing whitish structureless areas on a pale background; yellow to brownish comedo-like openings are visible.

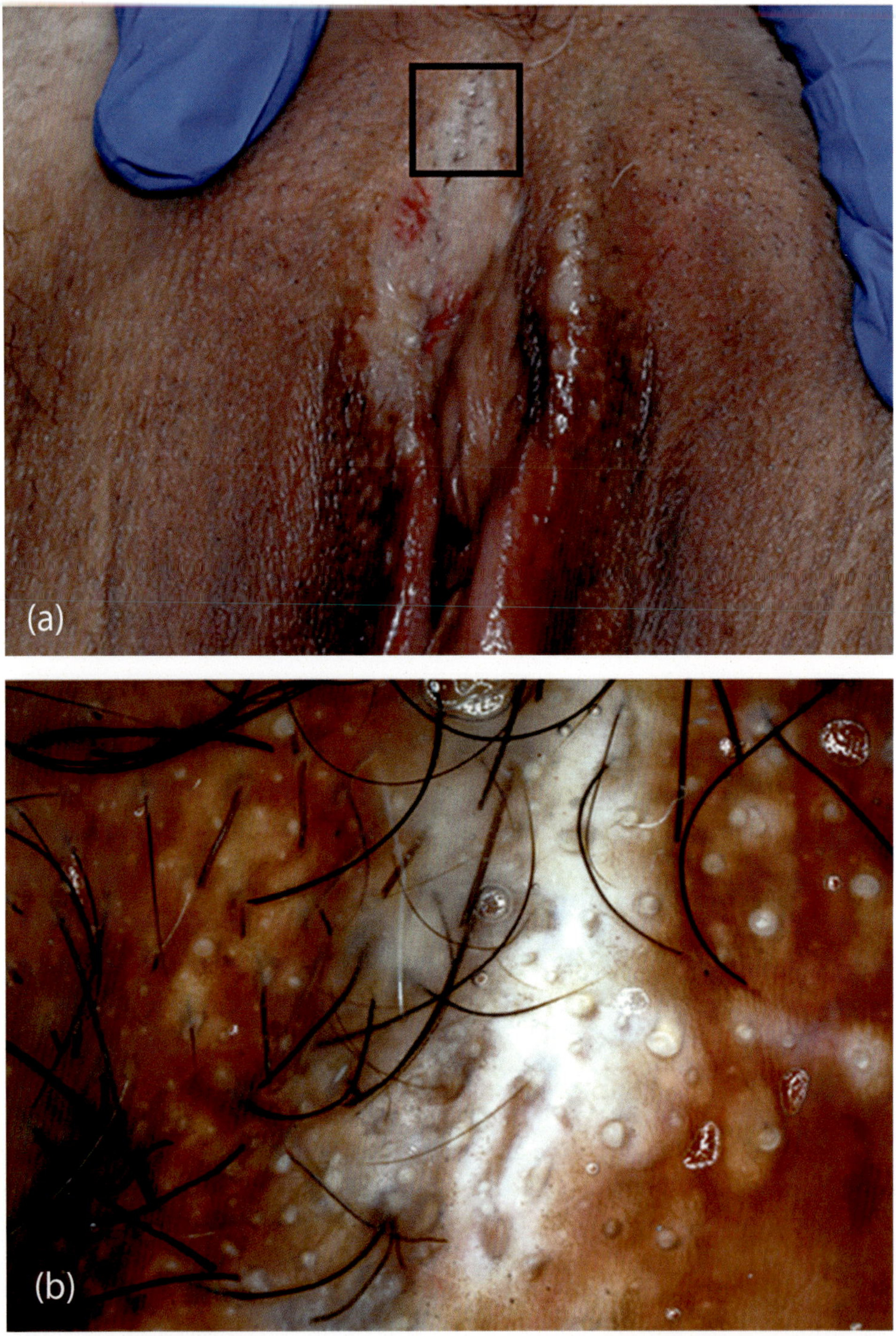

Figure 9.4 (a) Vulvar lichen sclerosus involving labia minora and majora, inter-labial sulci, clitoral hood and fourchette. The square indicates the area where dermoscopy was performed. (b) Dermoscopy (×20) showing typical white structureless areas and comedo-like openings; the latter are surrounded by white pigmentation, configuring the so-called white spot disease.

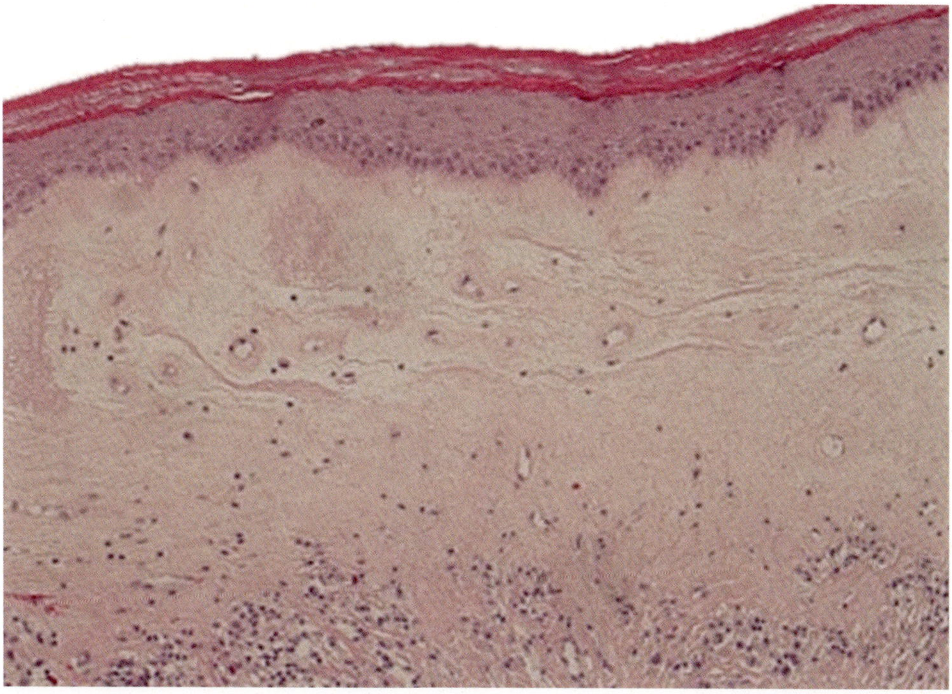

Figure 9.5 Histopathology of genital lichen sclerosus showing effacement of the epidermal rete ridge and homogenization of the papillary dermis above patchy lymphoid infiltrate (H&E, ×100).

CHAPTER 10

Lichen Simplex Chronicus

Alessandro Borghi MD, Alberto Monti MD, Pierantonia Zedde MD, Roberta Gafà MD, and Monica Corazza MD

DEFINITION

Anogenital lichen simplex chronicus (LSC) is a chronic, itching and extremely uncomfortable disorder characterized by lichenification, with varying degrees of excoriations caused by scratching and rubbing.

EPIDEMIOLOGY

Anogenital LSC is a quite common disorder, with an estimated prevalence of about 0.5% in Caucasians. Its highest prevalence peaks at 30–50 years of age and the disease is more common in females than in males (1). Vulvar LSC was found to comprise up to 35% of patient visits to vulvar specialty clinics (2).

ETIOLOGY

Anogenital LSC occurs in two settings. It can arise *de novo* on healthy, muco-cutaneous tissue (primary or idiopathic LSC) or as a consequence of pre-existing, underlying itching dermatitis, mainly psoriasis, lichen sclerosus, contact dermatitis, candidiasis, and tinea cruris (secondary LSC). These two subtypes differ substantially in their major triggers. In fact, primary LSC may be exacerbated by either psychological factors, such as depression, anxiety, and obsessive-compulsive disorder, or environmental ones, such as heat, sweat retention, rubbing of clothing, excessive use of cleansers, and application of irritating topical products (1). On the other hand, secondary LSC is triggered by itch from the underlying dermatological diseases mentioned above. Abnormal peripheral stimulation of type C sensory nerve fibres leads to the chronic perception of itching in LSC patients. Upregulation of some major histocompatibility complex molecules and increased skin infiltration of Langerhans and T cells seem to predispose to LSC and its chronic course (3). Regardless of etiology, a common pathomechanism underlies LSC development, namely the perpetuation of the itch-scratch cycle which leads in turn to the clinical-histological features of the disease. Both atopy and atopic dermatitis are thought to be important predisposing factors for both subtypes of LSC.

DOI: 10.1201/9781003007166-10

CLINICAL FEATURES

Patients with anogenital LSC report intense and intractable pruritus that may disturb sleep, disrupt social life, work life, and sex life. The skin responds to the persistent itch-scratch cycle by thickening progressively with more prominent skin markings, turning slightly grayish-brown, and becoming coarse and rough (lichenification) [Figures 10.1(a), 10.2(a), and 10.3(a)]. Scales, abrasions and fissures are frequently present within these well-demarcated, lichenified plaques. Hypopigmented and sometimes atrophic scars may be observed too. Due to disruption of the normal skin barrier, impetiginization can occur. Anogenital LSC is usually bilateral, but may be asymmetrical or even unilateral, probably because of a preferential scratching with the dominant hand. Vulvar LSC commonly involves the labia majora and, to a lesser extent, labia minora and vestibule. The vagina is spared (1, 2, 4, 5). In men, the scrotum is the most frequently involved site, but the proximal portion of the penis is commonly affected too. The upper inner thighs are occasionally involved. Perineum and perianal area are typical affected sites in both sexes. Chronic, paroxystic scratching may lead to irreversible architectural damages, especially in female LSC. Anogenital LSC does not seem to be associated with a higher risk of squamous cell cancer (6).

DIFFERENTIAL DIAGNOSIS

The main differential diagnoses include candidiasis, psoriasis, tinea cruris, contact dermatitis, and lichen sclerosus. Lice, scabies, warts, and neoplasia are further conditions that may mimic anogenital LSC. In secondary LSC, when it is superimposed on another underlying disease, discriminating between the two concurrent conditions may be particularly difficult (7).

DIAGNOSIS

The diagnosis of LSC is usually based on patient history and physical examination, but a skin biopsy can aid in equivocal cases (8). In cases of LSC superimposed on another condition, two concurrent histological processes are observable in a single biopsy specimen.

DERMOSCOPY

On dermoscopical examination, anogenital LSC shows a pink background topped with white-grayish structureless patches, varying in size and with tendency to coalesce [Figure 10.1(b)] (9). In cases of noticeable lichenification, a surface showing a pattern of gyri and sulci may be observed [Figure 10.2(b)]. The follicular openings appear surrounded by a bright white, circular halo, which is absent around those located on adjacent unimpaired skin [Figures 10.1(b) and 10.3(b)]. The pinkish-whitish background is characterized by a dense vascularization, mainly composed of both linear, serpentine and dotted vessels, arranged diffusely within the affected surfaces. This rich vascularization allows to differentiate LSC from lichen sclerosus, in which vessels are usually sparse (10). The whitish patches observed in LSC do not appear arranged in the dermoscopic patterns described for Wickham striae (11). In genital psoriasis dotted vessels are regularly distributed over a pale red, pinkish background and eczematous lesions, especially in acute forms, show dotted vessels distributed in a patchy pattern, together with yellow crusts, which correspond to spongiotic process and exudation (12).

HISTOPATHOLOGICAL CORRELATION

Histological examination of genital LSC shows compact hyperorthokeratosis with foci of parakeratosis, psoriasiform or pseudoepitheliomatous hyperplasia, hypergranulosis with no cell atypia, prominent fibroblasts, which appear enlarged and may be multinucleated with stellate cytoplasm, mild spongiosis, perivascular and interstitial lymphocytic inflammation with occasional eosinophils (Figure 10.4). Presence of zones of pale epithelium is a histopathologic feature associated with vulvar LSC and refers to clusters of pale squamous cells within different levels of the epithelium/epidermis (8). Mucosa affected by LSC may be indistinguishable from skin due to aberrant development of the granular layer and keratinization.

The white-grayish patches presumably correspond to the orthokeratotic epidermal hyperplasia found on histopathological examination. The bright circular haloes surrounding the follicular openings are likely the dermoscopic sign of acanthosis and hyperkeratosis around the hair canal at the level of the infundibulum (13).

REFERENCES

1. Lynch PJ. Lichen simplex chronicus (atopic/neurodermatitis) of the anogenital region. Dermatol Ther 2004;17:8–19.
2. Fruchter R, Melnick L, Pomeranz MK. Lichenoid vulvar disease: a review. Int J Womens Dermatol 2017;3:58–64.
3. Feng X, Yang M, Yang Z, et al. Abnormal expression of the co-stimulatory molecule b7-h3 in lichen simplex chronicus is associated with expansion of Langerhans cells. Clin Exp Dermatol 2020;45:30–5.
4. Stewart KM. Clinical care of vulvar pruritus, with emphasis on one common cause, lichen simplex chronicus. Dermatol Clin 2010;28:669–80.
5. Chibnall R. Vulvar pruritus and lichen simplex chronicus. Obstet Gynecol Clin North Am 2017;44:379–88.
6. Moyal-Barracco M, Wendling J. Vulvar dermatosis. Best Pract Res Clin Obstet Gynaecol 2014;28:946–58.
7. van der Meijden WI, Boffa MJ, Ter Harmsel WA, et al. 2016 European guideline for the management of vulval conditions. J Eur Acad Dermatol Venereol 2017;31:925–41.
8. Chan MP, Zimarowski MJ. Vulvar dermatoses: a histopathologic review and classification of 183 cases. J Cutan Pathol 2015;42:510–8.
9. Borghi A, Virgili A, Corazza M. Dermoscopy of inflammatory genital diseases: practical insights. Dermatol Clin 2018;36:451–61.
10. Borghi A, Corazza M, Minghetti S, et al. Dermoscopic features of vulvar lichen sclerosus in the setting of a prospective cohort of patients: new observations. Dermatology 2016;232:71–7.
11. Borghi A, Corazza M, Minghetti S, et al. Preliminary study on dermoscopic features of vulvar lichen planus: new insights for diagnosis. J Eur Acad Dermatol Venereol 2016;30:1063–5.
12. Lallas A, Zalaudek I, Argenziano G, et al. Dermoscopy in general dermatology. Dermatol Clin 2013;31:679–94.
13. Quaresma MV, Mariño Alvarez AM, Miteva M. Dermatoscopic-pathologic correlation of lichen simplex chronicus on the scalp: 'broom fibres, gear wheels and hamburgers'. J Eur Acad Dermatol Venereol 2016;30:343–5.

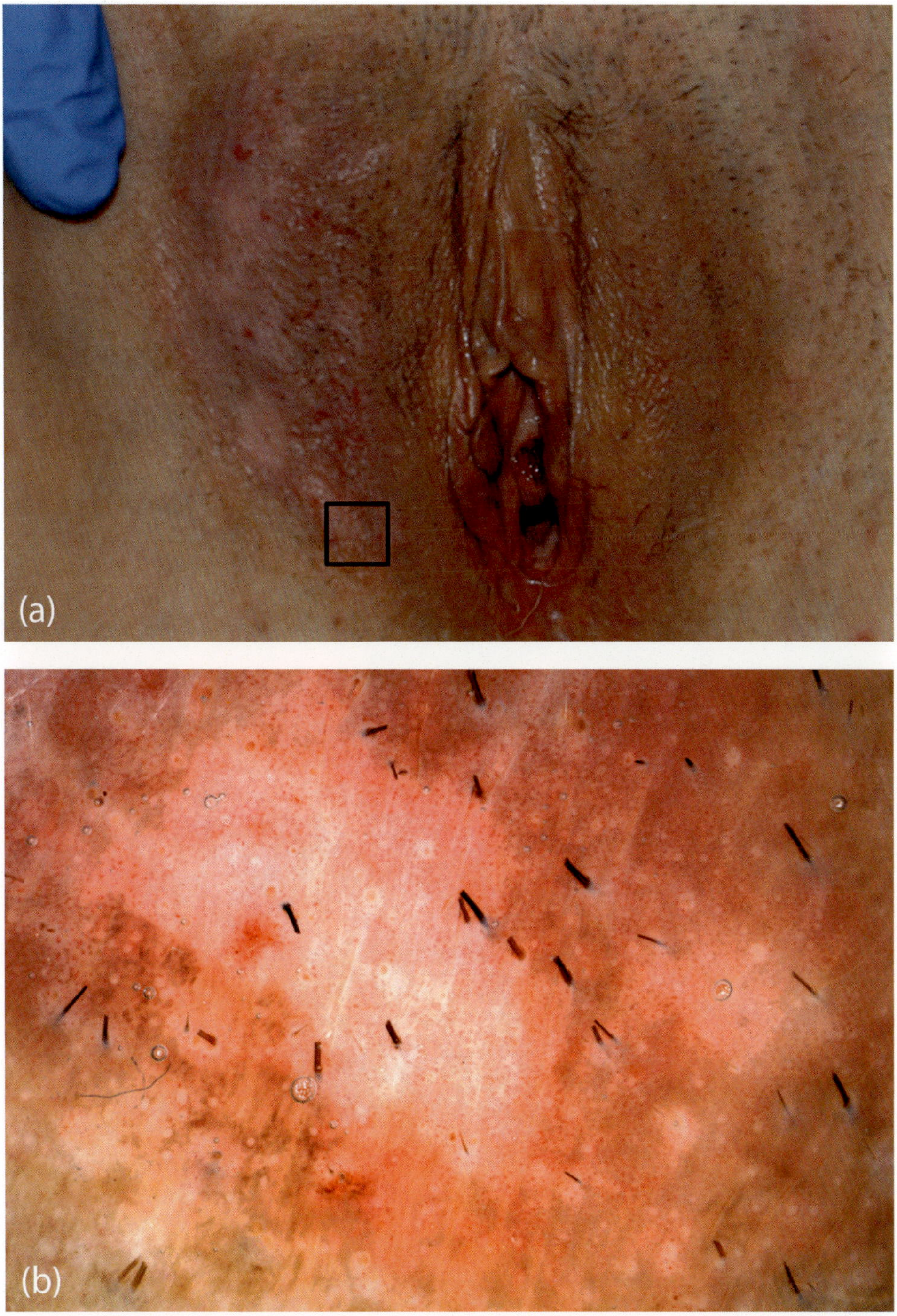

Figure 10.1 (a) Lichen simplex chronicus involving the right labium majus. The square indicates the area where dermoscopy was performed. (b) Dermoscopy (×20) showing a white-pinkish background with a thick vascularization, mainly composed by dotted vessels diffusely arranged. Bright circular haloes surrounding the follicular openings are visible within the affected surface.

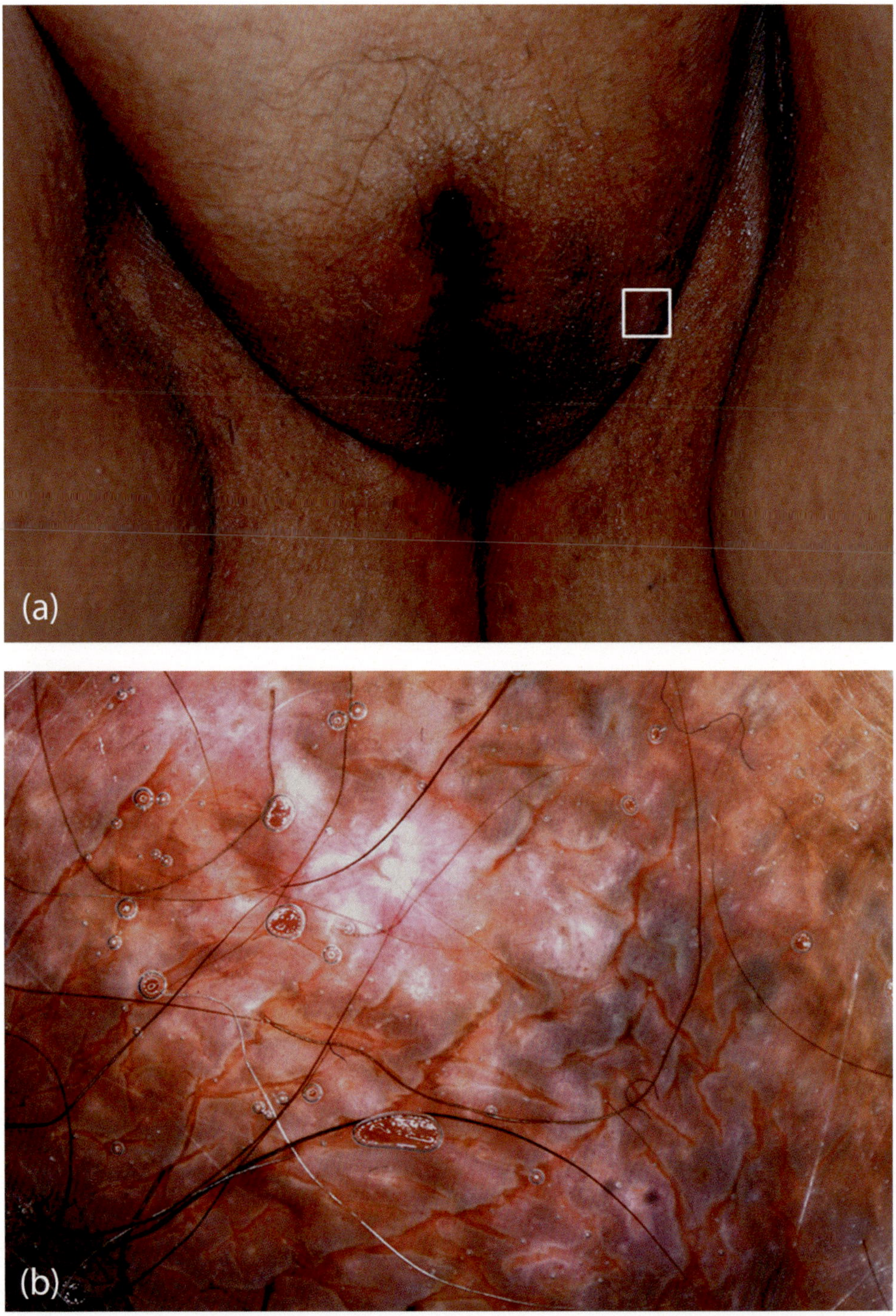

Figure 10.2 (a) Lichen simplex chronicus of the labia majora, with marked lichenification. The square indicates the area where dermoscopy was performed. (b) Dermoscopy (×20) showing a "gyri and sulci" pattern, milky-pinkish to grayish in color. Dotted vessels are also observable.

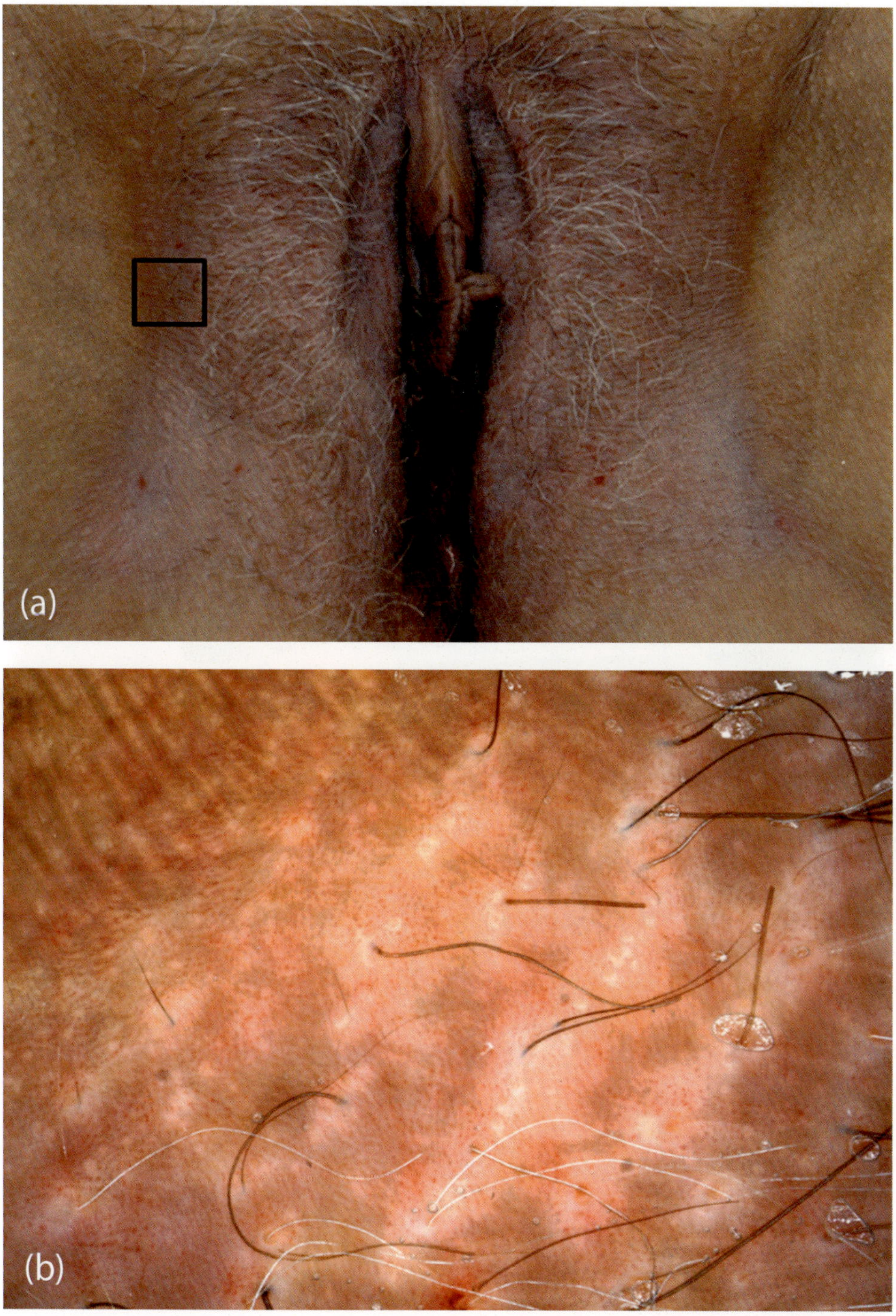

Figure 10.3 (a) Lichen simplex chronicus affecting the labia majora. The square indicates the area where dermoscopy was performed. (b) Dermoscopy (×20) showing whitish and grayish-pink background, with a rich vascularization, composed of linear and dotted vessels with diffuse arrangement.

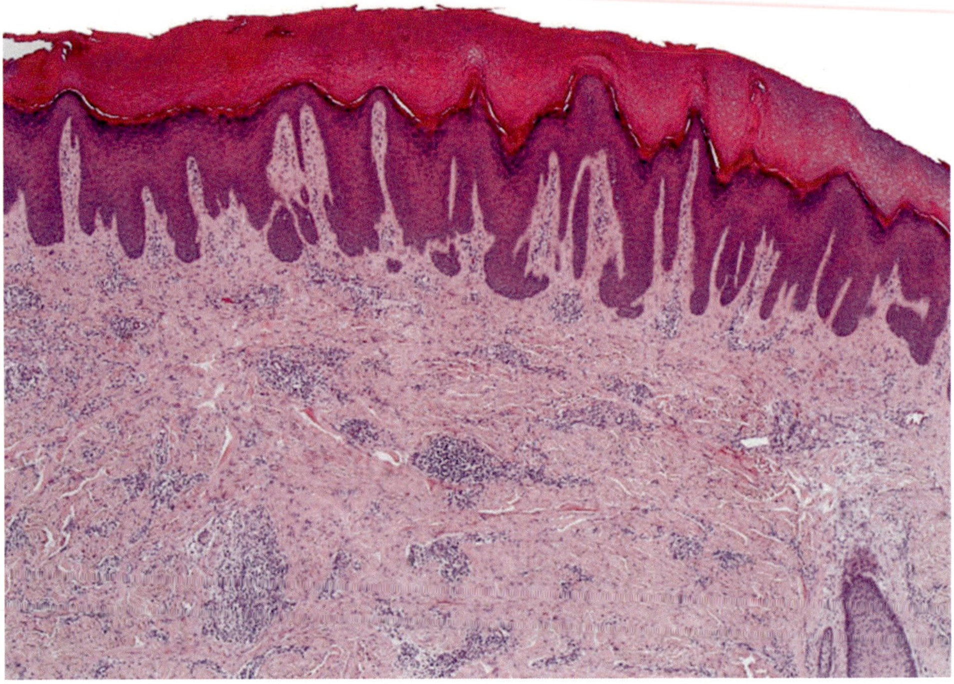

Figure 10.4 Histopathology of lichen simplex chronicus showing compact hyperkeratosis of the epidermis with acanthosis and thickened granular layer, fibrosis and sparse inflammatory infiltrate of the papillary dermis (H&E, ×40).

CHAPTER 11

Zoon Mucositis

Anna Elisa Verzì MD, Rosario Caltabiano MD, and Francesco Lacarrubba MD

DEFINITION

Zoon's plasma cell mucositis (ZM) is a benign inflammatory process that may involve the external genitalia with a chronic-relapsing course in males and females. It is called Zoon's plasma cell balanitis (ZB) or Zoon's plasma cell vulvitis (ZV), respectively.

EPIDEMIOLOGY

ZM is described as an infrequent entity but it is probably underreported or underdiagnosed. In particular, some studies found a prevalence of ZB ranging from 5% to 10% in patients who underwent examination for any genital issue (1, 2), whereas ZV has been rarely reported in the literature with less than 40 cases. ZM mainly involves middle-aged older males and females (3).

ETIOLOGY

The exact etiopathogenesis of ZM is unknown, but suggested predisposing factors include warmth, friction, poor hygiene, chronic irritation and/or infections (4–6). The retention of urine and smegma may contribute as ZB is mostly seen in uncircumcised men (4). It may explain why ZB undergoes to prolonged remission after circumcision (5). Another hypothesis includes chronic infection by *Mycobacterium smegmatis* or human papillomavirus (6). Moreover, a clinical and histopathological "zoonoid inflammation" is frequently encountered in genital dermatology as a corollary/consequence of other disorders, such as lichen sclerosus, lichen planus, genital penile intraepithelial neoplasia and squamous cell carcinoma (7, 8).

CLINICAL FEATURES

ZM clinically presents as single or multiple well-circumscribed, irregularly shaped, superficial, orange-red colored plaques [Figures 11.1(a), 11.2(a) and 11.3(a)]. Sometimes, multiple, pinpoint, red-brownish spots, also called "Cayenne pepper spots", may be detected on the background. In addition, ecchymotic areas due to mild traumas may be observed. Elective site of involvement in ZB is the glans, although the inner foreskin and coronal sulcus are frequently affected. In ZV,

DOI: 10.1201/9781003007166-11

labia minora and majora, clitoris, fourchette, urethral meatus and vaginal ostium may be involved. Lesions are usually asymptomatic but sometimes pruritus, dysuria, pain and burning sensation may be associated.

DIFFERENTIAL DIAGNOSIS

The diagnosis of ZM is often challenging due to clinical similarities with other genital dermatoses. In particular, the main differential diagnoses include erythroplasia of Queyrat, genital infections (candidiasis, syphilis, herpes), inflammatory diseases (lichen sclerosus, psoriasis, allergic contact dermatitis, Reiter's disease), bullous diseases (pemphigus vulgaris) and drug fixed eruption.

DIAGNOSIS

The diagnosis of ZM, in case of typical presentation, may be clinical and supported by dermoscopy. Recently, reflectance confocal microscopy (RCM) has been reported to assist the diagnosis of ZM (9–11) by revealing a normal nucleated epidermal honeycomb pattern, small bright cells, histologically corresponding to the inflammatory infiltrate in the upper dermis, and tortuous vessels running parallel to the surface at the epithelium–lamina propria junction. In some cases, an incisional biopsy for histopathological examination may be necessary to assess the definitive diagnosis.

DERMOSCOPY

Dermoscopy of ZM is characterized by two main features: focal or diffuse orangish structureless areas and fairly focused curved vessels [Figures 11.1(b), 11.2(b) and 11.3(b)] (12). These vessels may show different aspects as serpentine, convoluted, spermatozoa-like, chalice-shaped (13–16). Vessel configuration has been reported to allow the distinction of ZB from erythroplasia of Queyrat (that shows glomerular vessels), psoriasis (that is characterized by regular dotted/glomerular vessels), and also from nonspecific balanitis (usually revealing linear, irregular, unspecific vessels) (12).

HISTOPATHOLOGICAL CORRELATION

Histopathology of ZM is characterized by a subacute spongiotic mucositis with flattened epidermis and an underlying dense plasmacytic infiltrate. The main dermoscopic findings, consisting of focal or diffuse orange-yellow structureless areas and fairly focused curved vessels, histopathologically correspond to hemosiderin deposition and vascular dilatation/proliferation, respectively (Figure 11.4) (12, 17). Moreover, microhaemorrhages and erythrocyte extravasation correspond to the clinically evident "Cayenne pepper spots".

REFERENCES

1. Kumar B, Sharma R, Rajagopalan M, Radotra BD. Plasma cell balanitis: clinical and histopathological features—response to circumcision. Genitourin Med 1995;71(1):32–4.
2. Pearce J, Fernando I. The value of a multi-specialty service, including genitourinary medicine, dermatology and urology input, in the management of male genital dermatoses. Int J STD AIDS 2015;26(10):716–22.
3. Dayal S, Sahu P. Zoon balanitis: a comprehensive review. Indian J Sex Transm Dis AIDS 2016; 37(2):129–38.
4. Lepe K, Salazar FJ. Balanitis Circumscripta Plasmacellularis (Plasma Cell Balanitis, Zoon Balanitis). StatPearls [Internet]. Treasure Island, FL: StatPearls Publishing; 2020.
5. Retamar RA, Kien MC, Chouela EN. Zoon's balanitis: presentation of 15 patients, five treated with a carbon dioxide laser. Int J Dermatol 2003;42:305–7.
6. Pastar Z, Rados J, Lipozencic J, et al. Zoon plasma cell balanitis: an overview and role of histopathology. Acta Dermatovenerol Croat. 2004;12:268–73.
7. Bunker CB. Zoon balanitis-does it exist? J Eur Acad Dermatol Venereol 2020;34: e116–7.
8. Lacarrubba F, Borghi A, Verzì AE, et al. Dermoscopy of genital diseases: a review. J Eur Acad Dermatol 2020;34(10):2198–207.
9. Lacarrubba F, Verzì AE, Ardigò M, Micali G. Handheld reflectance confocal microscopy, dermatoscopy and histopathological correlation of common inflammatory balanitis. Skin Res Technol 2018;24(3):499–503.
10. Lacarrubba F, Ardigò M, Di Stefani A, et al. Dermatoscopy and reflectance confocal microscopy correlations in nonmelanocytic disorders. Dermatol Clin 2018;36(4):487–501.
11. Arzberger E, Komericki P, Ahlgrimm-Siess V, et al. Differentiation between balanitis and carcinoma in situ using reflectance confocal microscopy. JAMA Dermatol 2013;149(4):440–5.
12. Errichetti E, Lallas A, Di Stefani A, et al. Accuracy of dermoscopy in distinguishing erythroplasia of Queyrat from common forms of chronic balanitis: results from a multicentric observational study. J Eur Acad Dermatol Venereol 2019;33(5):966–72.
13. Errichetti E, Lacarrubba F, Micali G, Stinco G. Dermoscopy of Zoon's plasma cell balanitis. J Eur Acad Dermatol Venereol 2016;30(12):e209–10.
14. Chessa MA, Sechi A, Baraldi C, et al. Zoon's plasma cell balanitis: clinical and dermoscopic features in pediatric patients. Int J Dermatol 2018;57(11):e142–4.
15. Corazza M, Toni G, Virgili A, Borghi A. Plasma cell vulvitis: further confirmation of the diagnostic utility of dermoscopy. Int J Dermatol 2018;57(12):e164–5.
16. Marasca C, Annunziata MC, Cacciapuoti S, et al. Zoon balanitis in an immune-competent teenager. G Ital Dermatol Venereol 2019;154(2):221–3.
17. Weyers W, Ende Y, Schalla W, Diaz-Cascajo C. Balanitis of Zoon: a clinicopathologic study of 45 cases. Am J Dermatopathol 2002;24(6):459–67.

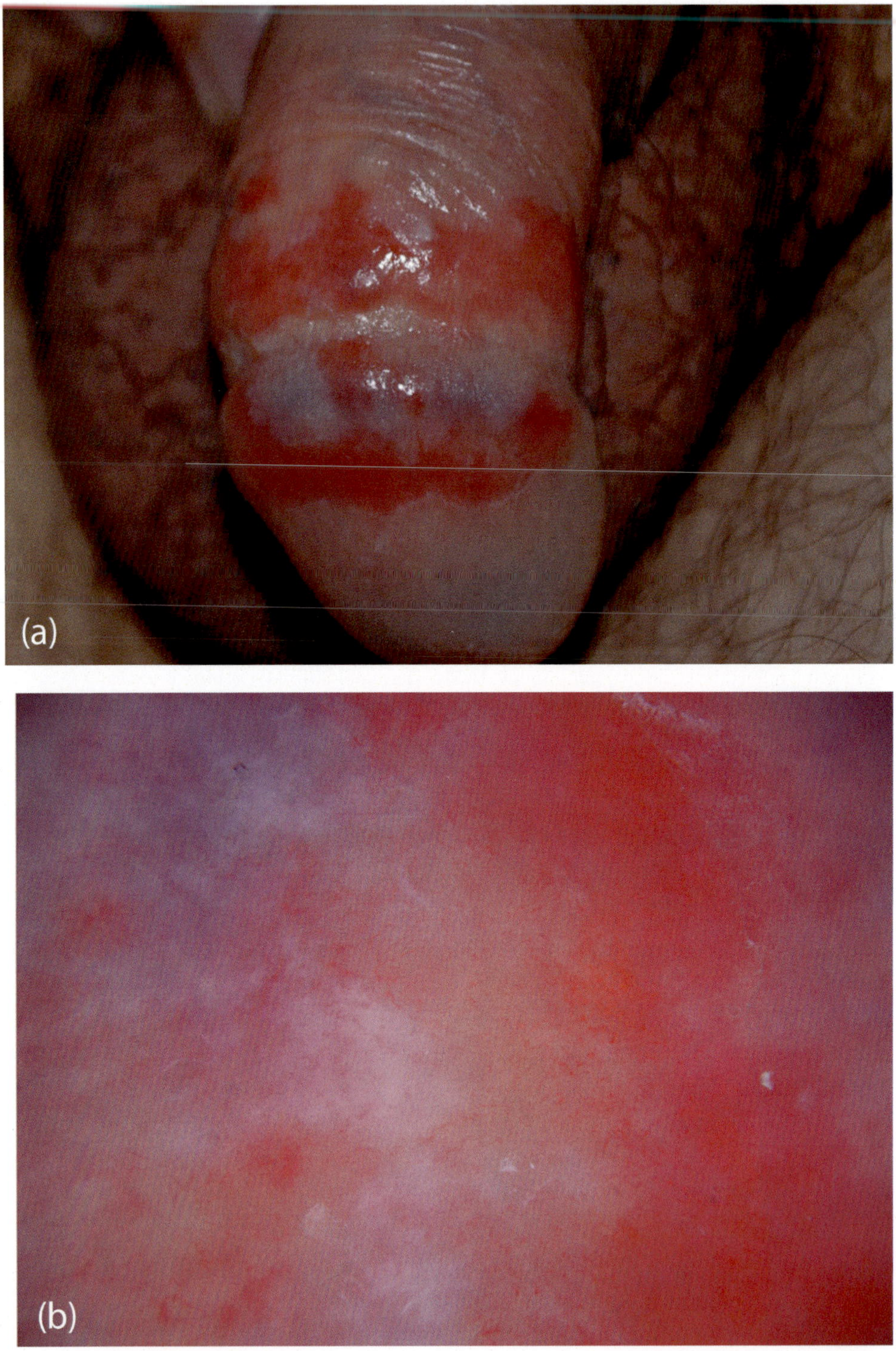

Figure 11.1 (a) Zoon's balanitis. Reddish macules involving the glans and the prepuce in a 42-year-old man. The patient had been unsuccessfully treated for candidiasis. (b) Dermoscopy (×10) showing orangish areas and sparse curved vessels.

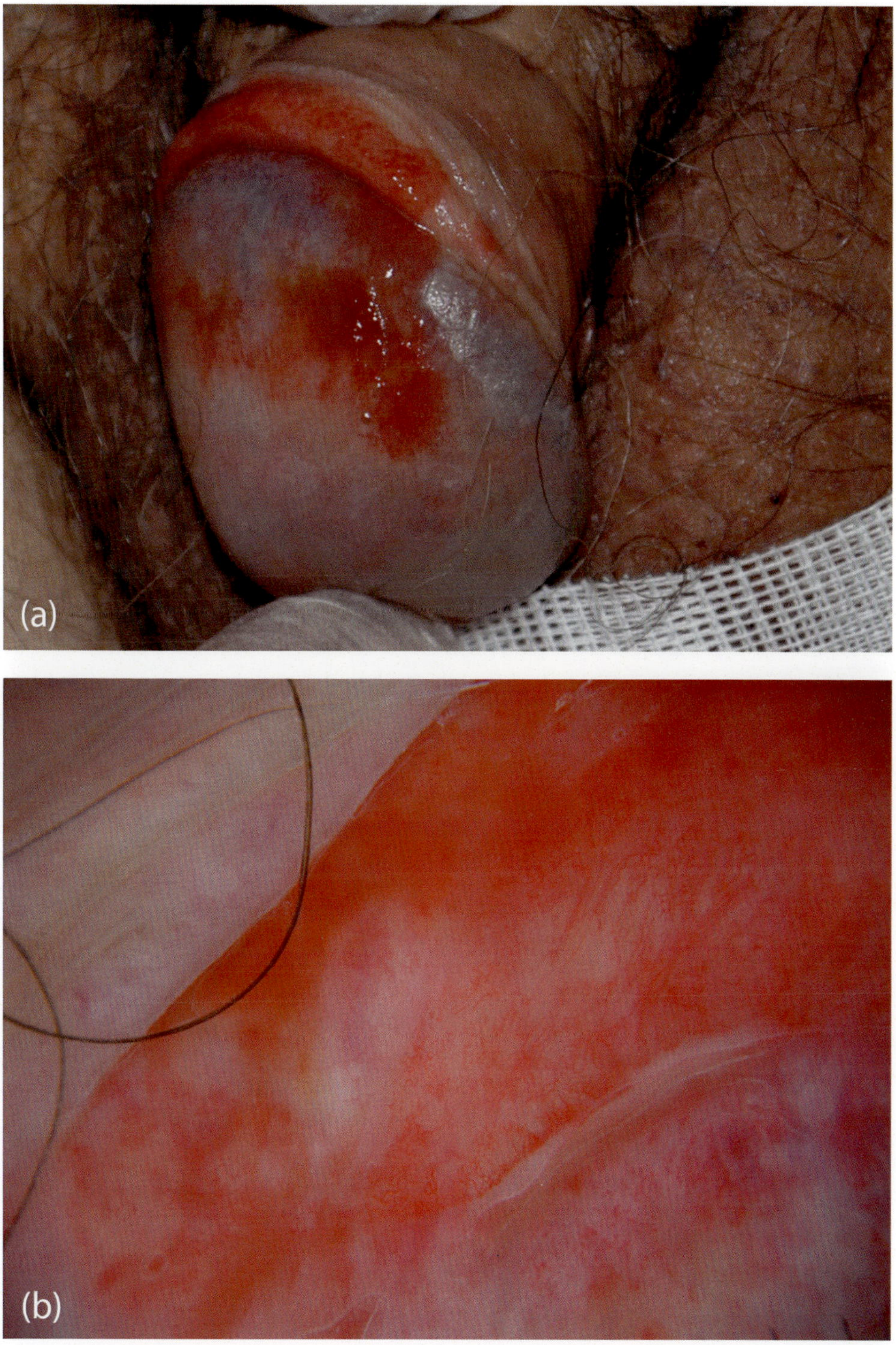

Figure 11.2 (a) Zoon's balanitis. Well-circumscribed, irregularly shaped, orange-red macules involving the glans and the prepuce in a 53-year-old man. (b) Dermoscopy (×10) showing an intense orange color and curved vessels.

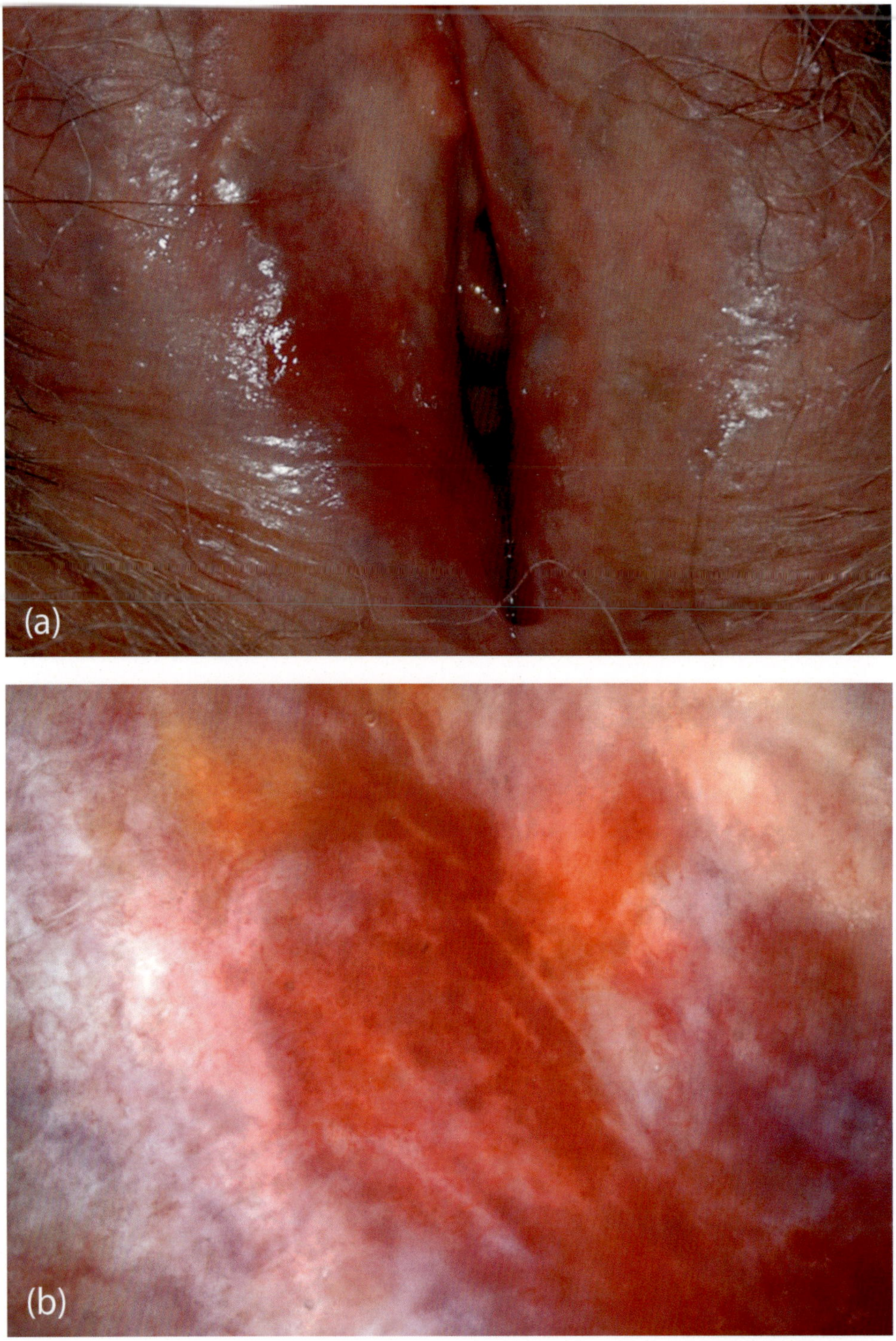

Figure 11.3 (a) Zoon's vulvitis. Irregularly shaped, reddish macules of the vulva, more evident on the right labium, in a 58-year-old woman. The lesions were asymptomatic. (b) Dermoscopy (×10) showing diffuse orange-yellow structureless areas and fairly focused curved vessels.

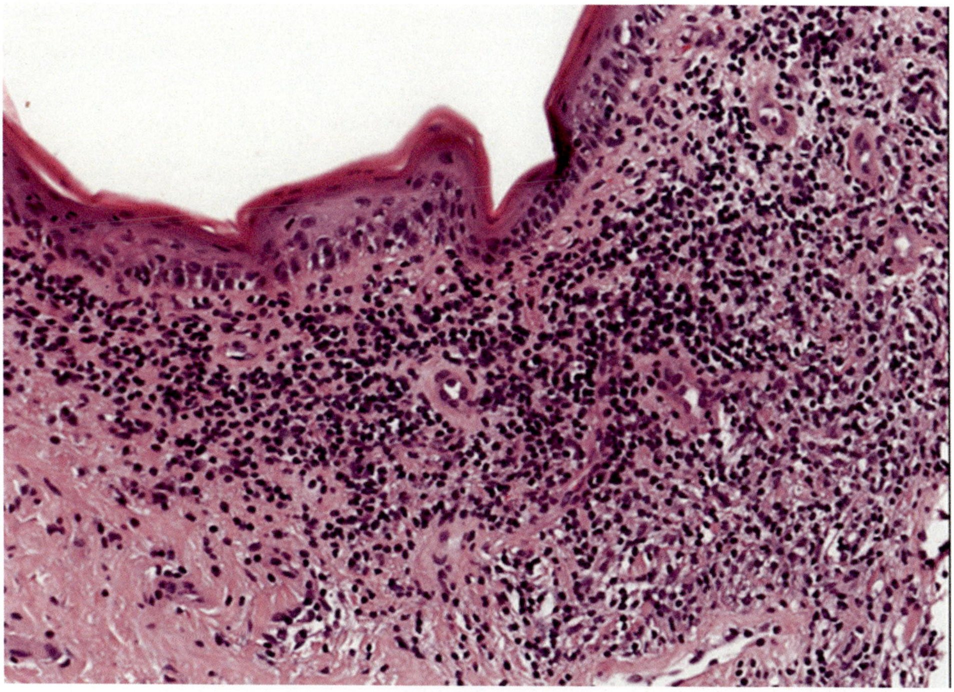

Figure 11.4 Histopathology of Zoon's balanitis showing epidermal attenuation with absent granular layer, sparse dyskeratosis and spongiosis. In the dermis, there is a dense band of inflammatory infiltrate with many plasma cells. Extravasated erythrocytes, hemosiderin and vascular proliferation are also present (H&E, ×100).

CHAPTER 12

Psoriasis

Maria Letizia Musumeci MD PhD, Giuseppe Broggi MD, and Giuseppe Micali MD

DEFINITION

Psoriasis is a chronic and immune mediated inflammatory skin disease (1). Genital involvement may be isolated or may be part of a more diffuse disease.

EPIDEMIOLOGY

Psoriasis affects 2–3% of the population, approximately. Genital psoriasis occurs in 30–60% of patients with plaque psoriasis and in up to 80% of patients with inverse psoriasis during the course of the disease (1). In 2–5% of cases, lesions involve the genital area only (1). Children and adults of both sexes may be affected.

ETIOLOGY

Psoriasis has multifactorial genetic and environmental causes (1). In the genital area, possible trigger factors are bacteria and yeasts colonization and skin injuries that result in Koebner phenomenon.

CLINICAL FEATURES

Psoriasis of the genitalia often appears as well-demarcated, brightly erythematous, thin plaques. Unlike plaque psoriasis, scaling is generally mild or absent and the surface appears as moist, smooth, and shiny [Figures 12.1(a) and 12.2(a)]. Maceration and fissuring, due to the combination of moisture, warmth, and friction, may occur and cause itch and/or pain (1). In male patients, both penis and scrotum may be involved, with glans most commonly affected. In children, the base of the penis may often represent the only localization. Vulvar psoriasis is generally symmetrical and may vary from silvery, scaly patches adjacent to the labia majora to moist, grayish plaques or glossy, red plaques without scaling in the skin folds [Figure 12.3(a)]. In infants, genital psoriasis appears as well-demarcated, erythematous, and sometimes silvery plaques in the diaper area, termed napkin psoriasis (1, 2).

DOI: 10.1201/9781003007166-12

DIFFERENTIAL DIAGNOSIS

Various disorders should be taken in consideration as possible differential diagnoses, including dermatophytosis and candidiasis, lichen planus, seborrheic dermatitis, contact dermatitis due to deodorants, perfumes and colored synthetics, erythroplasia of Queyrat, plasma cell balanitis or vulvitis, intertrigo, extramammary Paget's disease, fixed drug eruption, lichen sclerosus, lichen simplex chronicus, and Reiter's syndrome (balanitis circinata).

DIAGNOSIS

Genital psoriasis goes largely undiagnosed, especially in those cases exclusively localized in this area, even though it has a detrimental impact on quality of life and sexual health (3). The diagnosis is usually clinical, especially when genital lesions are part of a more generalized form of psoriasis. Dermoscopy and reflectance confocal microscopy, the latter showing dark dermal papillae filled with dilated and round vessels, are very useful to support the diagnosis (4), although histopathological examination is sometimes required.

DERMOSCOPY

The dermoscopic pattern of psoriasis has been extensively described in the literature (4–9). It is characterized, at low magnification (×10), by the presence of regularly distributed "red dots" (or "dotted capillaries") over a pale red background [Figures 12.1(b), 12.2(b), and 12.3(b)]. At high magnification (≥×100), the "red dots" appear as dilated, tortuous capillaries with a "bushy" aspect [Figure 12.2(c)]. In a study of 12 subjects with different types of balanitis, only patients with biopsy-proven psoriatic balanitis showed the presence of "bushy" capillaries (8). The typical vascular pattern in genital psoriasis is easily recognizable because of the lack of white scales, typically observed in cutaneous plaque psoriasis, that may hamper a correct visualization (10). Moreover, the value of dermoscopy is well known also in the therapeutic monitoring, with a number of studies reporting morphological modifications and loop changes after topical and systemic treatments (11).

HISTOPATHOLOGICAL CORRELATION

Histopathology of psoriasis is characterized by acanthosis, elongated rete ridges, hypogranulosis, parakeratosis, thinning of the suprapapillary plates and abscesses within the stratum corneum (Munro microabscesses). The dermoscopic vascular pattern typical of psoriasis ("red dots" and "bushy" capillaries) histologically corresponds to dilated, elongated, and tortuous capillary loops within the regularly elongated dermal papillae (Figure 12.4) (12).

REFERENCES

1. Meeuwis KA, de Hullu JA, Massuger LF, et al. Genital psoriasis: a systematic literature review on this hidden skin disease. Acta Derm Venereol 2011;91:5–11.
2. Beck KM, Yang EJ, Sanchez IM, Liao W. Treatment of genital psoriasis: a systematic review. Dermatol Ther (Heidelb) 2018;8(4):509–25.

3. Ryan C. Genital psoriasis: the failure of dermatologists to identify genital involvement. Br J Dermatol 2019;180(3):460–1.
4. Lacarrubba F, Verzì AE, Ardigò M, Micali G. Handheld reflectance confocal microscopy, dermatoscopy and histopathological correlation of common inflammatory balanitis. Skin Res Technol 2018;24(3):499–503.
5. Micali G, Verzì AE, Giuffrida G, et al. Inverse psoriasis: from diagnosis to current treatment options. Clin Cosmet Investig Dermatol 2019;12:953–9.
6. Woelber L, Prieske K, Mendling W, et al. Vulvar pruritus – causes, diagnosis and therapeutic approach. Dtsch Arztebl Int 2020;116(8):126–33.
7. Errichetti E, Lallas A, Di Stefani A, et al. Accuracy of dermoscopy in distinguishing erythroplasia of Queyrat from common forms of chronic balanitis: results from a multicentric observational study. J Eur Acad Dermatol Venereol 2019;33(5):966–72.
8. Lacarrubba F, Nasca MR, Micali G. Videodermatoscopy enhances diagnostic capability in psoriatic balanitis. J Am Acad Dermatol 2009;61:1084–6.
9. Lallas A, Apalla Z, Argenziano G, et al. Dermoscopic pattern of psoriatic lesions on specific body sites. Dermatology 2014;228(3):250–4.
10. Lacarrubba F, Borghi A, Verzì AE, et al. Dermoscopy of genital diseases: a review. J Eur Acad Dermatol 2020;34(10):2198–207.
11. Lacarrubba F, Pellacani G, Gurgone S, et al. Advances in non-invasive techniques as aids to the diagnosis and monitoring of therapeutic response in plaque psoriasis: a review. Int J Dermatol 2015;54(6):626–34.
12. Micali G, Lacarrubba F, Musumeci ML, et al. Cutaneous vascular patterns in psoriasis. Int J Dermatol 2010;49(3):249–56.

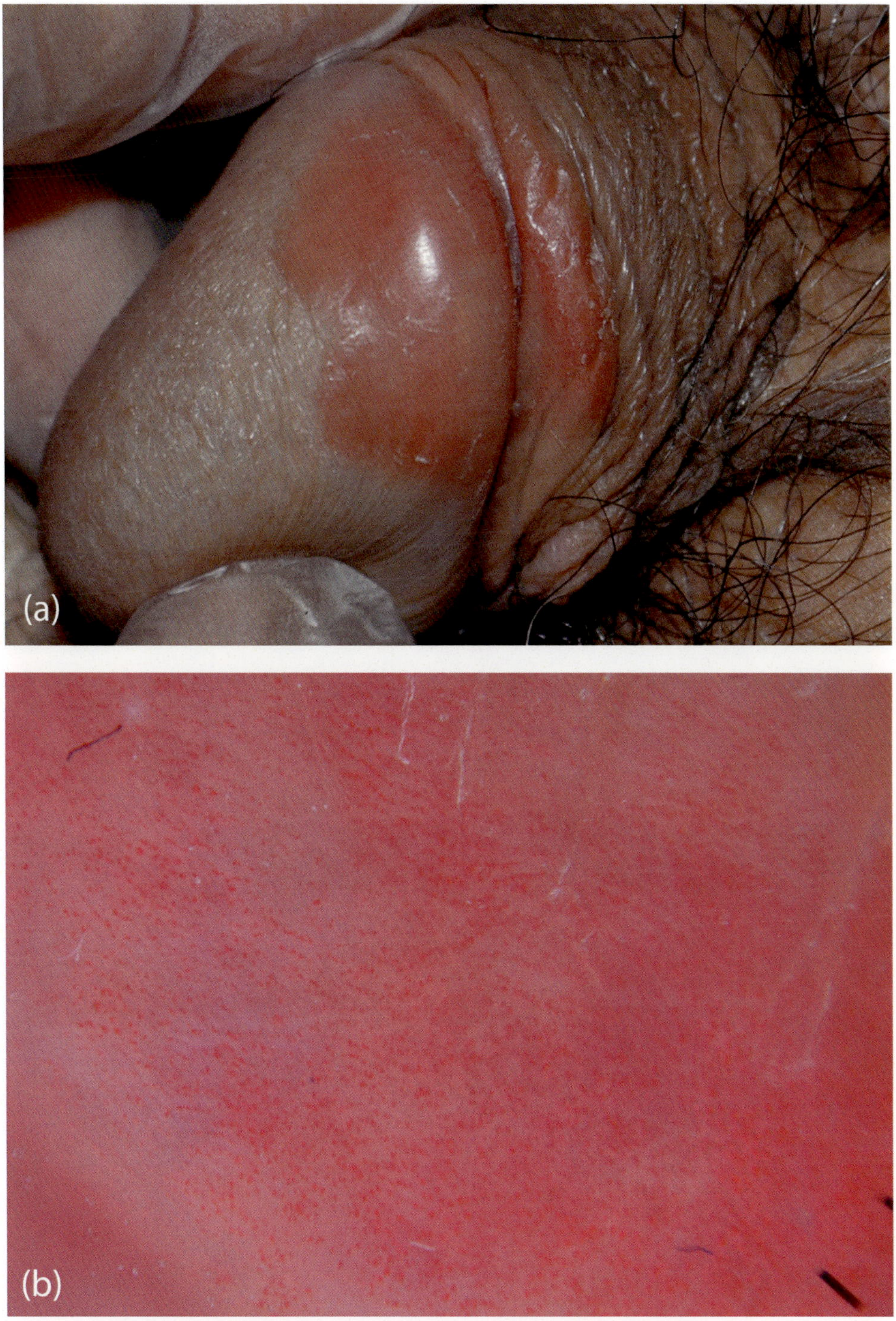

Figure 12.1 (a) Psoriatic balanitis. Well-defined, erythematous macule involving the glans and the prepuce in a 35-year-old man. Note the absence of scales. (b) Dermoscopy (×10) showing homogeneously distributed red dots ("dotted capillaries").

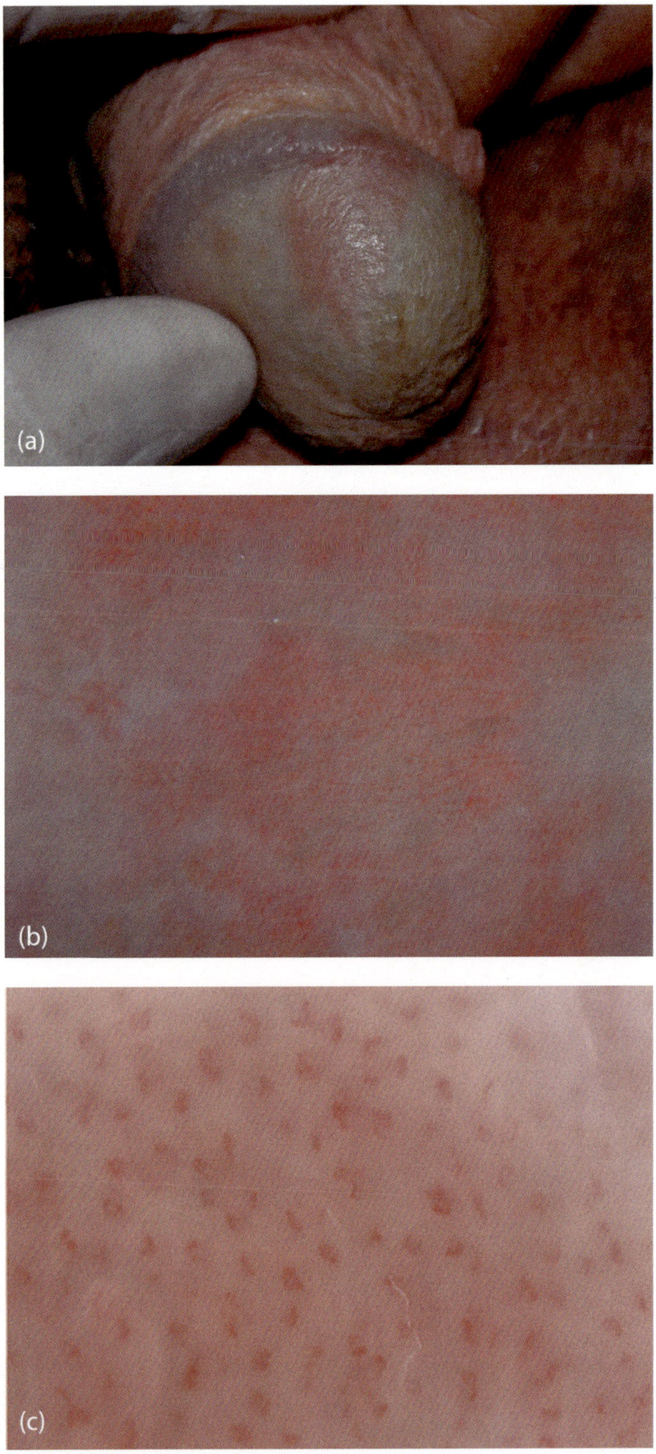

Figure 12.2 (a) Psoriatic balanitis. Minimal, erythematous macule of the glans in a 42-year-old man. (b) Dermoscopy (×10) showing homogeneously distributed red dots ("dotted capillaries"). (c) High-magnification dermoscopy (×100) of psoriasis of the glans showing regular, uniformly distributed, dilated and convoluted capillaries ("bushy" capillaries).

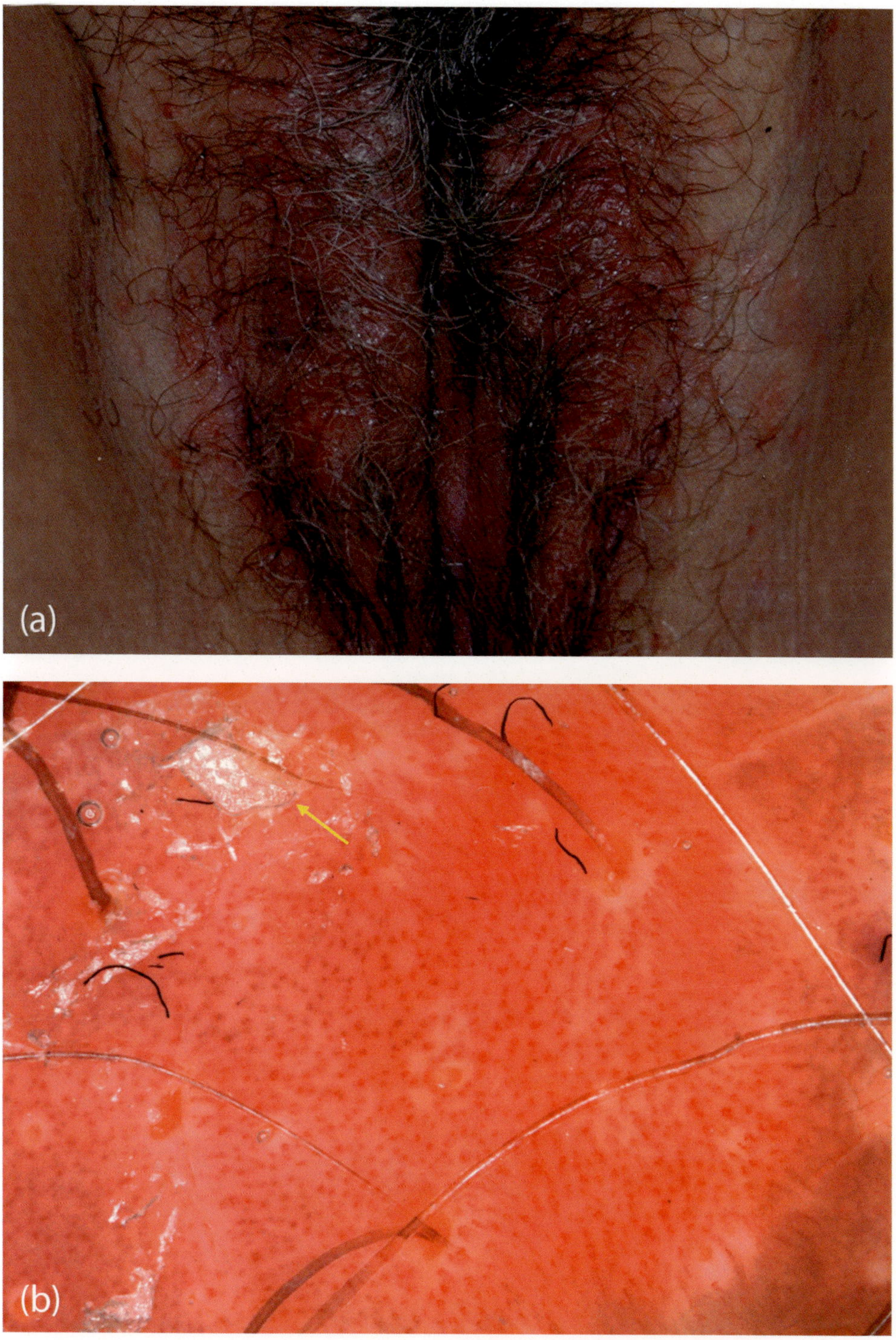

Figure 12.3 (a) Psoriatic vulvitis. Erythematous-desquamative plaque of the vulva. (b) Dermoscopy (×10) showing red dots ("dotted capillaries") associated with few whitish scales (arrow).

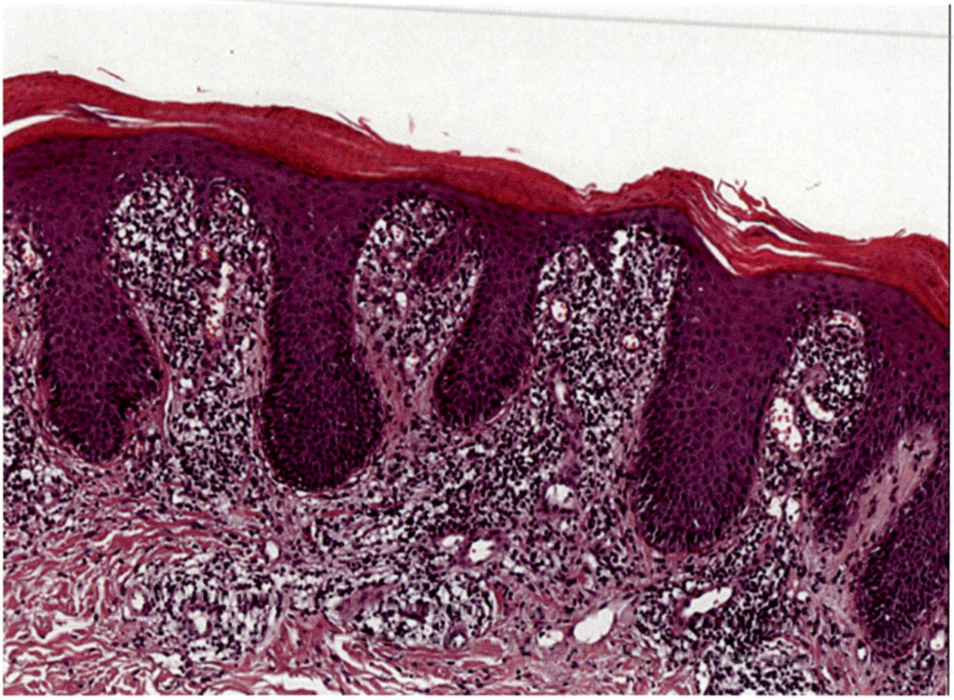

Figure 12.4 Histopathology of genital psoriasis showing parakeratosis, elongated rete ridges, and dilated, elongated, and tortuous capillary loops in the papillary dermis (H&E, ×100).

CHAPTER 13

Vitiligo

Giuseppe Broggi MD, Davide Francesco Puglisi MD, and Giuseppe Micali MD

DEFINITION

Vitiligo is a common acquired disorder characterized by depigmentation of the skin and/or mucous membranes.

EPIDEMIOLOGY

Vitiligo affects 0.5–2% of the world population, with an average age of onset of 20 years (1). The genitalia are a common site of involvement, although underreported. In a review of 1010 Indian patients, genital involvement was recorded in 6.7% of cases (2). In men over the age of 40 years seeking prostate screening in Brazil, 0.7% had genital vitiligo (3).

ETIOLOGY

Vitiligo is a multifactorial disorder with a complex pathogenesis (1, 4). The etiology is unknown, mainly involving genetic and autoimmune factors (5). Melanin pigment depletion likely results from an immune-mediated melanocyte damage, as suggested by the frequent association with other autoimmune disorders, such as Hashimoto thyroiditis, Graves' disease, Addison's disease, diabetes mellitus, alopecia areata, pernicious anemia, systemic lupus erythematosus, and inflammatory bowel disease. Some cases have been reported to be induced by imiquimod cream for the treatment of genital warts (6).

CLINICAL FEATURES

Vitiligo is a benign disorder with a chronic relapsing course. Typical lesions consist of well-demarcated, white amelanotic macules or patches of variable size [Figures 13.1(a) and 13.2(a)]. They are usually roundish, with convex, irregular borders, and centrifugally enlarging. Multiple and confluent lesions may be observed. Common sites of localization are the back of the hands, axillae, genitalia, periorificial areas of the face, and extensor body areas subject to trauma. Hairs may lose their pigmentation. The involvement of the genital area, that may include the mucosa, often causes an impairment of the quality of life both in males and females (7–9).

DOI: 10.1201/9781003007166-13

DIFFERENTIAL DIAGNOSIS

The most common differential diagnoses in the genital area include lichen sclerosus and post-inflammatory hypopigmentation.

DIAGNOSIS

The diagnosis of vitiligo is generally clinical, and Wood's lamp examination may enhance unnoticed lesions. Biopsy is occasionally performed in selected cases to rule out other hypopigmentary disorders.

DERMOSCOPY

Dermoscopy may be useful in differentiating depigmentation disorders (10). The most common dermoscopic feature of vitiligo consists of depigmented, glowing areas [Figures 13.1(b) and 13.2(b)] (11–13). Perifollicular hyperpigmentation is more frequently seen in progressing or repigmenting lesions than stable lesions (Figure 13.3) (11–15). It has been suggested that retention or loss of the perifollicular pigment is an important dermoscopic marker of vitiligo activity, with perifollicular hyperpigmentation typifying unstable vitiligo and perifollicular depigmentation suggesting stable disease (13–15). Other frequent features of vitiligo are represented by perilesional hyperpigmentation and depigmented hairs (leukotrichia) [Figures 13.2(b) and 13.3). Interfollicular pigmentation, a pigmentary network within the lesions, and lesional and perilesional telangiectasia may also be observed. Dermoscopy is very useful for the differential diagnosis with post-inflammatory hypopigmentation that shows poorly defined, hypopigmented areas alternating with normal skin [Figure 13.4(a) and (b)].

HISTOPATHOLOGICAL CORRELATION

Histopathology of vitiligo is characterized by absence of melanocytes and melanin granules in the basal layer (Figure 13.5) that may be highlighted by Fontana-Masson staining and that is responsible for the depigmented, glowing areas observed at dermoscopy. Occasional lymphocytes may be noted at the advancing border of the lesions (16, 17).

REFERENCES

1. Tarlé RG, Nascimento LM, Mira MT, Castro CC. Vitiligo – part 1. An Bras Dermatol 2014;89(3): 461–70.
2. Vora RV, Patel BB, Chaudhary AH, et al. A clinical study of vitiligo in a rural set up of Gujarat. Ind J Comm Med 2014;39:143–6.
3. Romero FR, Romero AW, Almeida RM, et al. Prevalence and risk factors for penile lesions/anomalies in a cohort of Brazilian men ≥40 years of age. Int Braz J Urol 2013;39:55–62.
4. Picardo M. Vitiligo: new insights. Br J Dermatol 2012;166:472–3.
5. Miniati A, Weng Z, Zhang B, et al. Neuro-immuno-endocrine processes in vitiligo pathogenesis. Int J Immunopathol Pharmacol 2012; 25:1–7.
6. Li W, Xin H, Ge L, et al. Induction of vitiligo after imiquimod treatment of condylomata acuminata. BMC Infect Dis 2014;14:329.
7. Bhandarkar SS, Kundu RV. Quality-of-life issues in vitiligo. Dermatol Clin 2012;30:255–68.
8. Kim do Y, Lee J, Oh SH, et al. Impact of genital involvement on the sexual lives of vitiligo patients. J Dermatol 2013;40:1065–7.

9. Morales-Sánchez MA, Vargas-Salinas M, Peralta-Pedrero ML, et al. Impact of vitiligo on quality of life. Actas Dermosifiliogr 2017;108(7):637–42.
10. Al-Refu K. Dermoscopy is a new diagnostic tool in diagnosis of common hypopigmented macular disease: a descriptive study. Dermatol Reports 2018;11(1):7916.
11. Meng R, Zhao G, Cai RK, et al. Application of polarized light dermoscopy in the early diagnosis of vitiligo and its differential diagnosis from other depigmented diseases. Chin J Dermatol 2009;42: 810–3.
12. Thatte SS, Khopkar US. The utility of dermoscopy in the diagnosis of evolving lesions of vitiligo. Indian J Dermatol Venereol Leprol 2014;80:505–8.
13. Jha AK, Sonthalia S, Lallas A. Dermoscopy as an evolving tool to assess vitiligo activity. J Am Acad Dermatol 2018;78(5):1017–9.
14. Kumar Jha A, Sonthalia S, Lallas A, Chaudhary RKP. Dermoscopy in vitiligo: diagnosis and beyond. Int J Dermatol 2018;57(1):50–4.
15. Errichetti E, Zelin E, Pinzani C, et al. Dermoscopic and clinical response predictor factors in nonsegmental vitiligo treated with narrowband ultraviolet B phototherapy: a prospective observational study. Dermatol Ther (Heidelb) 2020;10(5):1089–98.
16. Faria AR, Tarlé RG, Dellatorre G, et al. Vitiligo – Part 2 – classification, histopathology and treatment. An Bras Dermatol 2014;89(5):784–90.
17. Bergqvist C, Ezzedine K. Vitiligo: a review. Dermatology 2020;236(6):571–92.

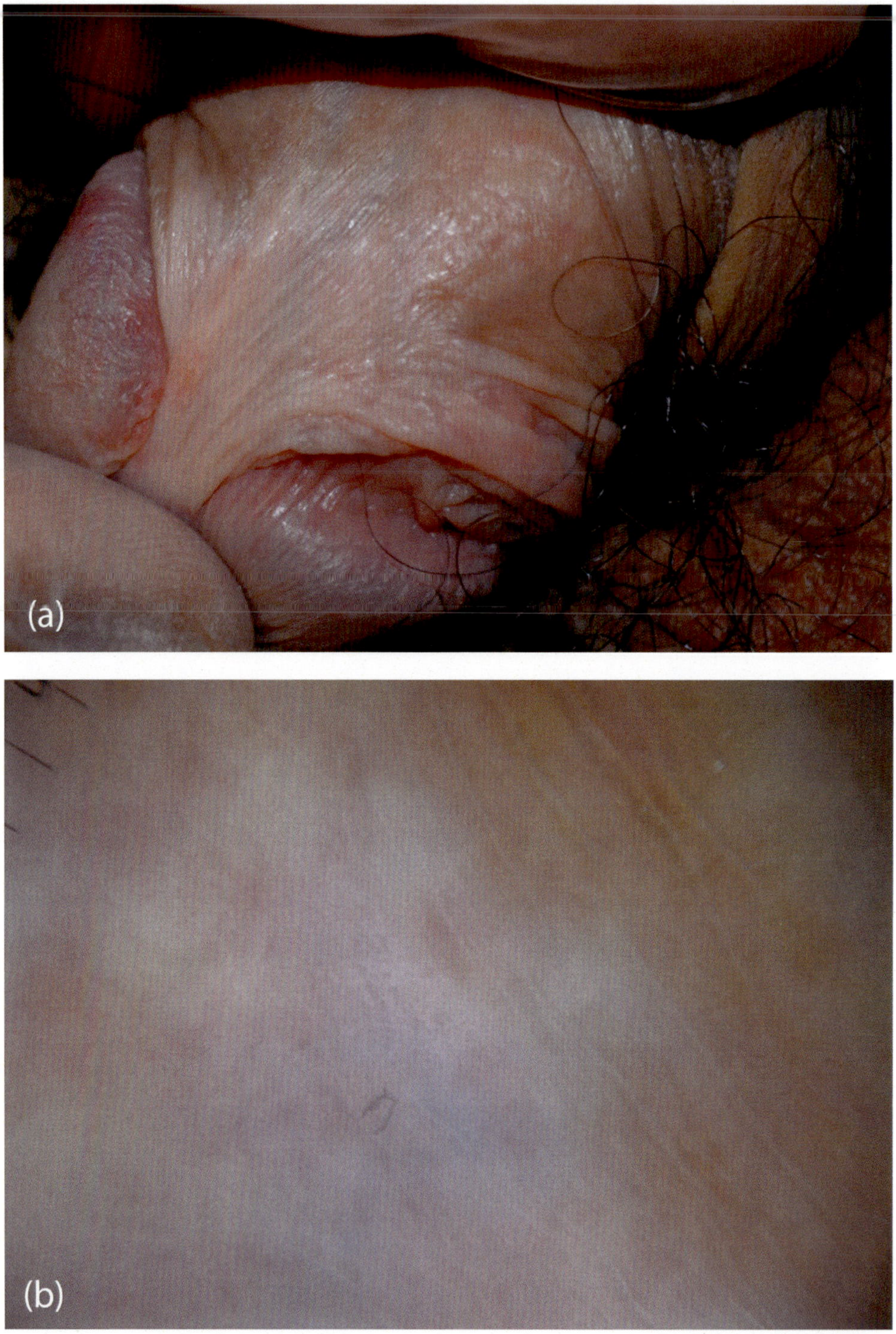

Figure 13.1 (a) Vitiligo. Well-demarcated, white macule involving the prepuce and the frenulum in a 44-year-old man. (b) Dermoscopy (×10) showing a depigmented, glowing area, expression of stable disease.

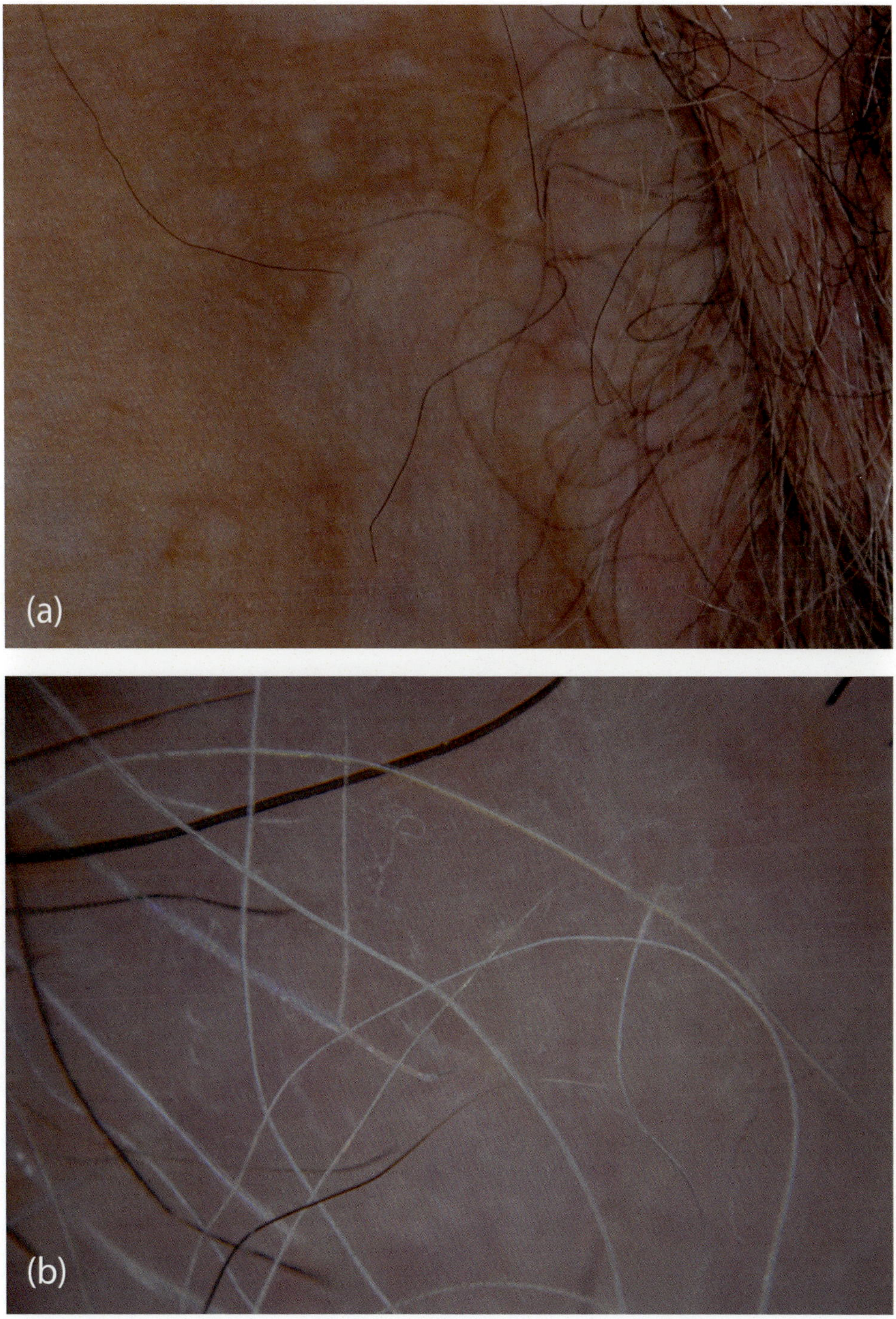

Figure 13.2 (a) Vitiligo. Multiple, well-demarcated, white macules of the genital area in a 49-year-old woman. (b) Dermoscopy (×10) showing a depigmented, glowing area, and depigmented hairs (leukotrichia).

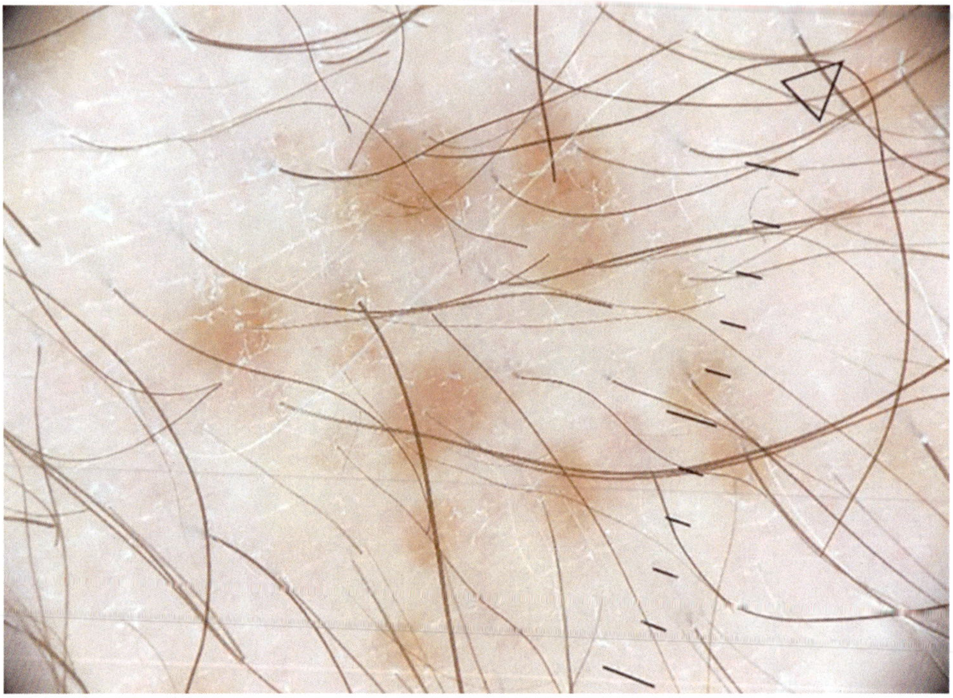

Figure 13.3 Vitiligo. Dermoscopy (×10) showing perifollicular hyperpigmentation, in this case expression of progressing disease. Leukotrichia is also visible.

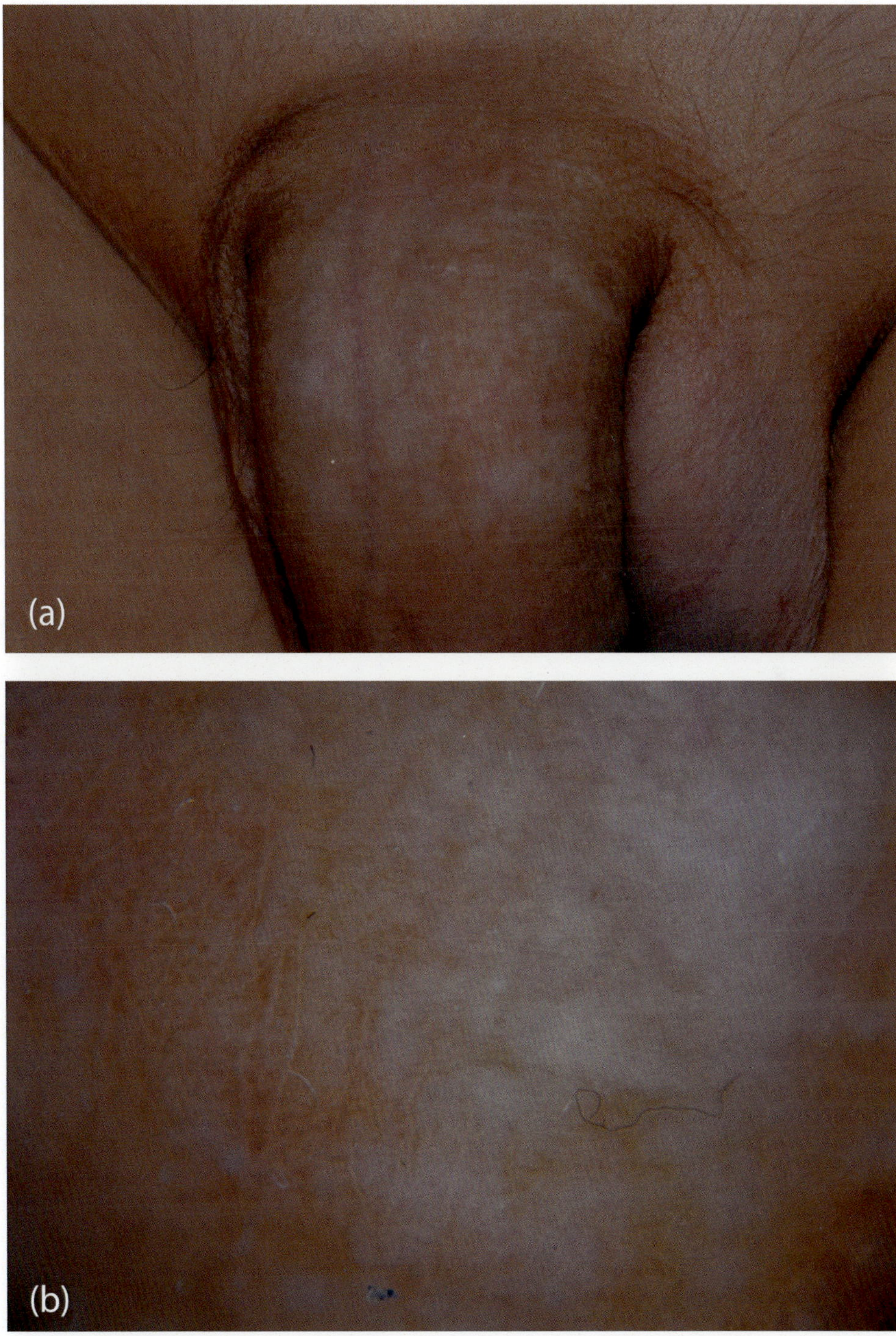

Figure 13.4 (a) Post-inflammatory hypopigmentation. Whitish macules of the penile shaft in a 7-year-old boy. The parents referred a previous treatment of eczematous lesions with topical steroids. (b) Dermoscopy (×10) showing poorly defined, hypopigmented areas alternating with normal skin.

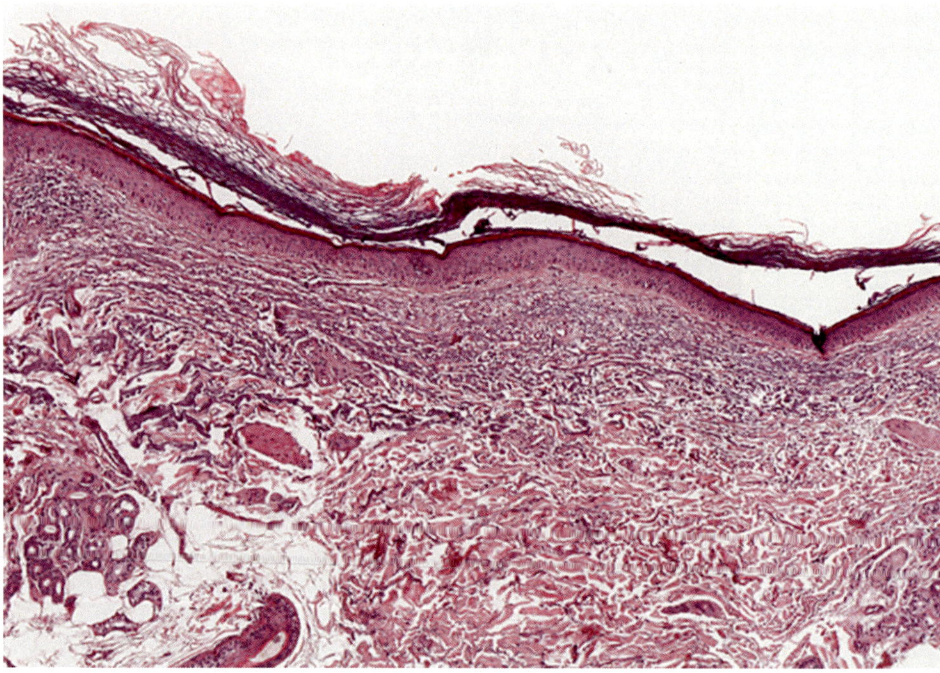

Figure 13.5 Histopathology of vitiligo showing total absence of basal melanocytes (H&E, ×100).

CHAPTER 14

Hidradenitis Suppurativa

Maria Letizia Musumeci MD PhD and Giuseppe Micali MD

DEFINITION

Hidradenitis suppurativa (HS), also known as Verneuil's disease or acne inversa, is a chronic inflammatory disease of the pilosebaceous unit affecting skin areas rich in apocrine glands and their surrounding tissues, with a strong negative impact on quality of life (1).

EPIDEMIOLOGY

The global prevalence of HS has been reported between 0.00033% and 4.1% depending on the studied populations (2). In Caucasians, the female/male ratio is 3:1. HS most commonly occurs in the third and fourth decades of life, and an average delay of 7–10 years has been reported between disease onset and diagnosis (2).

ETIOLOGY

The etiopathogenesis of HS is not completely understood. Three key processes have been implicated, namely follicular hyperkeratosis and dilatation, follicular rupture and subsequent inflammatory response, and chronic inflammation with architectural tissue changes (2).

CLINICAL FEATURES

HS is clinically characterized by the presence of deep-seated and painful nodules or abscesses, draining sinuses and prominent scarring (3) usually localized on the armpits, submammary folds, groin, and buttocks. The genital region, both in males and females, represents the area most frequently involved [Figures 14.1(a) and 14.2(a)]. Sometimes, a mild to severe genital lymphedema may occur as a complication (4).

Double- and multi-ended pseudocomedones, also defined as keratin-filled interconnected multipores, are also considered a typical clinical sign of HS (5) and appear as coupled or multiple blackheads. They are likely the results of keratinization of the residual stump of two adjacent follicles undergoing cicatricial rearrangements (5).

DOI: 10.1201/9781003007166-14

Another feature commonly observed in HS patients is represented by roundish, atrophic scars that are the result of follicular dilation and rupture following inflammatory outbreaks and subsequent subcutaneous remodeling. They appear as well demarcated areas deeper than the surrounded skin, with wide base and irregular margins (3).

DIFFERENTIAL DIAGNOSIS

The main differential diagnoses of HS include bacterial/fungal infections, erysipelas, Crohn's disease, lymphogranuloma venereum, and granuloma inguinale. In addition, double- and multi-ended pseudocomedones should be differentiated from secondary comedones that may be observed in acne conglobata (6).

DIAGNOSIS

No pathognomonic tests exist, and the diagnosis is primarily clinical, although ultrasound imaging can further define lesional morphology and depth (2). Based on the modified Dessau definition, three diagnostic criteria should be met: presence of typical lesions, typical locations, and chronicity (2).

DERMOSCOPY

Dermoscopy examination may be useful to enhance the diagnostic accuracy of HS, allowing a better visualization of double-ended pseudocomedones and atrophic scars (3). Double-ended pseudocomedones typically appear at dermoscopy as coupled deepening hollows presenting large, irregular openings with undermined borders and a superficially located or deep-seated keratin mass [Figures 14.1(b) and (c) and 14.2(b)]. They are observed in the context of a whitish scarred tissue of variable depth and morphology (atrophic, bridging, and/or circinate scars) and are sometimes connected by a bluish tract detectable through a translucent, cicatricial tissue (3, 4). Dermoscopy may also be useful to highlight the undermined borders of HS scars and the presence of variable scar depth levels likely due to long-lasting wax and wane tissue repair during the relapsing course of the disease (Figures 14.3 and 14.4). Linear fibrotic bands may be interposed between adjacent atrophic scars (3). The recognition of these aspects may lead to the diagnosis in the case of minimal/mild HS.

HISTOPATHOLOGICAL CORRELATION

Histopathology of HS may show infundibular lymphocytic infiltrate, follicular epidermal hyperplasia and hyperkeratosis, sinus tracts, tunnels, cysts, follicular rupture, and dermal fibrosis (2). The pseudocomedones correspond to large, multiloculated, superficially and horizontally oriented hollows with multiple dilated superficial openings (Figure 14.5). The cavities are lined by normal multilayered epithelium and filled with corneal lamellae, cellular debris, and amorphous material, without evidence of hair follicle (3). They are the result of keratinization of the residual follicular stump of two adjacent follicular units after multiple scarring rearrangements (3).

REFERENCES

1. Lacarrubba F, Dini V, Napolitano M, et al. Ultrasonography in the pathway to an optimal standard of care of hidradenitis suppurativa: the Italian Ultrasound Working Group experience. J Eur Acad Dermatol Venereol 2019;33(Suppl 6):10–4.
2. Nguyen TV, Damiani G, Orenstein LAV, et al. Hidradenitis suppurativa: an update on epidemiology, phenotypes, diagnosis, pathogenesis, comorbidities and quality of life. J Eur Acad Dermatol Venereol 2021;35(1):50–61.
3. Lacarrubba F, Musumeci ML, Martorell A, et al. Role of the imaging techniques in the diagnosis and staging of hidradenitis suppurativa. G Ital Dermatol Venereol 2018;153(3 Suppl 2):20–5.
4. Musumeci ML, Scilletta A, Sorci F, et al. Genital lymphedema associated with hidradenitis suppurativa unresponsive to adalimumab treatment. JAAD Case Rep 2019;5(4):326–8.
5. Lacarrubba F, Musumeci ML, Nasca MR, et al. Double-ended pseudocomedones in hidradenitis suppurativa: clinical, dermoscopic, and histopathological correlation. Acta Derm Venereol 2017;97(6):763–4.
6. Lacarrubba F, Dall'Oglio F, Musumeci ML, et al. Secondary comedones in a case of acne conglobata correlate with double-ended pseudocomedones in hidradenitis suppurativa. Acta Derm Venereol 2017;97(8):969–70.

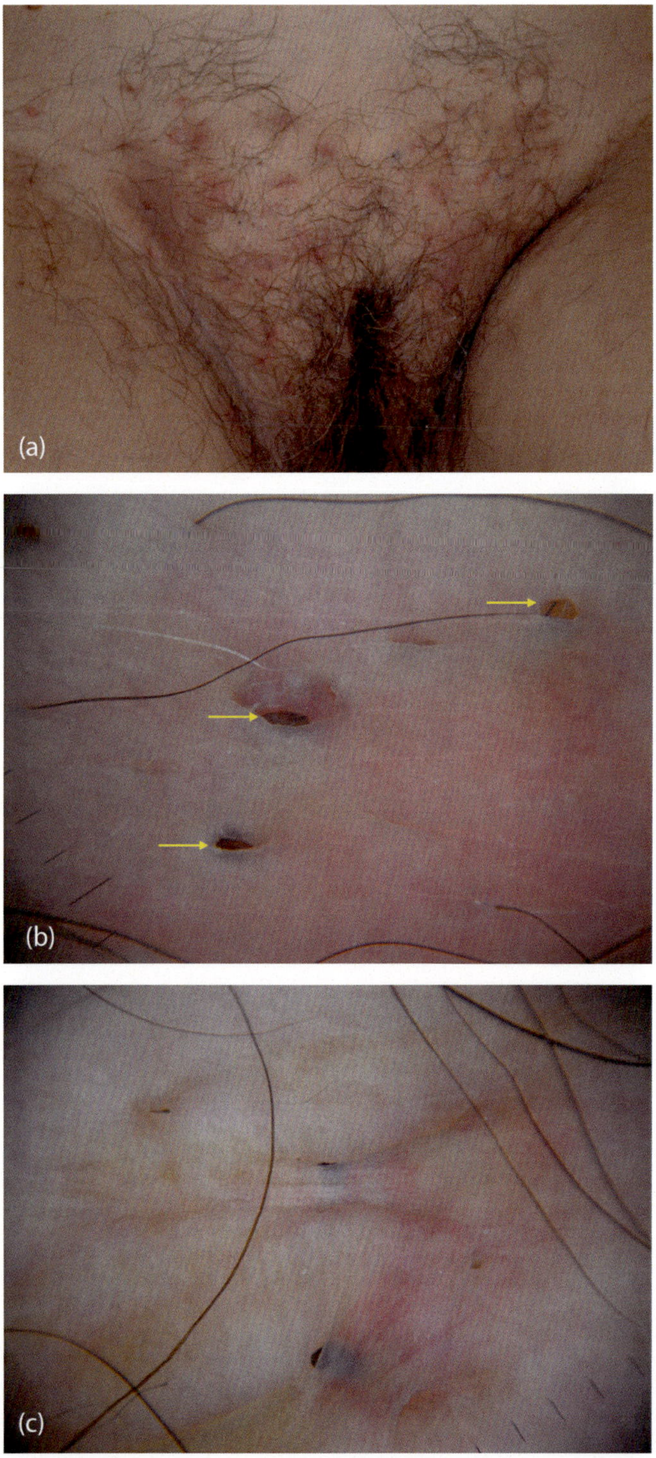

Figure 14.1 (a) Hidradenitis suppurativa. Multiple, mild inflammatory lesions and scars of the genital area in a 34-year-old woman. (b) Dermoscopy (×10) showing multiple double-ended pseudocomedones: deepening hollows presenting large, irregular openings with undermined borders and superficially located keratin masses (arrows). (c) Dermoscopy (×10) showing double-ended pseudocomedones in the context of bridging scars.

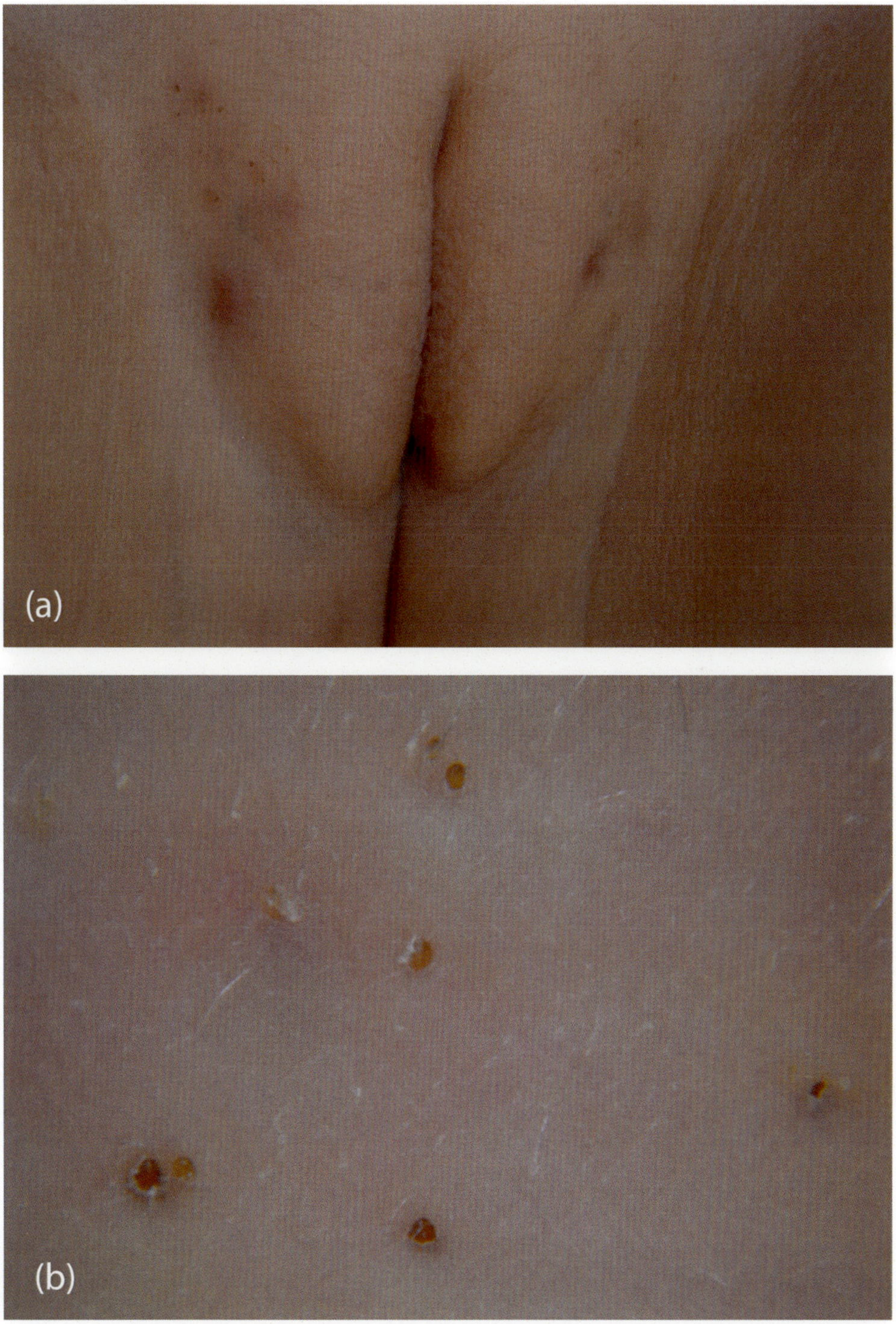

Figure 14.2 (a) Hidradenitis suppurativa. Minimal lesions in a 5-year-old girl. (b) Dermoscopy (×10) showing multiple double-ended pseudocomedones.

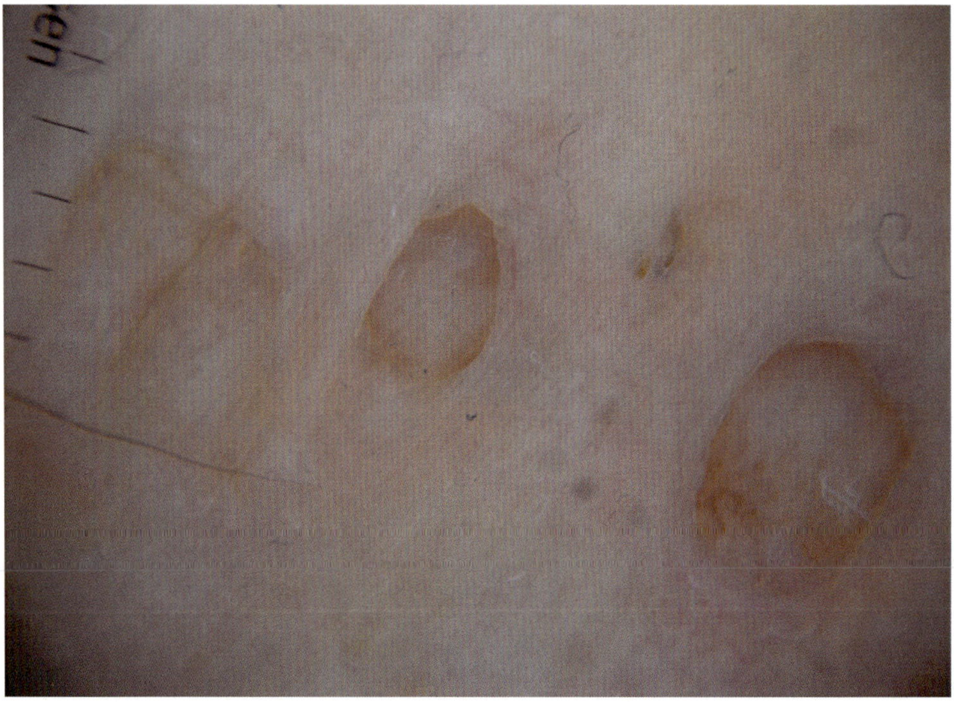

Figure 14.3 Hidradenitis suppurativa. Dermoscopy (×10) showing multiple round scars with undermined borders.

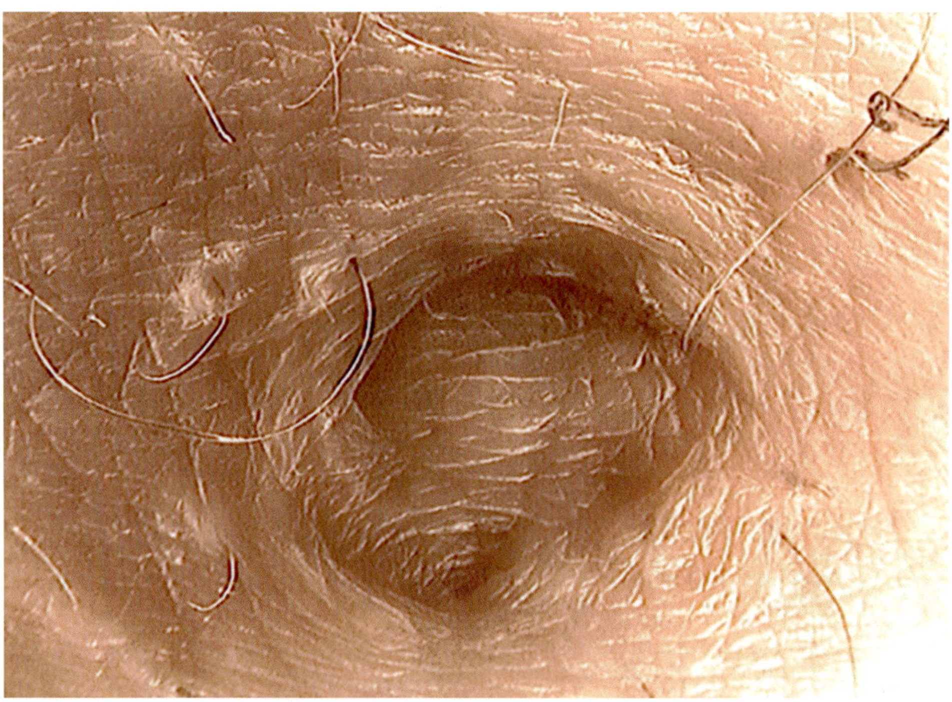

Figure 14.4 Hidradenitis suppurativa. Incident light dermoscopy (×20) showing a scar with variable depth levels likely due to long-lasting wax and wane tissue repair during the relapsing course of the disease.

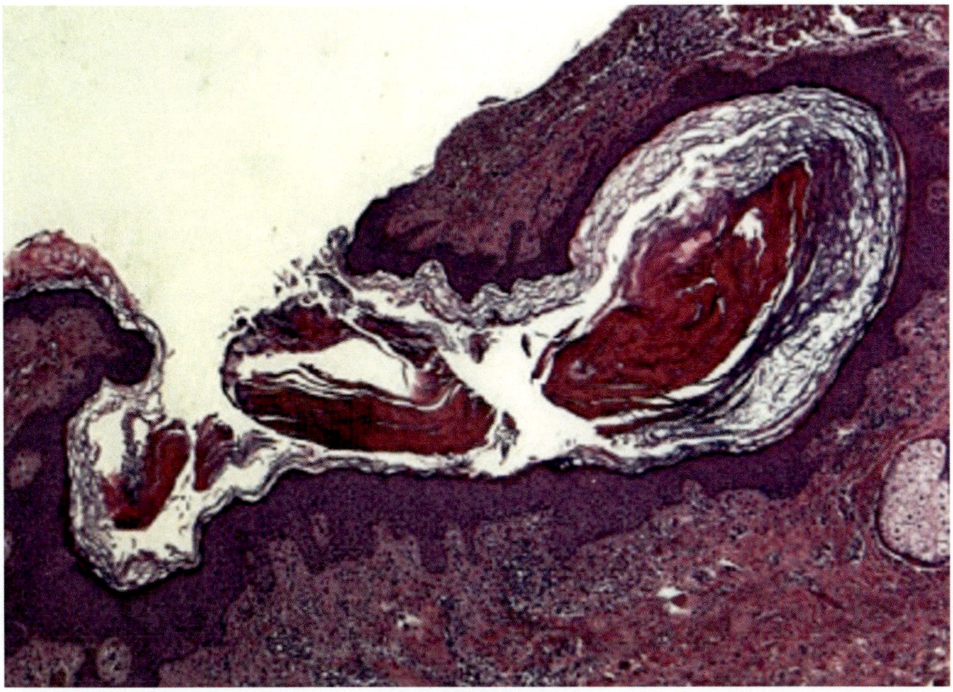

Figure 14.5 Histopathology of a pseudocomedo: large, horizontally oriented hollow lined by normal multilayered epithelium and filled with corneal lamellae, cellular debris and amorphous material, without evidence of hair follicle.

CHAPTER 15

Melanosis

Giuseppe Stinco MD, Aimilios Lallas MD, and Enzo Errichetti MD

DEFINITION

Genital melanosis (GM) is a relatively frequent, asymptomatic and benign pigmentation of the genitalia seen in both males and females (1, 2). It is often referred to as genital lentigo, genital melanotic macules, or genital hypermelanosis.

EPIDEMIOLOGY

It is estimated that about 10–12% of women and 3% of men are affected by GM, even though some studies have reported the incidence to be as low as 0.011% of patients presenting to a general dermatology. GM may be present in males and females of all ages, albeit it is more commonly observed in adulthood. No racial or ethnic predilection has been reported.

ETIOLOGY

GM is generally considered to be idiopathic, although several possible causes have been proposed. In particular, in a minority of cases, it has been associated with previous injury or irritation, treatment with anthralin or PUVA (psoralen and ultraviolet A) therapy. In women, hormonal influences (e.g., oral contraceptives and pregnancy) have also been suspected to play a possible role. Finally, in a subset of patients, GM may occur as a post-inflammatory pigmentation on the background of either lichen planus or lichen sclerosus.

CLINICAL FEATURES

GM presents as asymptomatic light brown to black-gray macules/patches having a size from 0.1 to 2 cm or more and irregular and poorly demarcated borders [Figures 15.1(a), 15.2(a), 15.3(a), and 15.4(a)] (1, 2). Although single lesions are possible, GM usually manifests as numerous, multifocal, confluent, and asymmetric lesions. It has a predilection for the mucosal surfaces rather than keratinized, hair-bearing skin of the external genitalia. In men, the glans penis is the most commonly involved area, followed by the prepuce, meatus, penile shaft, and perineum. In women, GM usually occurs on the mucosal labia majora, labia minora and clitoris, and, less frequently, on the vagina, cervix, introitus, mons pubis, and perineum.

DOI: 10.1201/9781003007166-15

DIFFERENTIAL DIAGNOSIS

Several conditions of genital areas may have similar appearance, including melanocytic nevi, atypical melanocytic nevi of the genital type, melanoma, physiologic hyperpigmentation and post-inflammatory hyperpigmentation, lentiginosis, angiokeratomas, seborrheic keratosis, squamous cell carcinoma, and pigmented basal cell carcinoma. GM may sometimes present as inhomogeneous pigmentation similar to melanoma and the differentiation may be challenging on clinical grounds. When numerous pigmented macules/patches are observed, it is important to take into account some genetic conditions, mainly including LEOPARD (multiple lentigines, ECG conduction abnormalities, ocular hypertelorism, pulmonic stenosis, abnormal genitalia, retardation of growth, and sensorineural deafness) syndrome, Peutz-Jeghers syndrome, NAME (nevi, atrial myxoma, myxoid neurofibroma, and ephelides) syndrome, and Carney complex (1).

DIAGNOSIS

The diagnosis is usually made by a physical examination and a complete medical history. Dermoscopy may be a useful aid for assisting the clinical recognition of GM (3–8). Additionally, reflectance confocal microscopy has also been showed to facilitate the diagnosis of GM and its differentiation from malignant pigmented lesions. In doubtful cases, a biopsy must be taken to perform histologic, immunohistochemical and ultrastructural features in order to achieve a definitive diagnosis (7).

DERMOSCOPY

Dermoscopy of GM has been widely studied in females, while only few case reports have been reported in males (3–6, 8). The most frequently detected patterns include the ring-like, the structureless and the parallel pattern. Other less common patterns are the globular-like, the cobblestone-like, the reticular-like, and the polycircular pattern.

The ring-like pattern is characterized by multiple white to tan roundish/oval structures having hyperpigmented well-defined circular borders, sometimes showing a grape-like arrangement [Figure 15.1(b)]. The structureless or homogeneous pattern is characterized by a homogenous light- to dark-brown pigmentation; a blue-gray hue is seen less commonly. The parallel pattern is typified by parallel linear and curved light- to dark-brown lines following the sulci of the skin/mucosal surface [Figure 15.2(b)]. The globular-like pattern features round to oval aggregated brownish globules, while the cobblestone-like pattern is characterized by globules that are bigger and polygonal [Figure 15.3(b)]. The reticular-like pattern shares similarities with the pigment network of melanocytic nevi, being typified by a regular and homogeneous reticular structure often ending abruptly at the edge of the lesion [Figure 15.4(b)]. Finally, the polycircular pattern is usually found only on the papillomatous surface of the outer edge of the labia minora and presents as polycircular brown pigmented areas. GM is usually devoid of vascular structures, even though milky-red areas and irregular vessels have been reported. Notably, globular-like, structureless, and parallel patterns are mainly observed in single lesions and were not associated with a specific genital site, while the ring-like, cobblestone-like, and reticular-like patterns are most frequently seen in multifocal macules located at specific anatomical sites, such as the labia majora and labia minora. Combined dermoscopic patterns are also seen not uncommonly.

HISTOPATHOLOGICAL CORRELATION

Histologically, GM shows an increase in melanin in the basal cell layer with either normal or slightly increased numbers of melanocytes, which are usually arranged solitarily in the basal layer without nests formation (Figure 15.5) (1, 2, 7). The melanocytes do not feature any atypia and they are not seen in stages of mitosis. Pigment incontinence in papillary dermis may be present. Melanocytes with longer dendrites at the dermo-epidermal junction are most frequent in men.

The ring-like pattern is correlated with the presence of hyperpigmentation in the epidermal basal layer and areas that lack pigmentation at the top of the dermal papillae, while the parallel pattern is correlated with elongated and clubbed rete ridges with hyperpigmentation of the basal layer without prominent melanocytic hyperplasia. The homogeneous pattern is characterized by the presence of melanin at all levels of the epidermis and/or the dermis. The reticular-like pattern is characterized by the presence of basal cell layer hyperpigmentation, acanthosis, and thick hyperpigmented epidermal crests blending at their base. Finally, the globular-like pattern corresponds to the variable distribution of the melanin pigment along the epidermal basal layer and clusters of melanophages in papillary dermis.

REFERENCES

1. Lenane P, Keane CO, Connell BO, et al. Genital melanotic macules: clinical, histologic, immunohistochemical, and ultrastructural features. J Am Acad Dermatol 2000;42:640–4.
2. Haugh AM, Merkel EA, Zhang B, et al. A clinical, histologic, and follow-up study of genital melanosis in men and women. J Am Acad Dermatol 2017;76:836–40.
3. Mannone F, De Giorgi V, Cattaneo A, et al. Dermoscopic features of mucosal melanosis. Dermatol Surg 2004;30:1118–23.
4. Ferrari A, Buccini P, Covello R, et al. The ringlike pattern in vulvar melanosis: a new dermoscopic clue for diagnosis. Arch Dermatol 2008;144:1030–4.
5. Ronger-Savle S, Julien V, Duru G, et al. Features of pigmented vulval lesions on dermoscopy. Br J Dermatol 2011;164:54–61.
6. Ferrari A, Zalaudek I, Argenziano G, et al. Dermoscopy of pigmented lesions of the vulva: a retrospective morphological study. Dermatology 2011;222:157–166.
7. Murzaku EC, Penn LA, Hale CS, et al. Vulvar nevi, melanosis, and melanoma: an epidemiologic, clinical, and histopathologic review. J Am Acad Dermatol 2014;71:1241–9.
8. Cengiz FP, Emiroglu N, Wellenhof RH. Dermoscopic and clinical features of pigmented skin lesions of the genital area. An Bras Dermatol 2015;90:178–83.

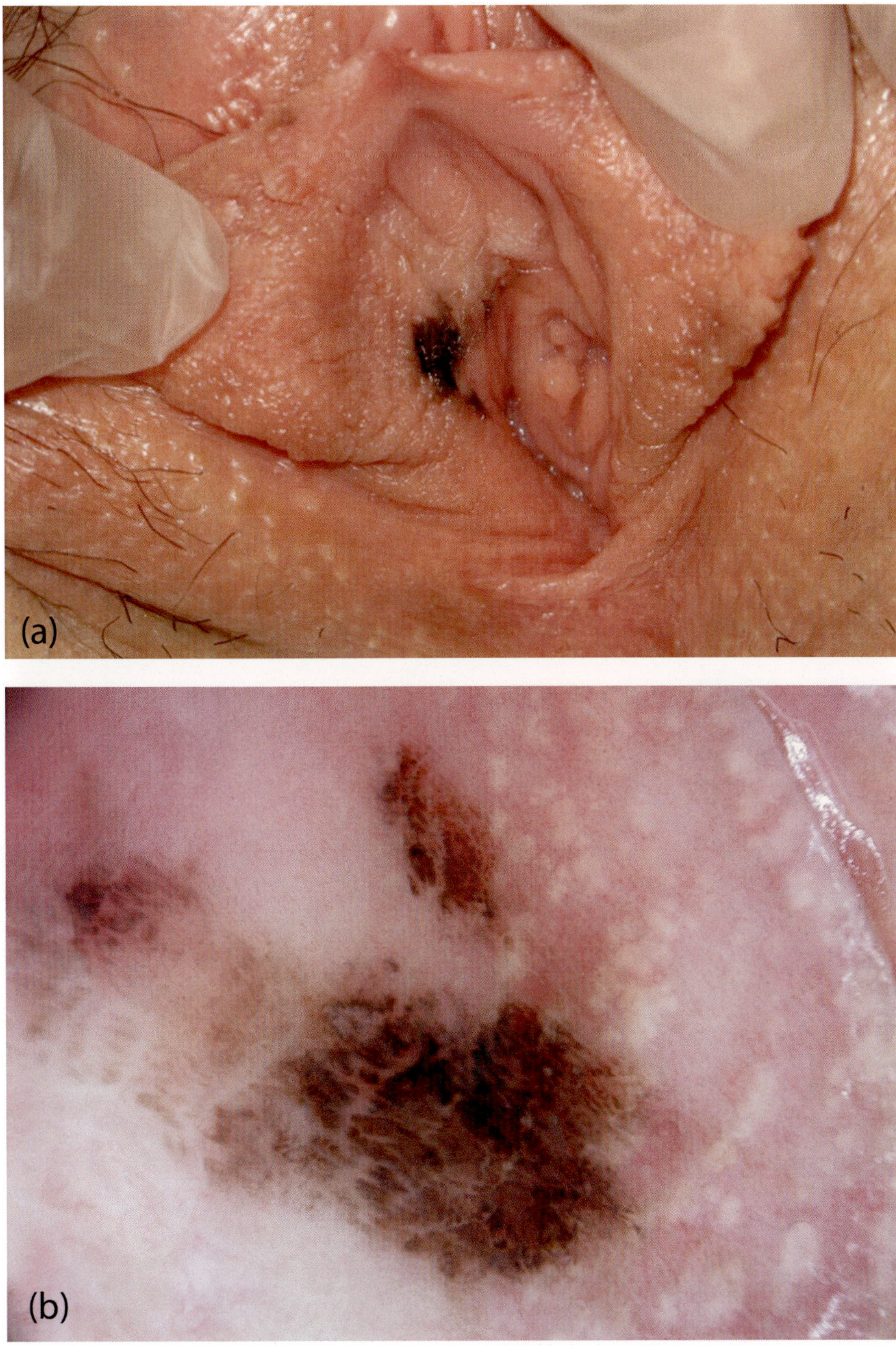

Figure 15.1 (a) Genital melanosis. A few dark-brown patches on the vaginal introitus. (b) Dermoscopy (×10) mainly showing a ring-like pattern with roundish/oval brown structures having hyperpigmented well-defined borders, with a sort of grape-like arrangement.

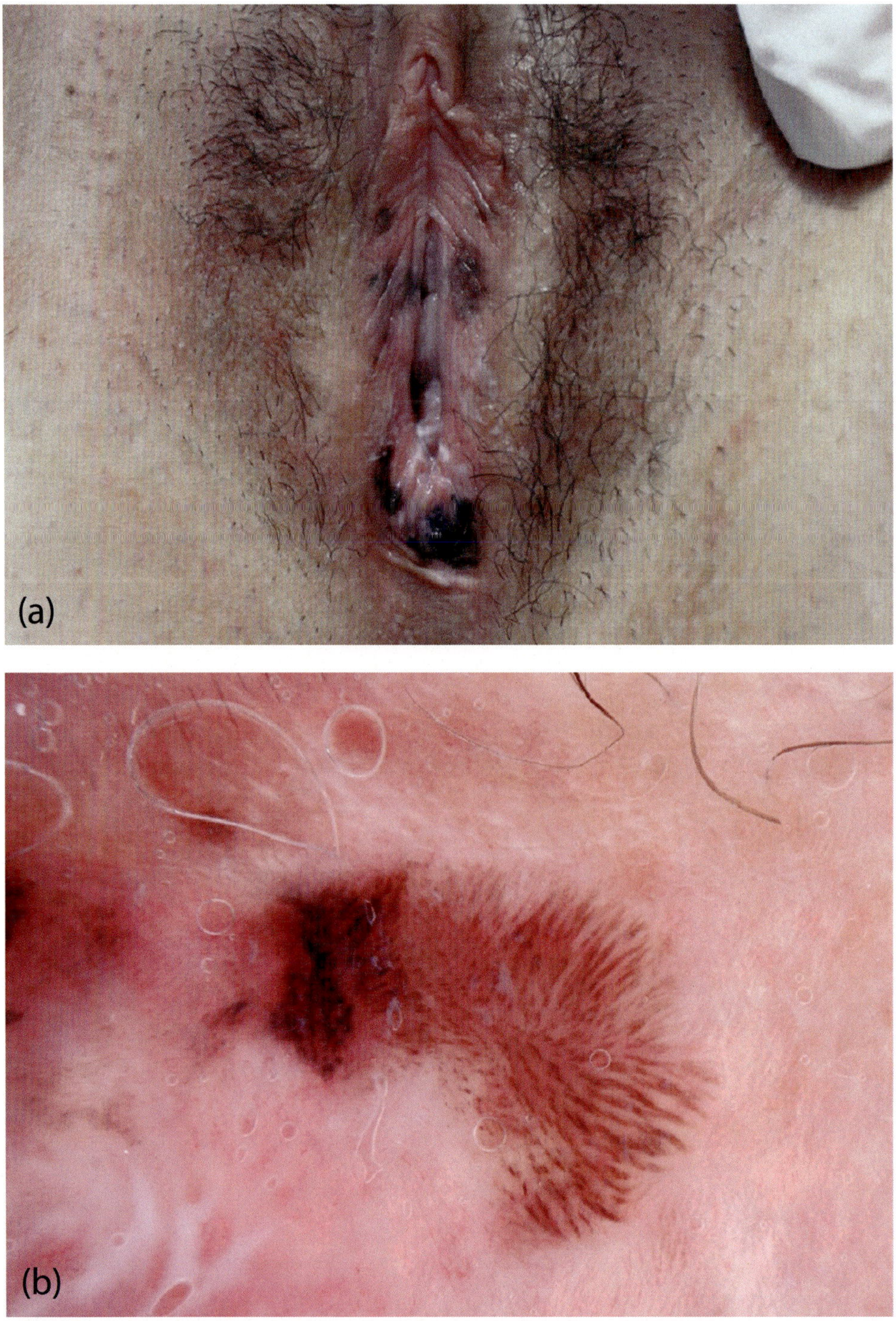

Figure 15.2 (a) Genital melanosis. Multiple dark-brown macules of the vulva. (b) Dermoscopy (×10) displaying a parallel pattern, consisting of parallel linear and curved light- to dark-brown lines.

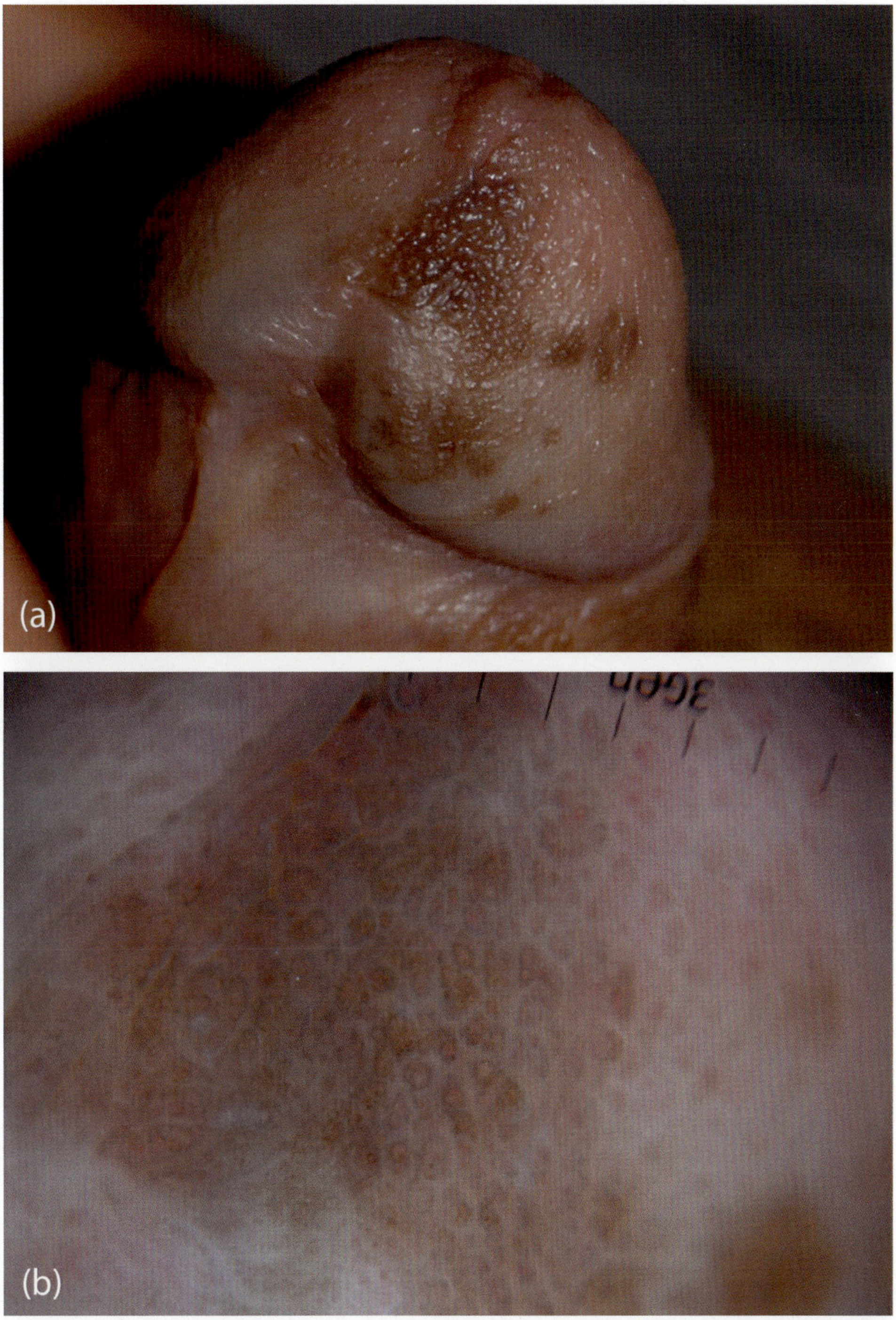

Figure 15.3 (a) Genital melanosis. Brownish, irregular macules of the glans. (b) Dermoscopy (×10) revealing a cobblestone-like pattern.

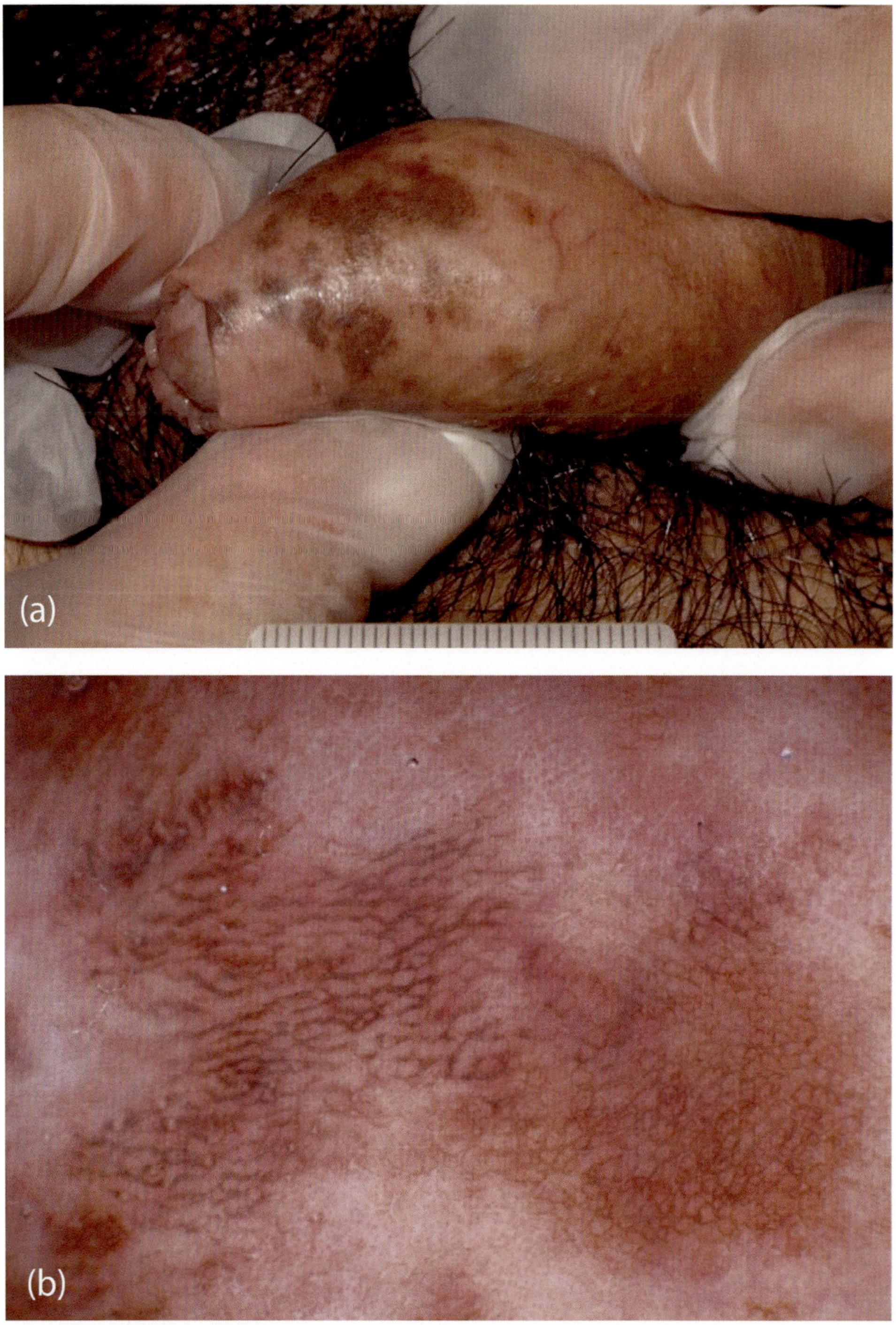

Figure 15.4 (a) Genital melanosis. Multiple brownish patches localized on the penile shaft. (b) Dermoscopy (×10) revealing a reticular-like pattern, with delicate and regular brown network-like structures.

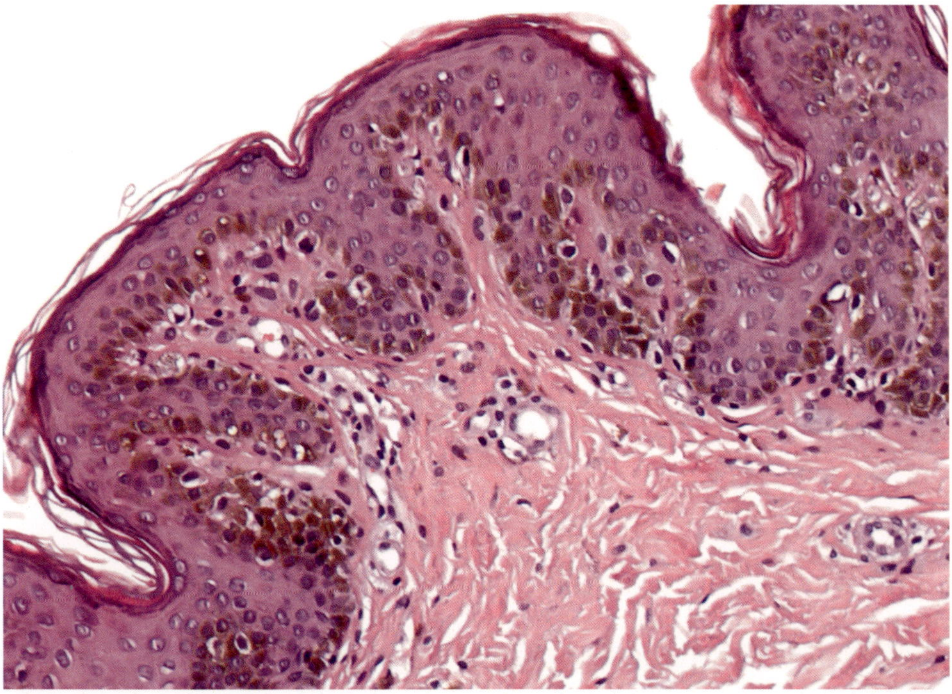

Figure 15.5 Histopathology of melanosis showing increased pigmentation of basal keratinocytes and melanocytes (H&E, ×100).

CHAPTER 16

Dowling-Degos Disease

Maria Rita Nasca MD PhD, Rosario Caltabiano MD, and Francesco Lacarrubba MD

DEFINITION

Dowling-Degos disease (DDD) is a genodermatosis characterized by acquired reticular hyperpigmentation in flexural sites that may associated with other cutaneous manifestations.

EPIDEMIOLOGY

DDD is a rare disorder usually of adult onset, although it may sometimes occur in childhood (1, 2). It has no racial predilection and seems to be more common in women than in men (3). Groin localization is mentioned fairly frequently, but specific involvement of genital involvement is unusual (3–9).

ETIOLOGY

DDD has an autosomal-dominant transmission with variable penetrance, but it can also occur sporadically. Heterogeneous mutations in genes involved in melanosome transfer and epidermal growth, such as the keratin 5 gene (KRT-5), have been implicated (10).

CLINICAL FEATURES

DDD is characterized by the presence of asymptomatic, reticulated macules varying in color from light brown to brown-black [Figures 16.1(a) and 16.2(a)]. They are typically localized on large body folds and flexures (such as axillae, antecubital fossae, neck, submammary region, and groins); however, genitalia, perineum, and perianal area may also be involved (3, 9–11). Other features of DDD include follicular hyperkeratotic papules, comedo-like lesions, pitted scars, and hypopigmentations (6, 7, 9, 12–13). Lesions are usually asymptomatic, although burning or itching may be reported. Onset of skin changes is typically after puberty, especially in the third to fourth decade of life (10), and the degree of pigmentation may increase with age.

DOI: 10.1201/9781003007166-16

DIFFERENTIAL DIAGNOSIS

The differential diagnosis of DDD in the genital area includes other disorders that may cause hyperpigmentation such as melanosis, acanthosis nigricans, seborrheic keratosis, melanoma, bowenoid papulosis and other genodermatoses such as Galli-Galli disease (an acantholytic variant of DDD), reticulate acropigmentation of Kitamura, and Peutz-Jeghers syndrome.

DIAGNOSIS

The diagnosis of DDD is classically based on the clinical presentation and histopathological features. Moreover, a detailed family history may be crucial (14). Genetic consultation may assist in a definitive and accurate diagnosis.

DERMOSCOPY

Dermoscopy of hyperpigmented macules shows the presence of brownish spots or reticular brownish pigmentation sometimes delimiting small, hypopigmented circles [Figures 16.1(b) and 16.2(b)]. A diffuse, light brown background may also be observed (12, 15, 16). Although this pattern is not specific of DDD, it is useful to rule out melanoma (3). In papular lesions, dermoscopy shows a star-like brown pattern on a reddish-brown background. Dermoscopy of hypopigmented lesions reveals an accentuation of the normal reticular pattern around the hypopigmented center (12, 15).

HISTOPATHOLOGICAL CORRELATION

The most notable feature of macular lesions in DDD is a striking filiform elongation of the rete ridges. Hyperpigmentation occurs mainly in the lower third of the rete ridges where it is variable in density but often quite intense (Figure 16.3). The number of melanocytes is not increased. The antler-like branching of rete ridges with basal hyperpigmentation is responsible for the irregular brownish projections at dermoscopy. The star-like brown pattern and the hypopigmented areas histopathologically correspond to follicular plugging and to epidermal atrophy with lack of pigment, respectively (12, 15).

REFERENCES

1. Rice AS, Cook C. Dowling Degos Disease. In: StatPearls [Internet]. Treasure Island, FL: StatPearls Publishing; 2020.
2. Zuo YG, Ho MG, Jin HZ, Wang BX. Case report: a case of newborn onset reticulate pigmented anomaly of the flexures in a Chinese female, J Eur Acad Dermatol Venereol 2008;22(7):901–3.
3. Coco V, Guerriero C, Esposito I, et al. A familial case of Dowling-Degos disease on the vulva. Clin Exp Dermatol 2019;44(8):921–3.
4. O'Goshi K, Terui T, Tagami H. Dowling-Degos disease affecting the vulva. Acta Derm Venereol 2001; 81(2):148.
5. Jafari R, T.M., Vakilzadeh F. Morbus Dowling-Degos in genitoperianal localisation in a mother and a daughter. Aktuelle Dermatologie 2003;29(6):240–2.
6. Massone C, Hofmann-Wellenhof R. Dermoscopy of Dowling-Degos disease of the vulva. Arch Dermatol 2008;144:417–8.

7. Taskapan O, Gokce E, Akin O, et al. Dowling-Degos disease with diffuse penile pigmentation. J Eur Acad Dermatol Venereol 2014;28(10):1405–6.
8. Zarzoso I, Bodet D, García-Patos V. A peculiar inheritance: the patient had a net-like pattern of pigmentation on her vulva and perianal skin. Am J Obstet Gynecol 2013;208(6):506.
9. Horner ME, Parkinson KE, Kaye V, Lynch PJ. Dowling-Degos disease involving the vulva and back: case report and review of the literature. Dermatol Online J 2011;17(7):1.
10. Strausburg M, Linos K, Staser K, Mousdicas N. Dowling-Degos disease co-presenting with Darier disease. Clin Exp Dermatol 2016;41(4):410–2.
11. McSweeney SM, Woolf RT, Calonje E, Lewis F. Just vulval lichen simplex? Clin Exp Dermatol 2020;45(2):232–4.
12. Nirmal B, Dongre AM, Khopkar US. Dermatoscopic features of hyper and hypopigmented lesions of Dowling Degos disease. Indian J Dermatol 2016;61(1):125.
13. Pickup T, Mutasim D. Dowling-Degos disease presenting as hypopigmented macules. J Am Acad Dermatol 2011;64;1224–5.
14. Wong LS, Yang YC. Dowling-Degos disease localized on vulva mimicking condyloma acuminata. Indian J Dermatol 2018;63(6):521–2.
15. Geissler S, Dyall-Smith D, Coras B, et al. Unique brown star shape on dermatoscopy of generalized Dowling-Degos disease. Australas J Dermatol 2011;52(2):151–3.
16. Errichetti E, Stinco G. Dermoscopy in general dermatology: a practical overview. Dermatol Ther (Heidelb) 2016;6(4):471–507.

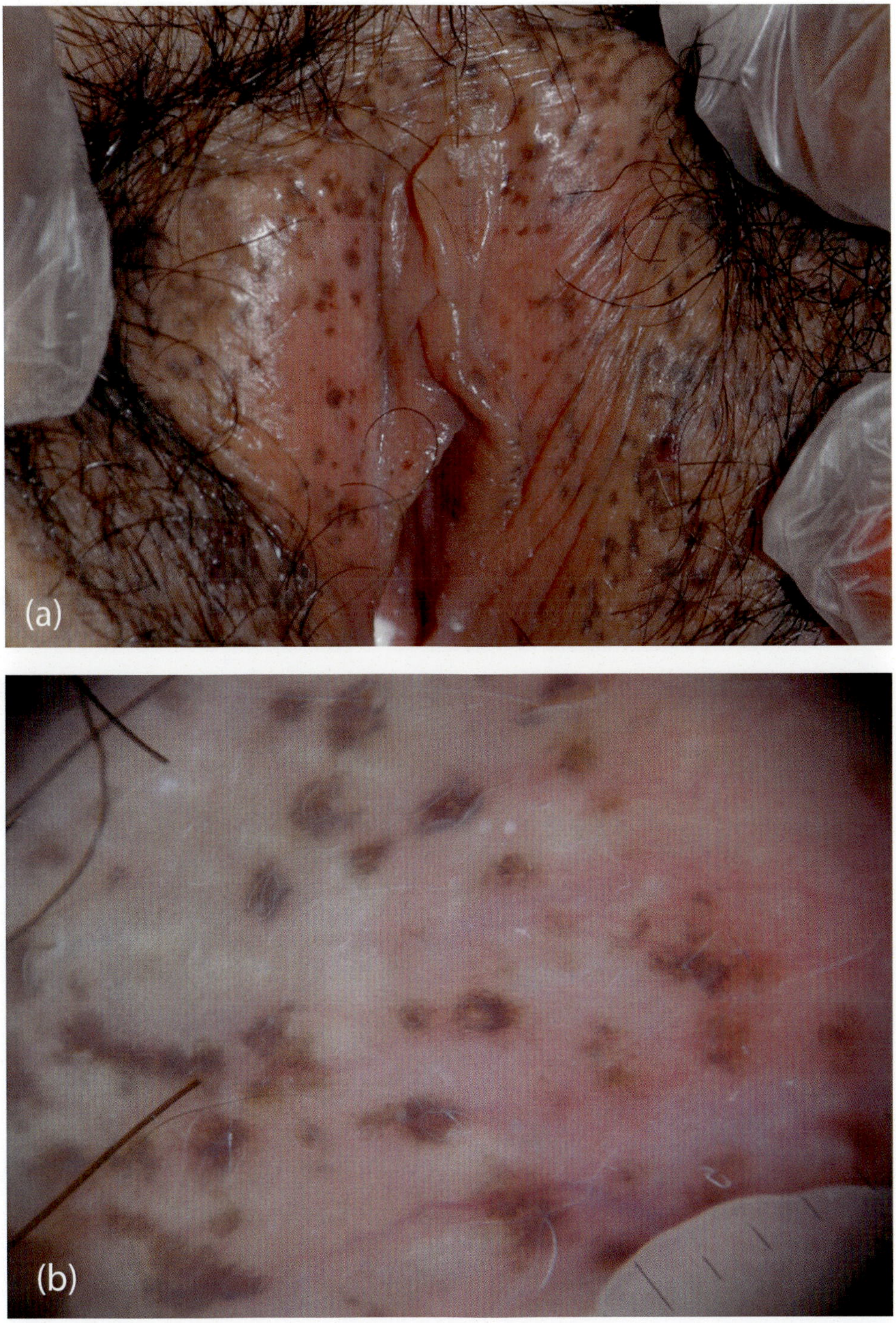

Figure 16.1 (a) Dowling-Degos disease. Multiple, hyperpigmented, macules of the vulva in a 32-year-old woman. (b) Dermoscopy (×10) showing roundish and irregular brownish spots.

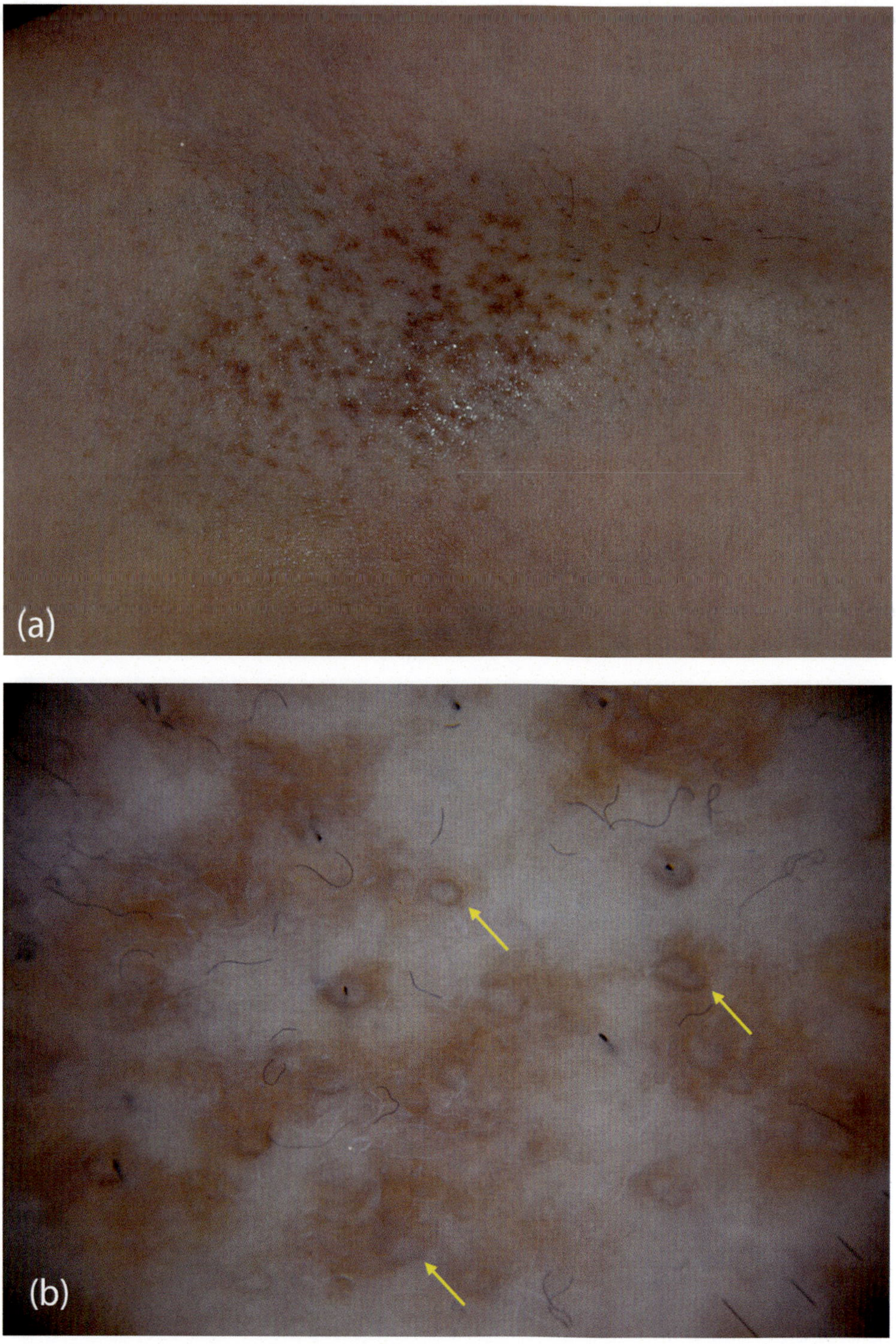

Figure 16.2 (a) Dowling-Degos disease. Multiple, hyperpigmented, reticulated macules of the right axilla in the same patient showed in Figure 16.1(a). (b) Dermoscopy (×10) showing a reticular, brownish pigmentation delimiting small, hypopigmented circles (arrows).

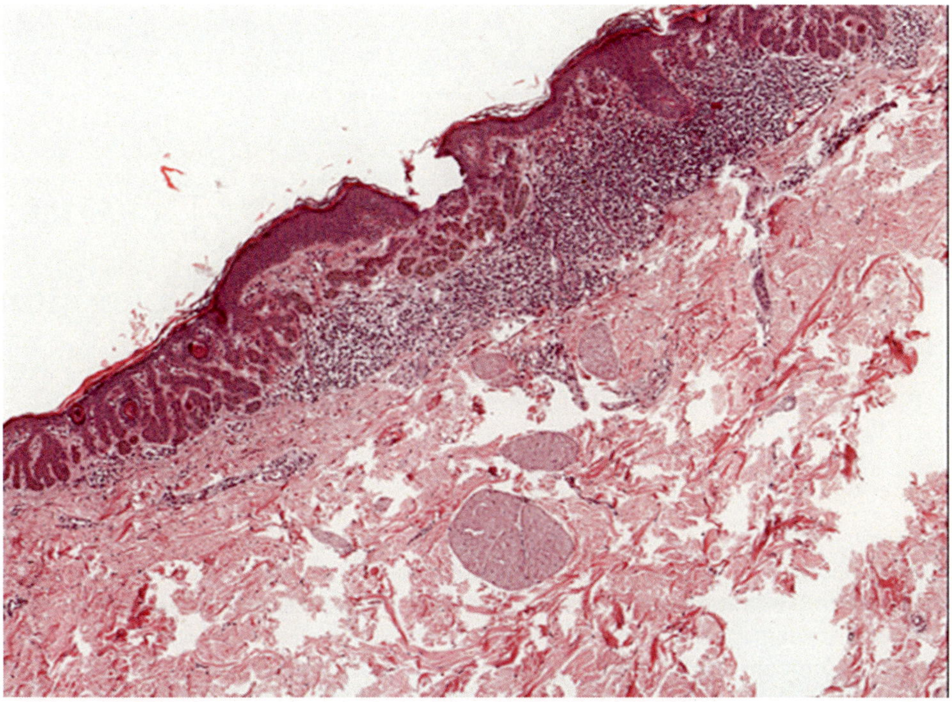

Figure 16.3 Histopathology of a macular lesion in Dowling-Degos disease showing hyperkeratosis with an epidermis of reduced thickness. Thin, filiform, pigmented, interconnecting epithelial strands grow down from the epidermis (H&E, ×100).

CHAPTER 17

Angiokeratoma

Anna Elisa Verzì MD, Livia Liguori MD, and Francesco Lacarrubba MD

DEFINITION

Angiokeratoma is a benign vascular proliferation composed of dilated capillaries in the upper dermis associated with epidermis overgrowth. Five clinical variants are recognized: angiokeratoma corporis diffusum (localized over the trunk and proximal extremities and associated with Fabry's disease), angiokeratoma of Mibelli (usually involving the hands and feet), angiokeratoma of Fordyce (limited to the scrotum and the vulva), angiokeratoma circumscriptum (present at birth in a unilaterally zosteriform shape and later enlarging and warty), and solitary and multiple angiokeratomas (the most common variant, localized on the whole body).

EPIDEMIOLOGY

Angiokeratomas are more frequent in men and affect approximately 0.16% among the general population (1). With regard to the genital area, they are quite common in the scrotum with an incidence increasing with age, whereas they are rare in the vulvar area, where they may be misdiagnosed with other more common benign and malignant lesions (2).

ETIOLOGY

The etiopathogenesis of angiokeratoma is still uncertain. In most cases, it appears spontaneously and without an apparent cause. Trauma, venous hypertension, vascular fragility, inguinal hernia and varicosities have been reported as possible etiopathogenetic factors (3). In females, angiokeratomas may often appear during pregnancy (4). Rarely, they can herald systemic disorders, such as Fabry's disease.

CLINICAL FEATURES

Angiokeratoma presents as an asymptomatic, reddish, roundish papule or nodule ranging in diameter from 2 to 10 mm with a different degree of hyperkeratosis [Figures 17.1(a), 17.2(a), 17.3(a) and 17.4(a)]. Single or multiple lesions may be observed. In case of accidental scratching or trauma, bleeding or change in color to dark purple or black (due to thrombosis) may occur and, in this case, patients may refer pain, discomfort and itch. Angiokeratomas generally occur in males on the scrotum and less often on the penis, in females on the labia majora and rarely on the labia minora or on the clitoris (5).

DOI: 10.1201/9781003007166-17

DIFFERENTIAL DIAGNOSIS

A variety of genital lesions may mimic angiokeratoma. They mainly include benign melanocytic nevi, Spitz-Reed nevi, melanoma, pigmented basal cell carcinoma, seborrheic keratosis, haemorrhagic spots, infectious lesions, such as molluscum contagiosum and viral warts, and other vascular lesions including haemangioma, pyogenic granuloma and Kaposi's sarcoma.

DIAGNOSIS

The diagnosis of angiokeratoma is generally clinical, and histopathological examination is rarely indicated. However, especially when the lesion appears dark purple or black, the diagnosis may be more difficult simulating a pigmented lesion.

DERMOSCOPY

Dermoscopy, that has been reported in both sexes (6–12), typically reveals six main structures: red lacunae (roundish red or red-blue structures corresponding to wide dilated vascular spaces in the upper/mid dermis), dark lacunae (roundish blue to black areas due to thrombosis of the vascular spaces), whitish veil (whitish, "ground-glass" areas), erythema and peripheral erythema (pinkish homogeneous areas) and haemorrhagic crusts (subsequent to trauma) [Figures 17.1(b), 17.2(b), 17.3(b) and 17.4(b)]. Based on the combination of these structures, three main dermoscopic patterns of angiokeratomas have been described: pattern 1 consists of dark lacunae and whitish veil; pattern 2 also includes peripheral erythema; and pattern 3 haemorrhagic crusts (1, 10).

HISTOPATHOLOGICAL CORRELATION

The histopathology of angiokeratoma is characterized by a dilatation of superficial dermal vessels associated with epidermal hyperplasia (Figure 17.5). The well-demarcated red/dark lacunae and the whitish veil seen at dermoscopy correspond to the wide dilated vascular spaces, that may be partially or completely thrombosed, and to hyperkeratosis and acanthosis, respectively.

REFERENCES

1. Zaballos P, Daufí C, Puig S, et al. Dermoscopy of solitary angiokeratomas: a morphological study. Arch Dermatol 2007;143:318–25.
2. Fogagnolo L, Cintra ML, Velho PE. Angiokeratoma of the vulva. An Bras Dermatol 2011;86(2):333–5.
3. Mittal R, Aggarwal A, Srivastava G. Angiokeratoma circumscriptum: a case report and review of the literature. Int J Dermatol 2005;44:1031–4.
4. Cohen PR, Young AW Jr, Tovell HM. Angiokeratoma of the vulva: diagnosis and review of the literature. Obstet Gynecol Surv 1989;44(5):339–46.
5. Imperial R, Helwig EB. Angiokeratoma of the vulva. Obstet Gynecol 1967;29(3):307–12.
6. Ferrari A, Zalaudek I, Argenziano G, et al. Dermoscopy of pigmented lesions of the vulva: a retrospective morphological study. Dermatology 2011;222(2):157–66.
7. Lacarrubba F, Dinotta F, Nasca MR, et al. Localized vascular lesions of the glans in patients with lichen sclerosus diagnosed by dermatoscopy. G Ital Dermatol Venereol 2012;147(5):510–1.
8. Oakley A. Dermatoscopic features of vulval lesions in 97 women. Australas J Dermatol 2016;57(1):48–53.
9. Jha AK, Sonthalia S, Jakhar D. Dermoscopy of angiokeratoma. Indian Dermatol Online J 2018; 9(2):141–2.
10. Micali G, Lacarrubba F. Augmented diagnostic capability using videodermatoscopy on selected infectious and non-infectious penile growths. Int J Dermatol 2011;50:1501–5.
11. Ramot Y, Tetro T, Soteriou L, et al. Solitary angiokeratoma of the vulva mimicking malignant melanoma. Cutis 2018;101(5):e6–e7.
12. Lacarrubba F, Borghi A, Verzì AE, et al. Dermoscopy of genital diseases: a review. J Eur Acad Dermatol 2020;34(10):2198–207.

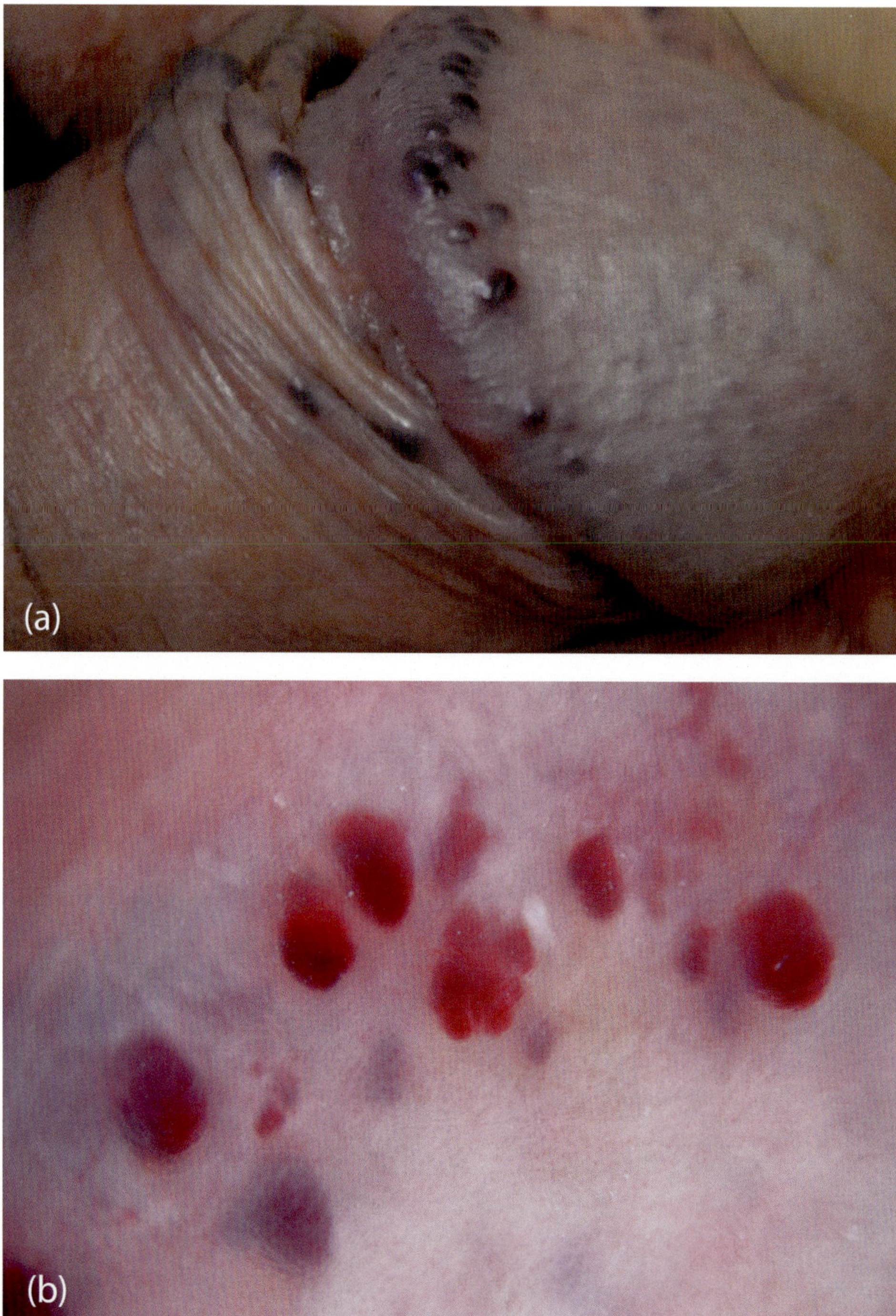

Figure 17.1 (a) Angiokeratomas. Multiple, violaceous, roundish papules involving the glans and the prepuce in a 41-year-old man. The patient complained of occasional bleeding. (b) Dermoscopy (×10) showing red lacunae and whitish veil.

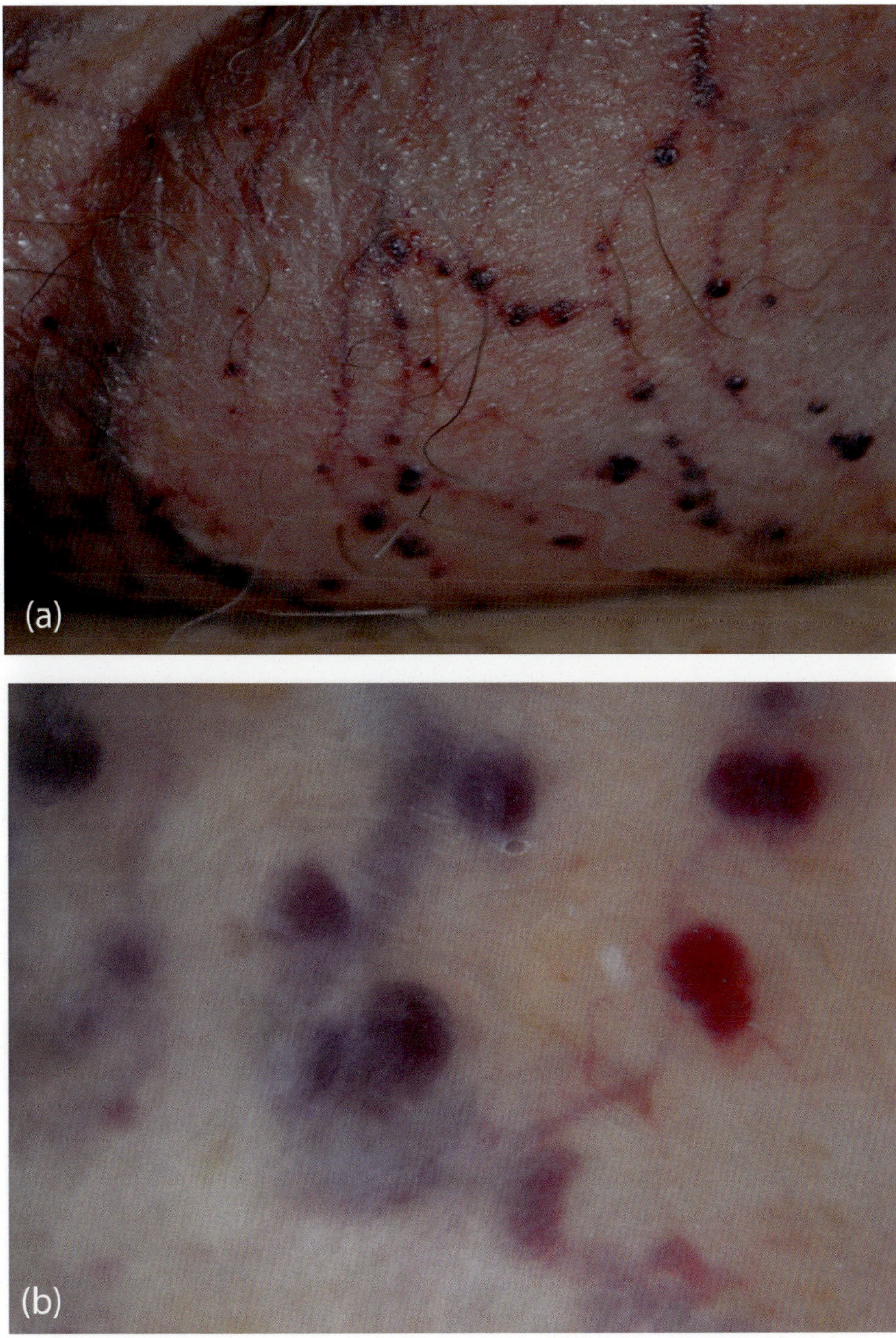

Figure 17.2 (a) Angiokeratomas. Multiple, reddish, roundish papules of the scrotum in a 38-year-old man. (b) Dermoscopy (×10) showing red lacunae, dark lacunae and whitish veil.

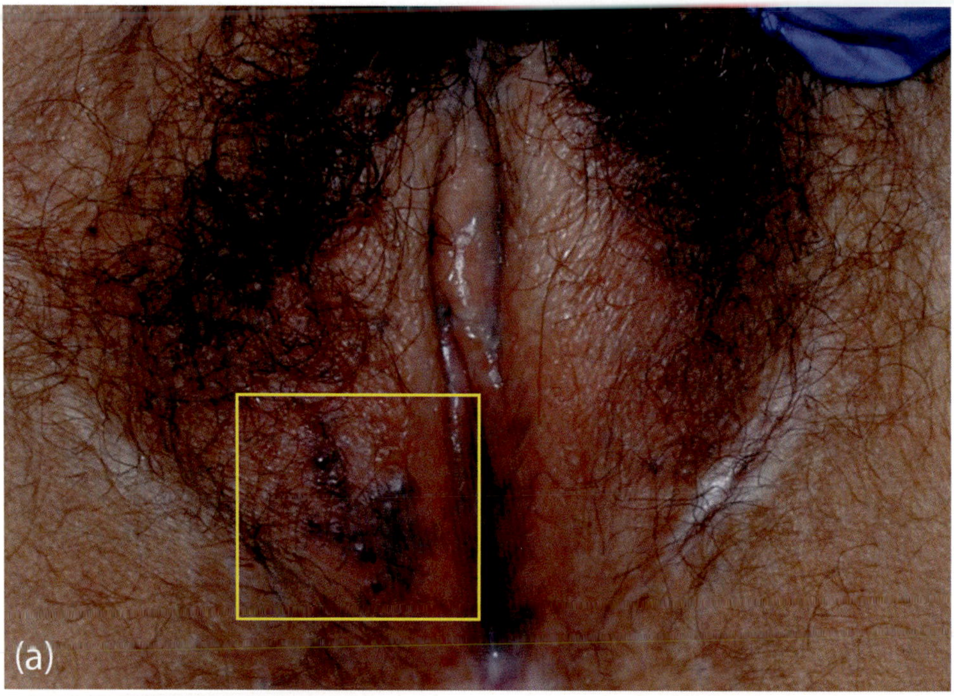

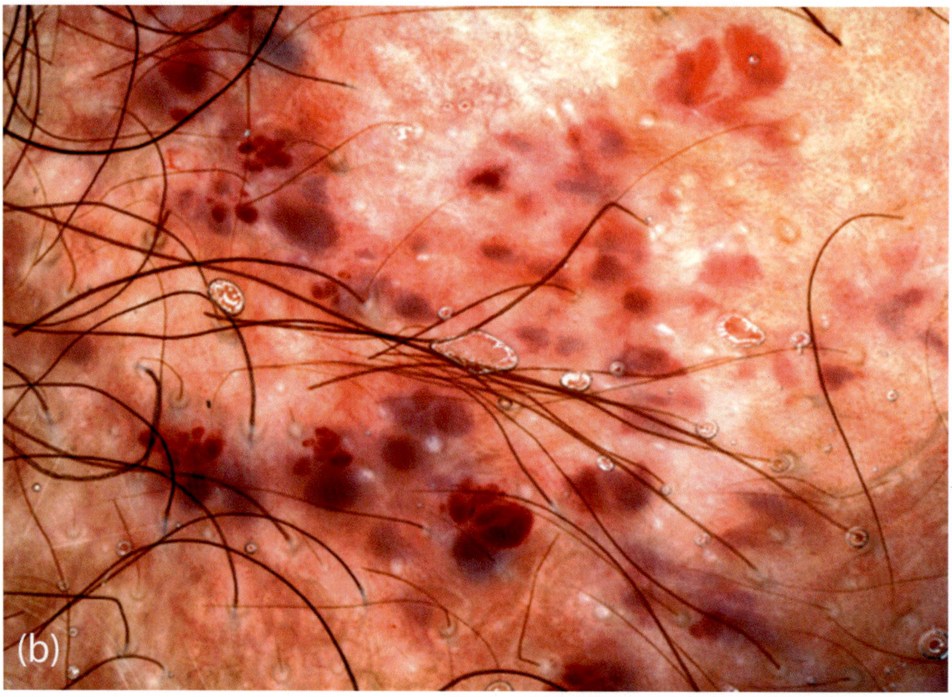

Figure 17.3 (a) Angiokeratomas. Multiple, dark papules of the vulva (square) in a 34-year-old woman. The patient was referred by her GP with a suspicion of melanoma. (b) Dermoscopy (×10) showing red lacunae and dark lacunae.

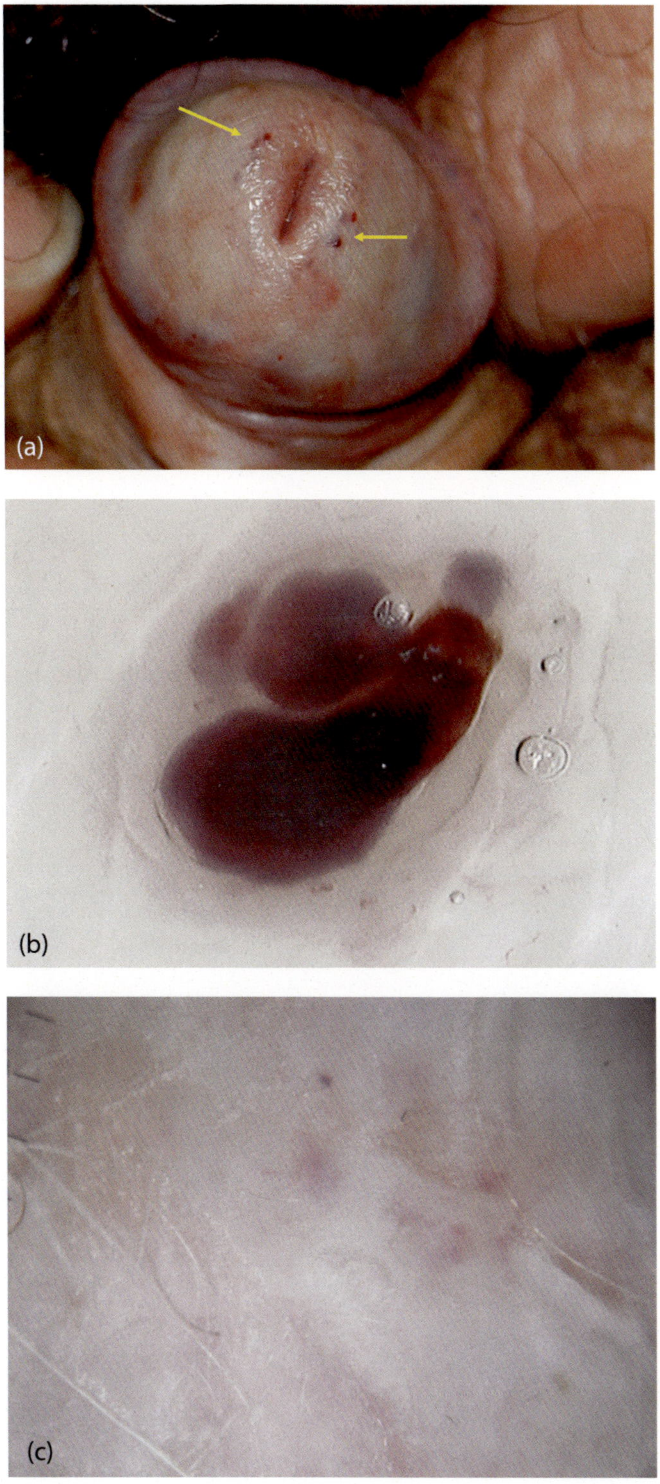

Figure 17.4 (a) Angiokeratomas in an adult patient with typical lichen sclerosus affecting the glans. Small, dark papules that were previously diagnosed as haemorrhagic spots of lichen sclerosus may be seen around the meatus (arrows). (b) Dermoscopy (×20) of an angiokeratoma showing red lacunae and a whitish veil. (c) Dermoscopy (×10) of the glans showing the features of lichen sclerosus (see Chapter 9): whitish structureless areas and red dots and globules corresponding to ecchymosis.

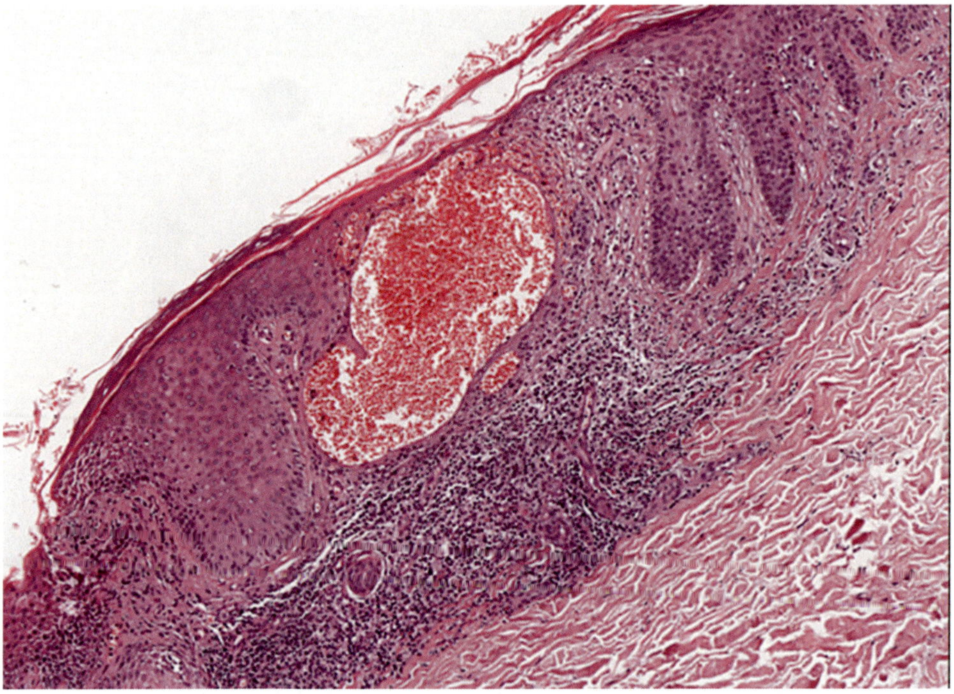

Figure 17.5 Histopathology of angiokeratoma showing dilated superficial vessels (H&E, ×100).

CHAPTER 18

Lymphangioma Circumscriptum

Federica Dall'Oglio MD PhD, Alice Sgrò MD, and Francesco Lacarrubba MD

DEFINITION

The term lymphangioma circumscriptum includes congenital and acquired (also referred as lymphangiectasias) benign cystic dilatations involving the superficial lymphatic vessels (1).

EPIDEMIOLOGY

The incidence of both congenital and acquired forms of lymphangioma circumscriptum in the genital region is low (2, 3). The scrotum and the vulva are the areas more frequently involved (1, 3).

ETIOLOGY

Lymphangioma circumscriptum may be caused by a congenital developmental anomaly of lymphatic vessels that leads to enlargement and sequestration of lymph fluid. Acquired lymphangiectasias of the genitalia result from damage and/or obstruction of previously normal lymphatic vessels of the pelvic area, usually developing as a result of malignancies, Crohn disease, surgery, radiotherapy, hidradenitis suppurativa and/or infections (4, 5).

CLINICAL FEATURES

Lymphangioma circumscriptum of external genitalia generally appears as multiple or clustered, flesh-colored vesicular lesions containing clear lymphatic fluid [Figures 18.1(a) and 18.2(a)]. The surface may be translucent, resembling a gelatinous mass of "frog spawn" over the skin, or verrucous, due to hyperkeratosis, resembling genital warts. Some lesions may turn purple due to the presence of red blood cells. With time, lesions may increase in size (2, 6). Patients may be asymptomatic or, rarely, may present pruritus or pain.

DIFFERENTIAL DIAGNOSIS

Lymphangioma circumscriptum of the genital area may resemble different disorders, such as genital warts, molluscum contagiosum, herpes simplex, and angiokeratoma (7–9).

DOI: 10.1201/9781003007166-18

DIAGNOSIS

The diagnosis of lymphangioma circumscriptum is generally clinical. Dermoscopy and reflectance confocal microscopy may be useful to confirm the clinical suspect and ultrasound for pre-operative evaluation of the margins (10–12). Histopathology examination is rarely necessary to achieve final diagnosis.

DERMOSCOPY

Dermoscopy of lymphangioma circumscriptum is characterized by two patterns: yellow lacunae circumscribed by pale septa, and reddish areas/red lacunae [Figures 18.1(b), 18.2(b), and 18.3] (9, 10, 12). Sometimes, the two aspects may coexist, with the reddish areas below, due to the high density of blood corpuscles, and pale area above, configuring the "hypopyon-like" appearance (10).

HISTOPATHOLOGICAL CORRELATION

The histopathology of lymphangioma circumscriptum is characterized by saccular dilations and ectatic lymphatic vessels lined by a single layer of endothelial cells in the papillary/reticular dermis, and filled with hypocellular fluid (Figure 18.4) (12). These aspects are responsible of the dermoscopic yellow lacunae. The reddish areas/red lacunae observed in some lesions reflect the inclusion of blood cells within the lymphatic vessels (12).

REFERENCES

1. Chang MB, Newman CC, Davis MD, Lehman JS. Acquired lymphangiectasia (lymphangioma circumscriptum) of the vulva: clinicopathologic study of 11 patients from a single institution and 67 from the literature. Int J Dermatol 2016;55(9):e482–7.
2. Adikari S, Philippidou M, Samuel M. A rare case of acquired lymphangioma circumscriptum of the penis. Int J STD AIDS 2017;28(2):205–7.
3. Kurude AA, Phiske MM, Kolekar KK, Nayak CS. Lymphangiomas: rare presentations in oral cavity and scrotum in pediatric age group. Indian J Dermatol Venereol Leprol 2020;86(2):230.
4. Yoon G, Kim HS, Lee YY, et al. Clinical outcomes of primary surgical treatment for acquired vulvar lymphangioma circumscriptum. Arch Gynecol Obstet 2016;293(1):157–62.
5. Piernick DM 2nd, Mahmood SH, Daveluy S. Acquired lymphangioma circumscriptum of the genitals in an individual with chronic hidradenitis suppurativa. JAAD Case Rep 2017;4(1):64–6.
6. Vatopoulou A, Anagnostopoulos A, Sujeewa F. Congenital lymphangioma circumscriptum of the vulva. J Obstet Gynaecol Res 2019;45(10):2137–8.
7. Sharma C, Bhardwaj A, Khanuja E, Singh G. Congenital vulvar lymphangioma mimicking genital wart – a rare case. J Obstet Gynaecol 2016;36(4):522–3.
8. Bonini J, Ducharme O, Ponroy B, et al. Acquired lymphangioma circumscriptum of the penis treated by electrocoagulation. Case Rep Dermatol 2019;11(3):260–3.
9. Massa AF, Menezes N, Baptista A, et al. Cutaneous lymphangioma circumscriptum – dermoscopic features. An Bras Dermatol 2015;90(2):262–4.
10. Jha AK, Lallas A, Sonthalia S. Dermoscopy of cutaneous lymphangioma circumscriptum. Dermatol Pract Concept 2017;7(2):37–8.
11. Sun Y, Su J, Li SS, Cui LG. The possible role of color Doppler and pulse wave Doppler ultrasound in the diagnosis of cutaneous lymphangioma circumscriptum. J Craniofac Surg 2020;31(1):e73–5.
12. Verzì AE, Lacarrubba F, Tedeschi A, Micali G. Localized acquired lymphangiectasias after breast surgery: enhanced non-invasive diagnosis using dermoscopy and reflectance confocal microscopy. Skin Res Technol 2020;26(2):205–8.

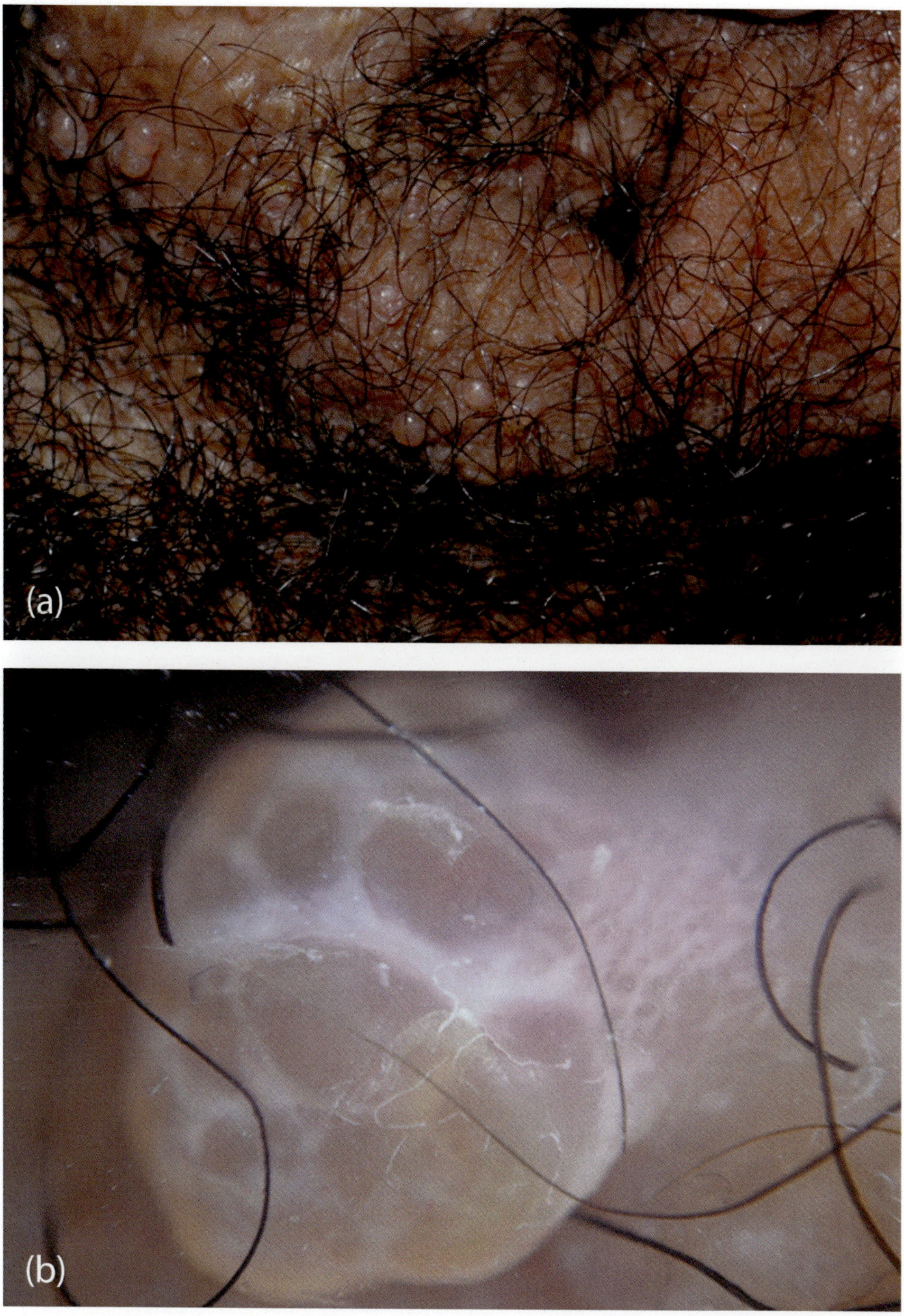

Figure 18.1 (a) Lymphangioma circumscriptum. Multiple, flesh-colored, translucent lesions of the scrotum in a 39-year-old man. Several lesions were previously treated as genital warts. (b) Dermoscopy (×10) showing yellow lacunae, reflecting the presence of lymphatic fluid, circumscribed by pale septa.

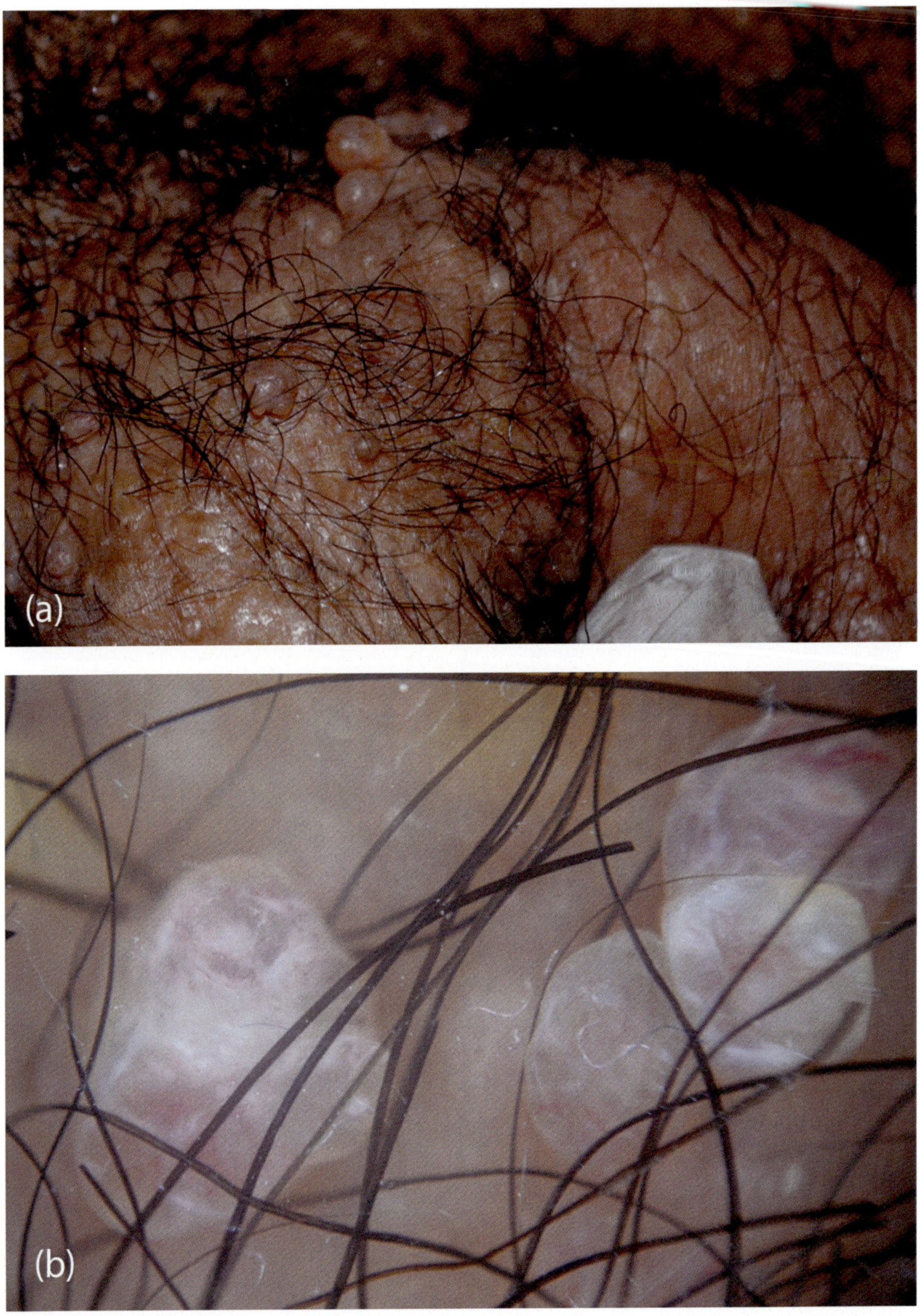

Figure 18.2 (a) Lymphangioma circumscriptum. Multiple, flesh-colored vesicular lesions of the scrotum. (b) Dermoscopy (×10) showing yellow lacunae circumscribed by pale septa.

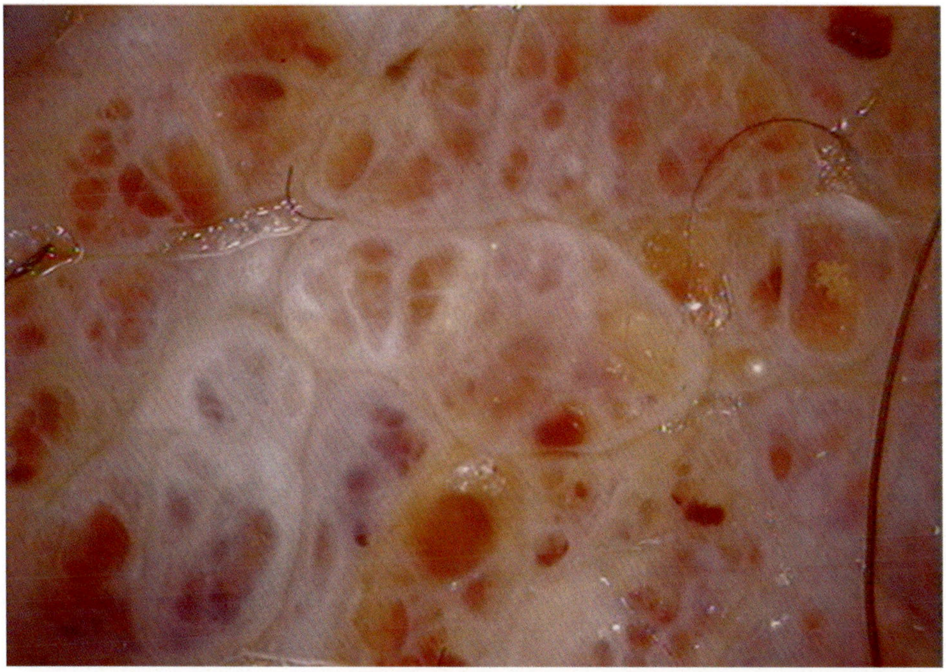

Figure 18.3 Lymphangioma circumscriptum. Dermoscopy (×10) showing yellow and reddish lacunae circumscribed by pale septa. The reddish lacunae reflect the inclusion of blood cells within the lymphatic vessels.

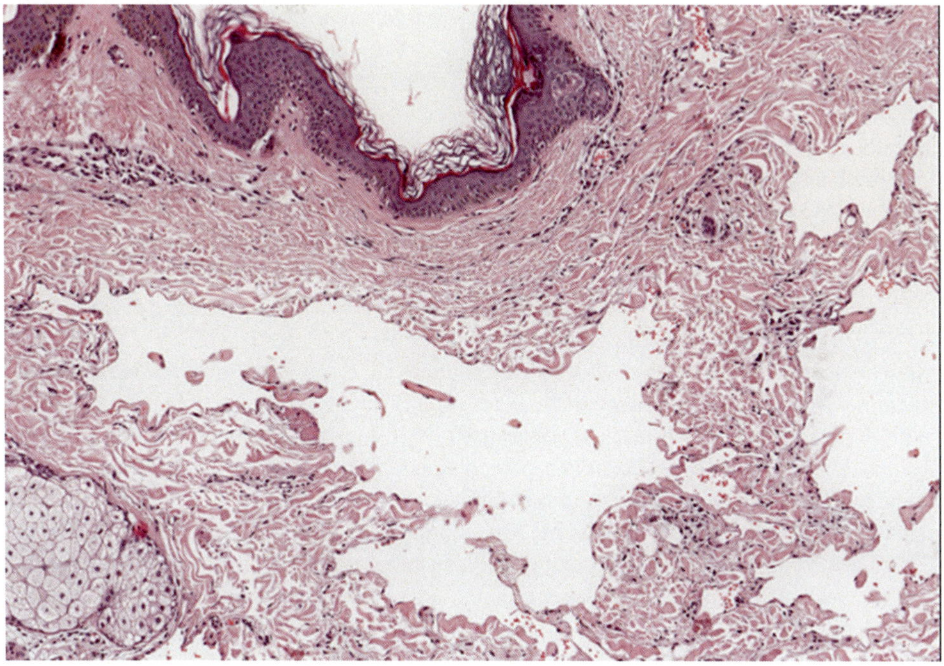

Figure 18.4 Histopathology of lymphangioma circumscriptum. showing thin-walled lymphatic channels in the reticular and papillary dermis (H&E, ×100).

CHAPTER 19

Melanocytic Nevi

Giuseppe Stinco MD, Aimilios Lallas MD, and Enzo Errichetti MD

DEFINITION

Genital melanocytic nevi are benign proliferations of melanocytes, which clinically appear as pink-tan to dark brown flat or elevated skin lesions. According to their age of onset, they are divided into congenital (presenting at the birth or within the first 2 years) and acquired nevi.

EPIDEMIOLOGY

The number of nevi increases with age reaching the maximum peak between 30 and 40 years. The prevalence of genital nevi among adult patients is about 3.5%, with an equivalent sex ratio.

ETIOLOGY

Nevus cells are a form of melanocyte that lack dendritic processes, with a tendency to aggregate into groups of cells. A complex interplay between genetic and environmental factors appears to play a key role in nevogenesis.

CLINICAL FEATURES

Common melanocytic nevi present as single, round/oval, symmetric/uniform macules, or flat-topped/dome-shaped papules with regular borders usually having a diameter of less than 1 cm; color ranges from pink to dark brown-black or, more rarely, blue [Figures 19.1(a), 19.2(a), and 19.3(a)] (1, 2).

Dysplastic nevi occur occasionally in genital area and manifest as irregular or asymmetric, flat macules of more than 5 mm in diameter having variable and indistinct borders and irregular pigmentation. A small subset of benign nevi named atypical melanocytic nevi of the genital type (AMNGT) occurs in young women or, more rarely, on male genitalia; they may have alarming clinical features, such as large size, irregular shape, and dark color (1, 2).

Genital nevi in females are more commonly located on the vulva (labia majora, minora, and clitoris), although they can also occur less frequently in the perineum and mons pubis. In males, they are usually located on the penis and scrotum. AMNGT are frequently located on the labia minora and have an equal distribution between mucosal surfaces and hair-bearing skin of

DOI: 10.1201/9781003007166-19

the external genitalia. In children younger than 10 years, AMNGT has a strong predilection for mucosal sites.

DIFFERENTIAL DIAGNOSIS

Macular or flat-topped nevi can be indistinguishable from flat pigmented warts and simple lentigines. A dome-shaped nevus can be confused with an angiokeratoma that is purple at closer examination. It is important to distinguish AMNGT from melanoma.

DIAGNOSIS

Melanocytic lesions of the genital area are usually diagnosed according to clinical findings and dermoscopy may help recognize them (3–8). Reflectance confocal microscopy has been reported to provide further information regarding the tissue and cell morphology. Nevi that appear atypical in any way require biopsy.

DERMOSCOPY

Genital melanocytic nevi generally exhibit dermoscopy features similar to nevi located on other parts of the body (3–8). Most genital naevi have a single dermoscopic pattern or two patterns Figures 19.1(b) 19.2(b), 19.3(b) and (c), although some lesions may display a multicomponent pattern. Both congenital and acquired nevi generally present a homogeneous brownish structureless or a globular pattern, yet a parallel pattern, homogeneous brown-gray pigmentation, a cobblestone pattern, and nonspecific patterns have also been described, with the last three presentations being seen more commonly in congenital lesions. A clear network-like pattern is found less commonly in genital areas due to a flatter epidermal-dermal junction (especially on mucosal surfaces). AMNGT usually show an atypical brown to black network and some irregular streaks or blotches at the periphery; mixed patterns (e.g., parallel lines together with a homogeneous brown-gray pigmentation or globules) have also been observed.

HISTOPATHOLOGICAL CORRELATION

The majority of common nevi located on genital areas has no peculiar histological characteristics. A benign nevus exhibits clusters of melanocytes in the basal layer of the epidermis, in the dermis, or both of them (Figures 19.4 and 19.5). More uncommon variants, mainly including dysplastic, blue, and Spitz nevi, have also rarely been reported. Dysplastic nevi show elongation and bridging of the rete ridges with nests of nevus cells, upper dermal lamellar fibrosis, variable chronic inflammatory infiltrate, and variable degrees of cellular atypia. AMNGT are proliferations of melanocytes that may have alarming histopathologic findings, such as cytologic atypia (melanocytes with larger and pleomorphic nuclei, sometimes with prominent nucleoli), skin adnexal involvement, growth as single cells with focal pagetoid spread, dense fibrosis in the papillary dermis, and inflammation. Globules on dermoscopy represent nests of melanin-containing nevus cells within the dermis or dermo-epidermal junction and a globular pattern corresponds to compound and intradermal nevi, while a pigmented network is related to melanin at the dermal-epidermal junction.

The asymmetry of colors and structures and the mixed globular-structureless pattern of AMNGT correspond to nests of atypical melanocytes that are spread unevenly along the rete ridges of the epidermis, focal pagetoid spread and fibrosis of the papillary dermis.

REFERENCES

1. Ribe A. Melanocytic lesions of the genital area with attention given to atypical genital nevi. J Cutan Pathol 2008;35:24–7.
2. Gleason BC, Hirsch MS, Nucci MR, et al. Atypical genital nevi. A clinicopathologic analysis of 56 cases. Am J Surg Pathol 2008;32:51–7.
3. Virgili A, Zampino MR, Marzola A, Corazza M. Vulvar melanocytic nevi: a dermoscopic investigation. Dermatology 2010;221:55–62.
4. Ronger-Savle S, Julien V, Duru G, et al. Features of pigmented vulval lesions on dermoscopy. Br J Dermatol 2011;164:54–61.
5. Hunt RD, Orlow SJ, Schaffer JV. Genital melanocytic nevi in children: experience in a pediatric dermatology practice. J Am Acad Dermatol 2014;70:429–34.
6. Murzaku EC, Penn LA, Hale CS, et al. Vulvar nevi, melanosis, and melanoma: an epidemiologic, clinical, and histopathologic review. J Am Acad Dermatol 2014;71:1241–9.
7. Cengiz FP, Emiroglu N, Wellenhof RH. Dermoscopic and clinical features of pigmented skin lesions of the genital area. An Bras Dermatol 2015;90:178–83.
8. Oakley A. Dermatoscopic features of vulval lesions in 97 women. Australas J Dermatol 2016;57:48–53.

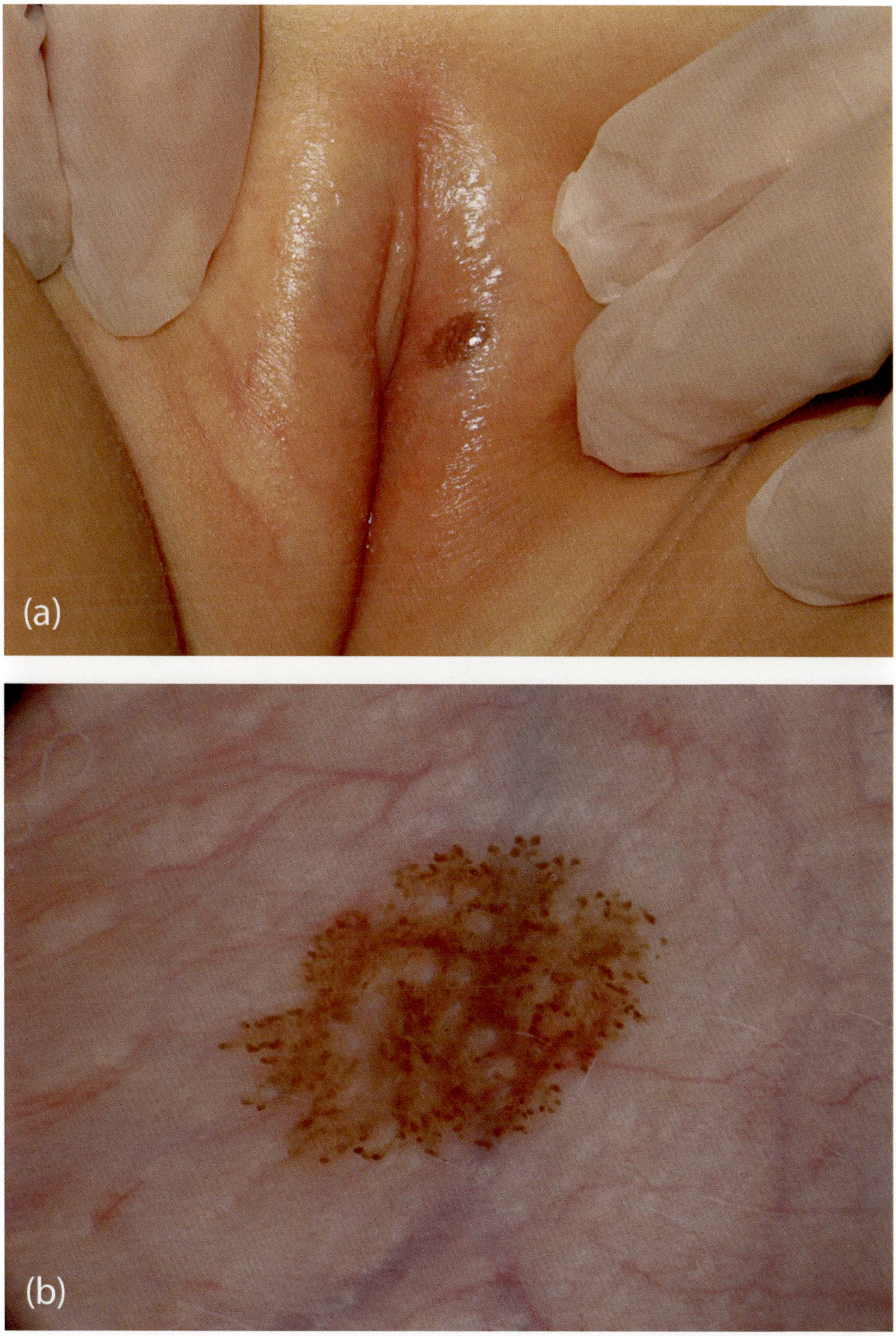

Figure 19.1 (a) Acquired melanocytic nevus of the vulva in a young girl. (b) Dermoscopy (×10) showing a globular pattern with a peripheral homogeneous rim of globules, which is a sign of nevus growth.

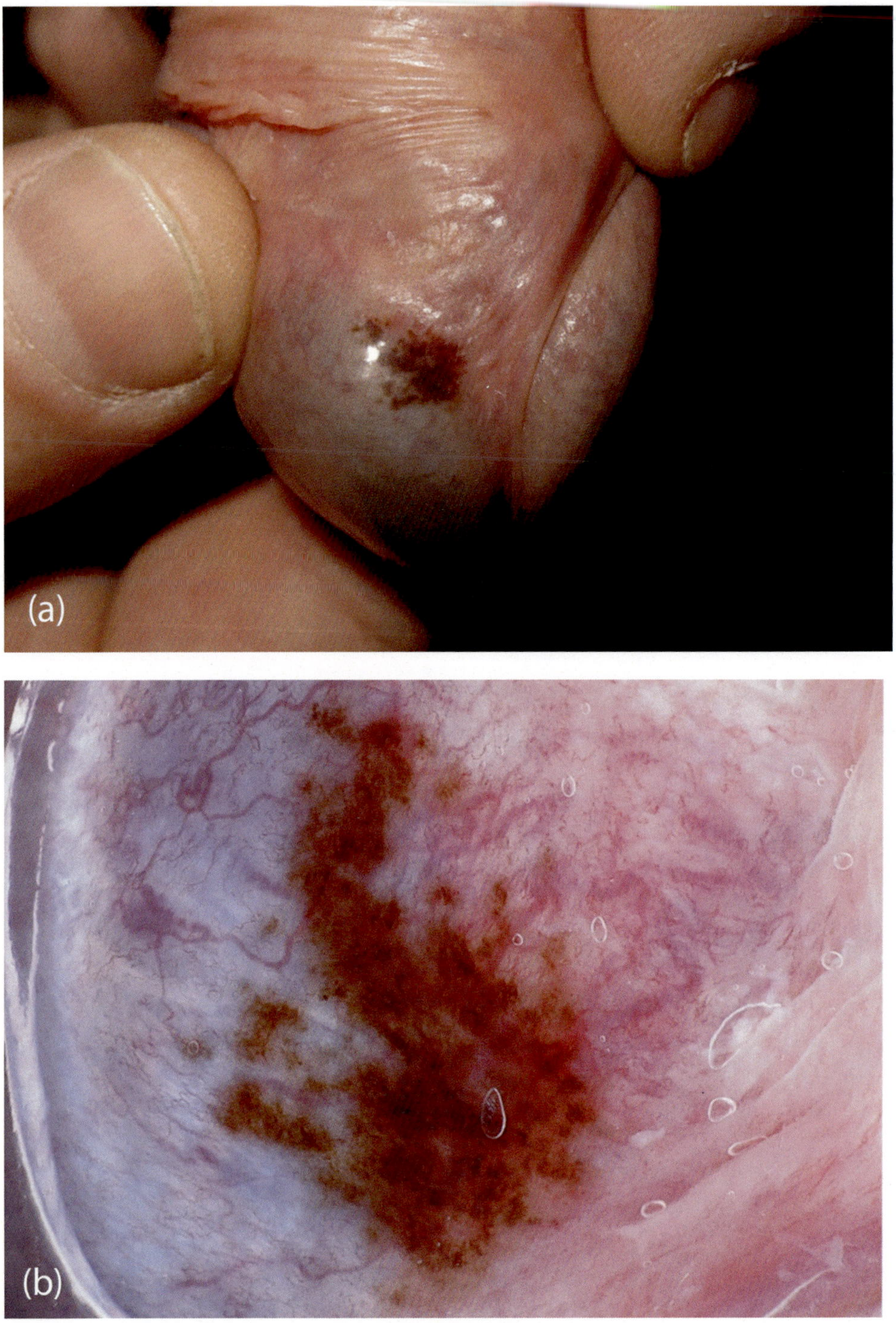

Figure 19.2 (a) Acquired melanocytic nevus of the glans. (b) Dermoscopy (×10) revealing multifocal brown structureless areas with sparse regular brown dots.

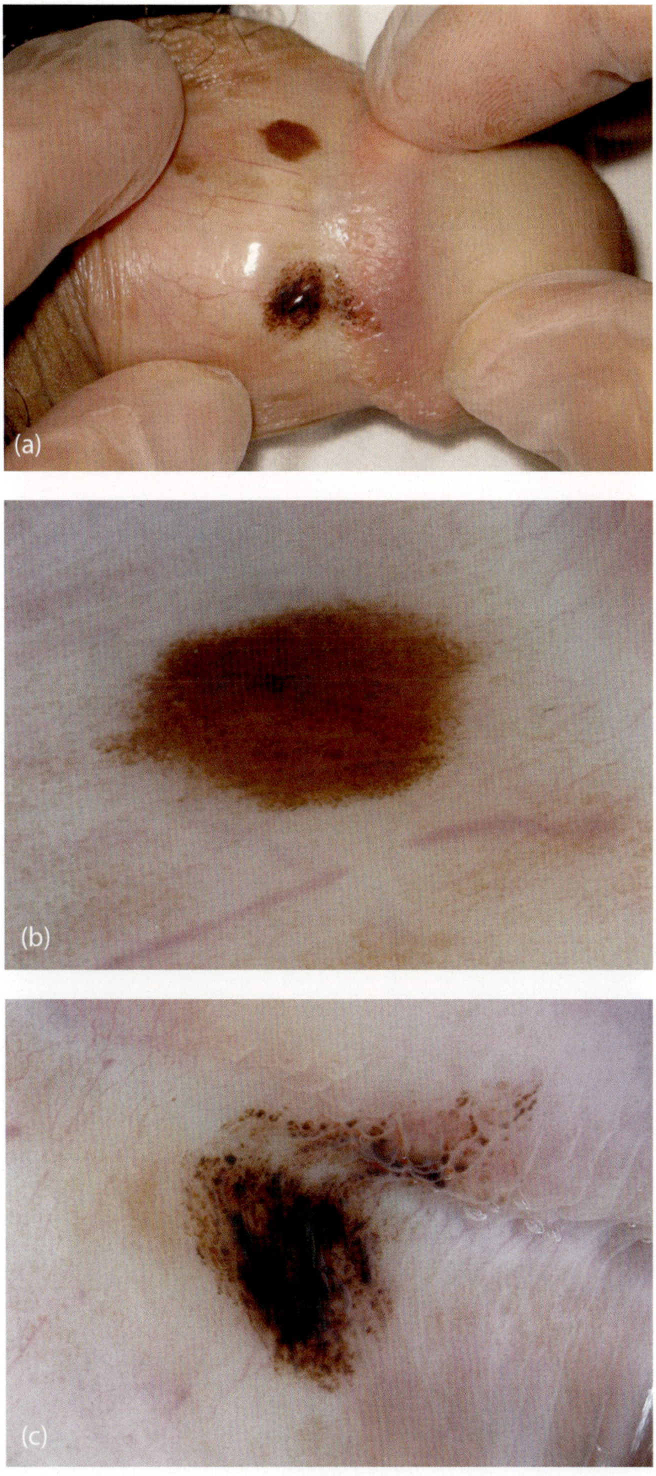

Figure 19.3 (a) Multiple melanocytic nevi of the penis. (b) Dermoscopy (×10) of the light brown lesion displaying regular brownish dots over a homogeneous brown background. (c) Dermoscopy (×10) of the darker lesion characterized by a globular pattern with regular brown and bluish globules.

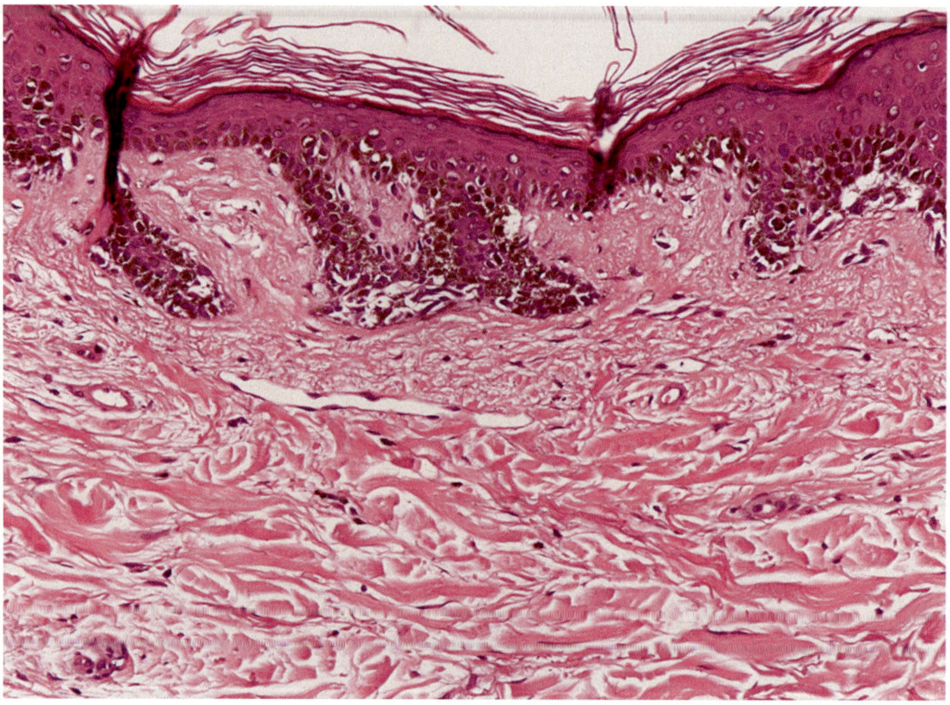

Figure 19.4 Histopathology of junctional nevus showing lentiginous and nested melanocytes. Nested melanocytes are large and fused between rete ridges (H&E, ×100).

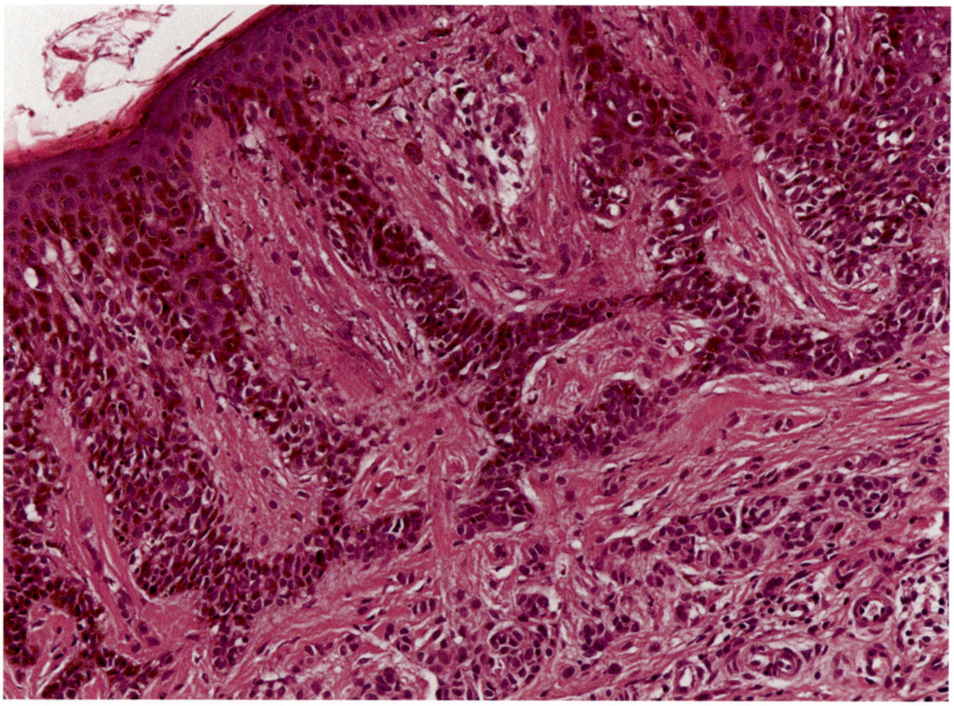

Figure 19.5 Histopathology of compound nevus showing dermal component composed of nevus cells which mature with depth (H&E, ×100).

CHAPTER 20

Seborrheic Keratosis

Giuseppe Stinco MD, Aimilios Lallas MD, and Enzo Errichetti MD

DEFINITION

Seborrheic keratosis (SK), also known as seborrheic wart, senile wart or basal cell papilloma, is the most common benign epidermal tumor of middle-aged or elderly people (1). It may arise anywhere on the skin, with the exception of the palms or soles and mucous membranes, and rarely occurs in the genital region (2–4).

EPIDEMIOLOGY

SK located on genital skin is relatively uncommon (about 2% of pigmented genital lesions) and seems to occur in a younger age group compared to classical localization. SK is observed worldwide across all racial and ethnic groups.

ETIOLOGY

The etiopathology of SK is still not completely understood, although a follicular origin has been proposed. Epidermal growth factor and/or its receptors have been implicated in the development of this type of lesion. Additionally, sun exposure, skin phenotype I and II, and a genetic predisposition with an autosomal dominant mode of inheritance have been considered risk factors in its development. It has also been suggested that the human papillomavirus (HPV) could play a role in the pathogenesis of SK, particularly of the genital region, but the causal relationship is controversial.

CLINICAL FEATURES

SKs of the genital area typically occur on the keratinized skin. In early developmental stages, SKs usually present as one or more well-demarcated, oval or round, skin-colored/brown/gray, flat macules, which then evolve into flat-topped, papules and plaques or polypoidal lesions (1–4). The surface often features a keratotic/verrucous or papillomatous appearance [Figures 20.1(a), 20.2(a), 20.3(a), 20.4(a), and 20.5(a)]. Very dark variants are also seen. They are usually asymptomatic, but itchiness may be present, especially in traumatized lesions.

DOI: 10.1201/9781003007166-20

DIFFERENTIAL DIAGNOSIS

SKs in the genital area are not uncommonly mistaken for human papillomavirus-associated lesions, but the clinical differential diagnosis of SK also includes malignant melanoma, melanocytic nevus, verruca vulgaris, acrochordons, epidermal nevus, actinic keratoses, extramammary Paget's disease, pigmented Bowen's disease, pigmented basal cell carcinomas, and squamous cell carcinomas.

DIAGNOSIS

SKs are usually recognized on clinical grounds according to their morphology, even though diagnosis may sometimes be challenging when classical clinical features are missing, especially on genitalia. In such cases, dermoscopy may help in supporting the diagnosis by showing peculiar findings (5–8). Reflectance confocal microscopy (RCM) has also been applied for non-invasive evaluation of SK, but, up to now, there is no data on RCM findings of genital SK. Histopathology is useful in doubtful cases.

DERMOSCOPY

The dermoscopic hallmarks of SK are often absent on genitalia due to the friction and maceration typical of this region. In fact, comedo-like openings are typically not seen in the vulvar area, while milia-like cysts are usually not affected by friction and maceration. The most common dermoscopic features of genital SKs include thick curved parallel fissures and ridges, irregularly distributed white, yellow and orange clods, and looped blood vessels [Figures 20.1(b), 20.2(b), 20.3(b), and 20.5(b)] (5–8). Milia-like cysts manifest as round, well-circumscribed, white to yellowish opalescent structures, while comedo-like openings, when present, appear as well-circumscribed round to oval craters of variable size with a dark brown, gray, or black color. Fissures and ridges present as thick linear, curvilinear, branched, or oval/circular lines whose colors vary from hypopigmented to brown, black, and blue. When spread throughout the lesion, such a finding gives rise to a brain-like or cerebriform appearance. Hairpin vessels or looped vessels present as two parallel linear vessels forming a half-looped or hairpin-like structure and are often surrounded by a whitish halo. In repeatedly traumatized SKs, the overlying hyperkeratosis often covers the underlying dermoscopic clues [Figure 20.4(b)], thus making their recognition more difficult.

HISTOPATHOLOGICAL CORRELATION

Histopatologically, SKs show variable degrees of acanthosis, pigmentation, horn cysts formation, hyperkeratosis, and papillomatosis. Invaginations of the horny layer form the characteristic cyst pockets or "horny pseudocysts" (Figure 20.6). Melanocyte proliferation and hyperpigmentation is quite common. Several different histological subtypes of SK have been described, i.e., acanthotic, adenoid, hyperkeratotic, clonal, irritated, and melanoacanthoma. Overlapping features are quite common. Morphological variants of SK involving genital area mainly include acanthotic or hyperkeratotic. The histopathologic counterpart of comedo-like opening consists of keratin-filled cysts in the epidermis that are opened to the surface of the lesion, milia-like cysts correspond to small intraepidermal horn cysts, and fissures/ridges correspond to the variation in epidermal surface height (papillomatosis). Finally, hairpin vessels are related to enlarged capillaries with a change in dermal papilla orientation.

REFERENCES

1. Hafner C, Vogt T. Seborrheic keratosis. J Dtsch Dermatol Ges 2008;6:664–77.
2. De Giorgi V, Massi D, Salvini C, et al. Pigmented seborrheic keratoses of the vulva clinically mimicking a malignant melanoma: a clinical, dermoscopic-pathologic case study. Clin Exp Dermatol 2005; 30:17–9.
3. Shenoy MM, Teerthanath S, Bhagavan KR. Genital and perianal melanoacanthomas. Indian J Dermatol 2007;52:109–10.
4. Livaoglu M, Karacal N, Gücer H, Arvas L. Giant genital seborrheic keratosis. Dermatol Surg 2007; 33:1357–8.
5. Grazzini M, Gori A, Rossari S, et al. Seborrheic keratosis of the vulva clinically mimicking a genital wart: a case study. Int J Dermatol 2013;52:1156–7.
6. Braun RP, Ludwig S, Marghoob AA. Differential diagnosis of seborrheic keratosis: clinical and dermoscopic features. J Drugs Dermatol 2017,16:835–842.
7. Minagawa A. Dermoscopy–pathology relationship in seborrheic keratosis. J Dermatol 2017;44:518–24.
8. Salim S, Bouhelab J, Benzekri A, Hassam B. Seborrheic keratoses of the penis: about a rare case. J Dermatol Res Ther 2018,4:062.

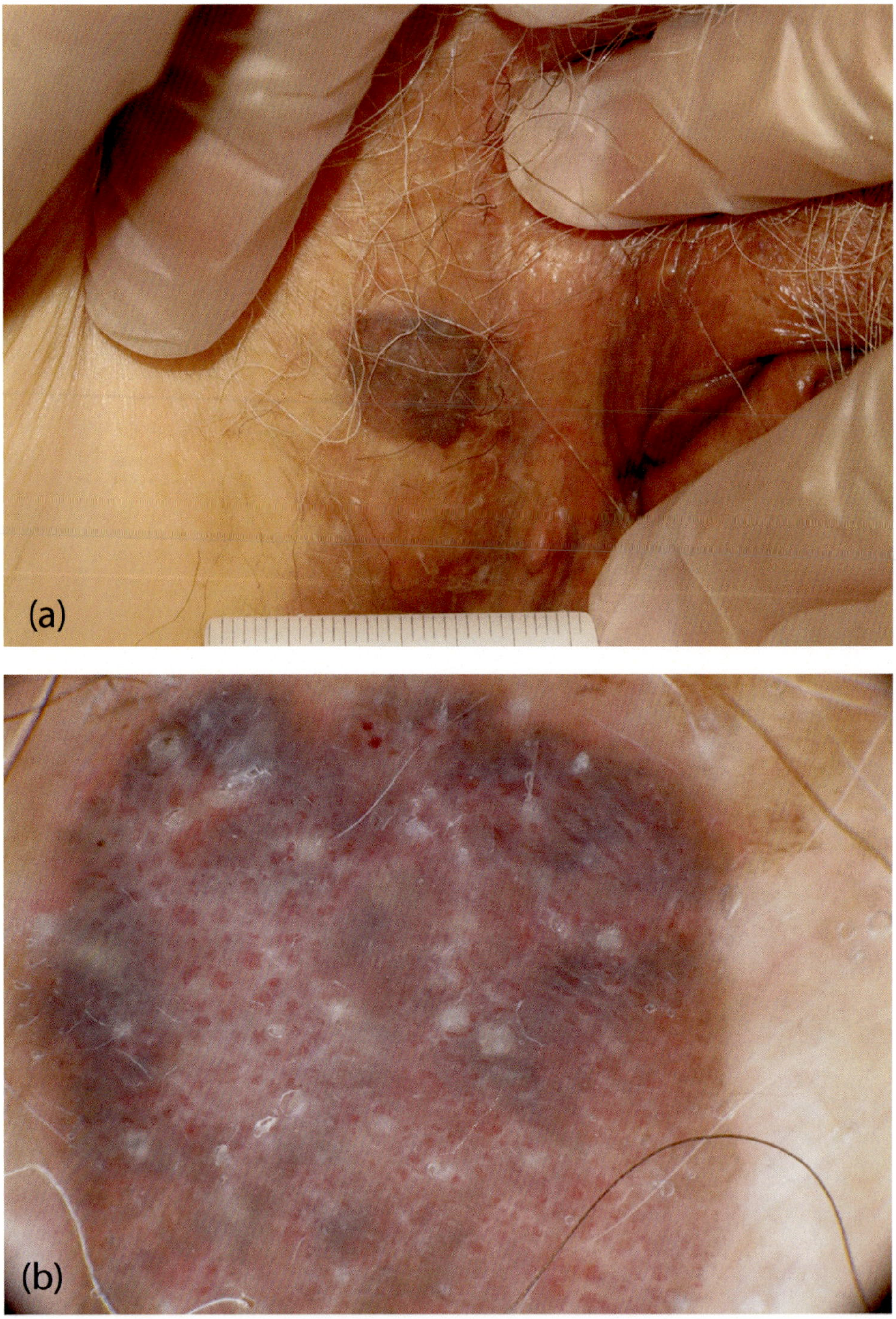

Figure 20.1 (a) Seborrheic keratosis. Brown, roundish lesion on the right labium majus. (b) Dermoscopy (×10) showing hairpin and convoluted vessels having a white halo, along with several milia-like cysts.

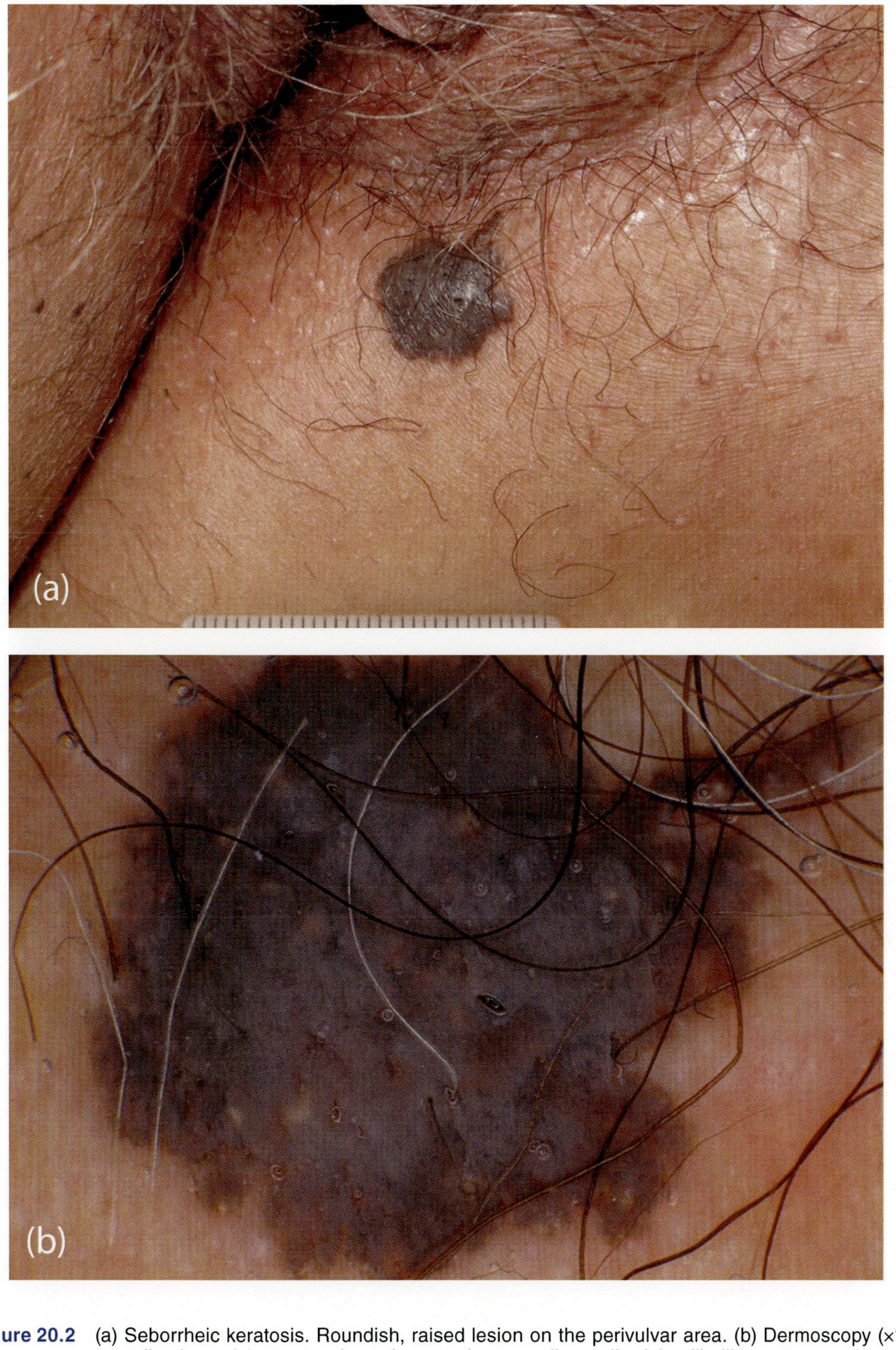

Figure 20.2 (a) Seborrheic keratosis. Roundish, raised lesion on the perivulvar area. (b) Dermoscopy (×10) revealing brownish structureless pigmentation as well as yellowish milia-like cysts.

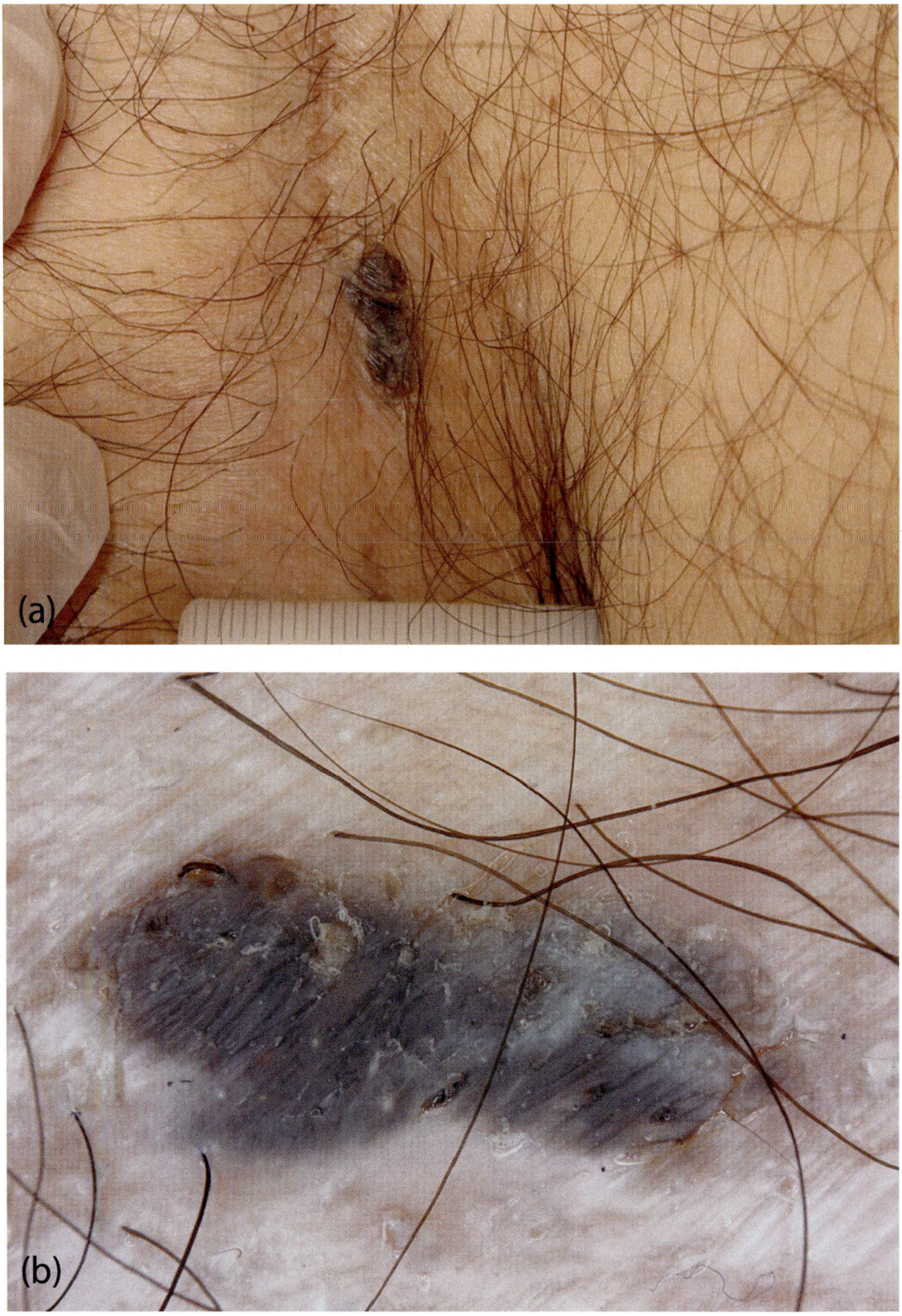

Figure 20.3 (a) Seborrheic keratosis. Elongated, grayish lesion on the inguinal crease. (b) Dermoscopy (×10) displaying milia-like cysts over a dark background.

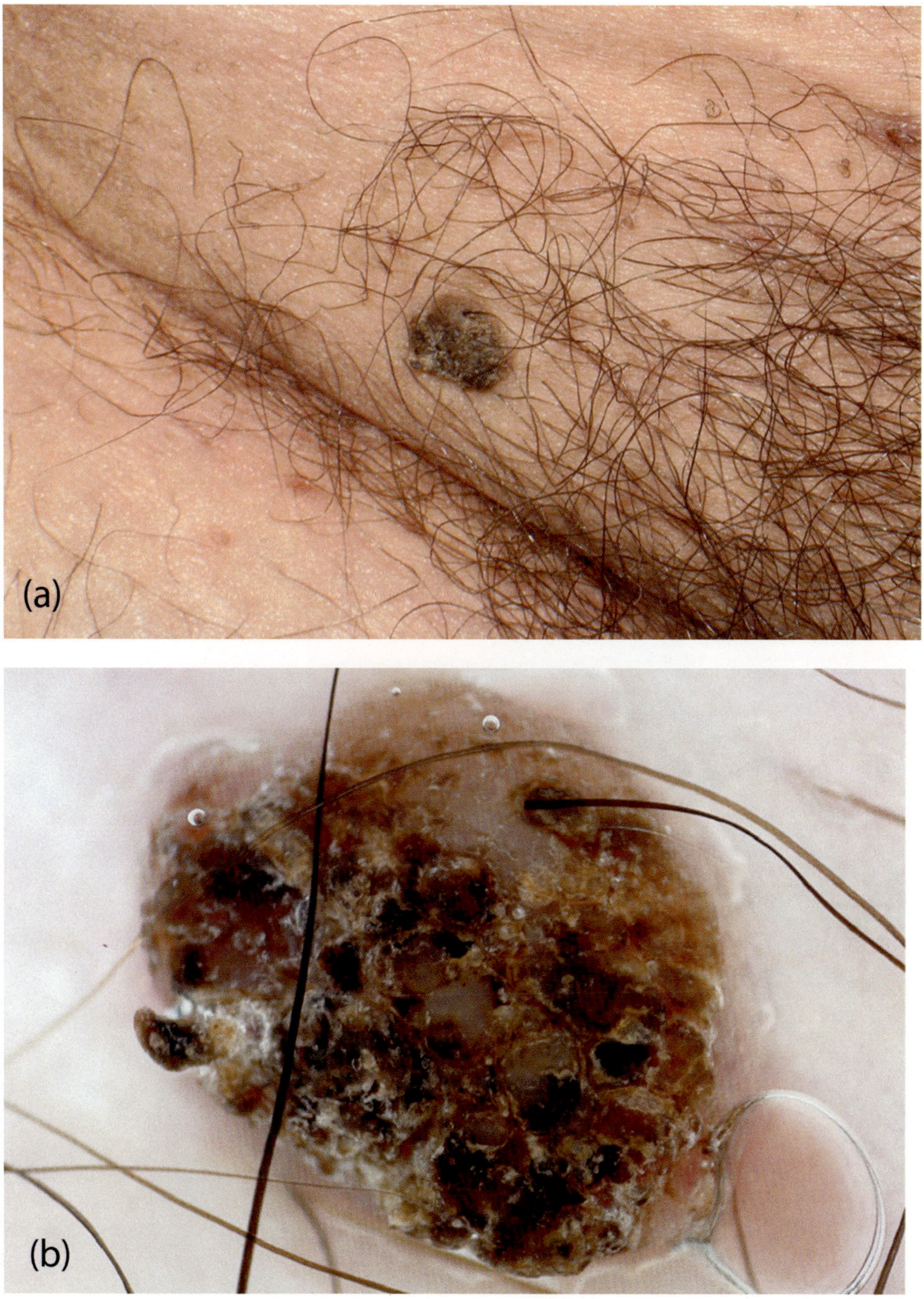

Figure 20.4 (a) Seborrheic keratosis. Hyperkeratotic lesion on the pubic area in a male. (b) Dermoscopy (×10) showing diffuse hyperkeratosis covering the underlying structures.

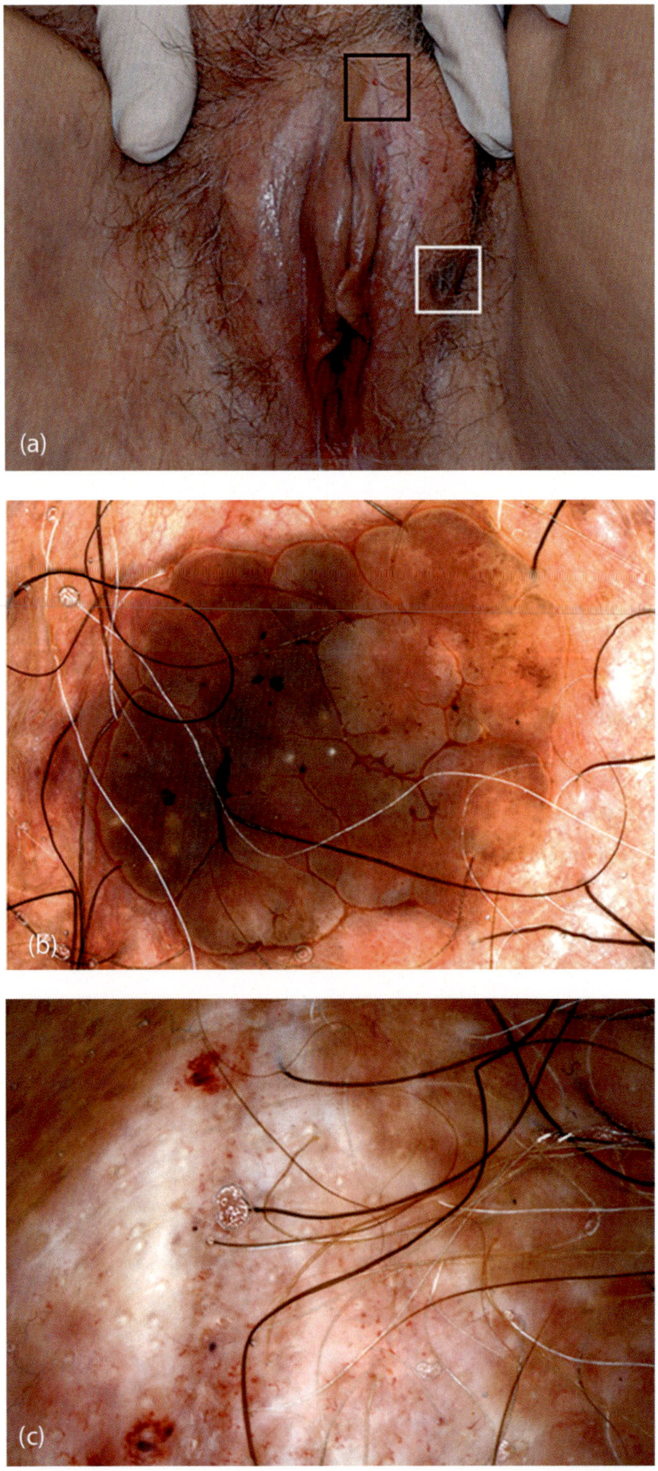

Figure 20.5 (a) Seborrheic keratosis of the left labium major in a patient with vulvar lichen sclerosus. The squares indicate the areas where dermoscopy was performed. (b) Dermoscopy (×7) of the white square showing the typical features of seborrheic keratosis: fissures and ridges, comedo-like openings, and milia-like cysts. (c) Dermoscopy (×10) of the black square showing the features of lichen sclerosus (see Chapter 9): whitish structureless areas, comedo-like openings and red to purpuric blotches.

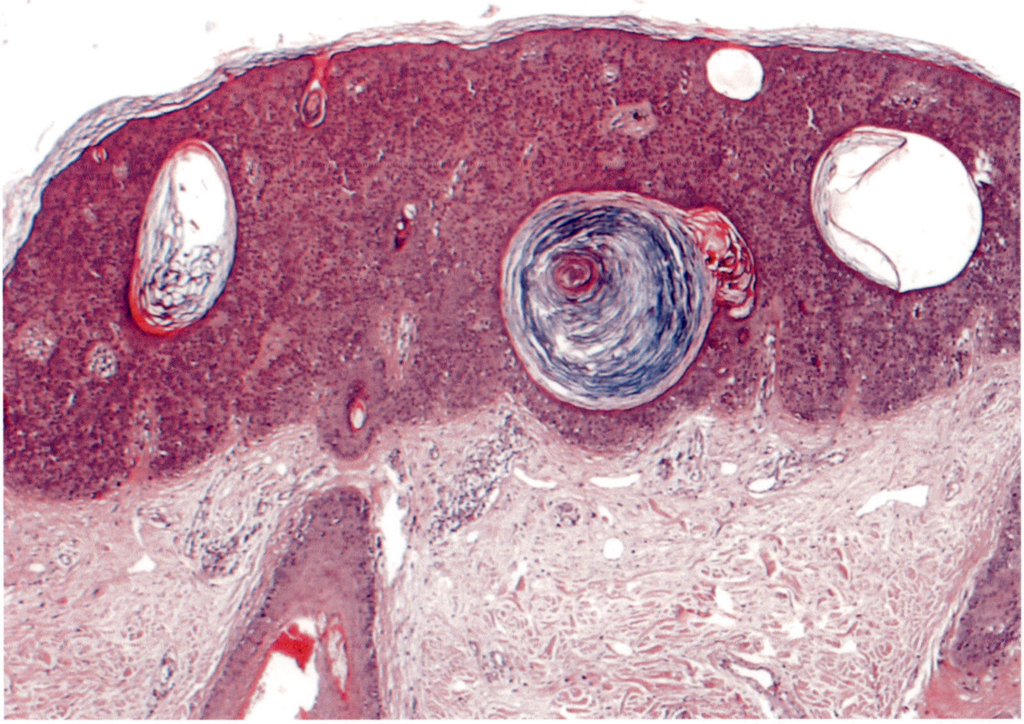

Figure 20.6 Histopathology of seborrheic keratosis showing acanthosis and intraepidermal keratin-filled cysts (H&E, ×100).

CHAPTER 21

Median Raphe Cyst

Aurora Tedeschi MD PhD, Nella Pulvirenti MD PhD, and Giuseppe Micali MD

DEFINITION

Median raphe cyst (MRC), also known as genitoperineal cyst of median raphe, mucoid cyst of penis, or apocrine cystadenoma/hydrocystoma of penis, represents a congenital developmental defect of the male genitalia (1).

EPIDEMIOLOGY

MRC is an uncommon lesion most commonly observed in the first decade of life. However, being often asymptomatic, it is probably underestimated and may be noticed later, during the second to third decades (1, 2).

ETIOLOGY

MRC reflects a developmental defect in male genitalia during embryogenesis, but the exact mechanism is not clear. It might result from tissue trapping during embryonic fusion of urethral folds for development of urethral groove, anomalous developmental of the periurethral glands of Littre, or aberrant blockage of the paraurethral duct (3).

CLINICAL FEATURES

MRC usually appears as a translucent, yellowish, cystic lesion of various sizes that may occur anywhere on the ventral side of the male genital area between urethral meatus, scrotum, perineum, and anus, along the midline/median raphe [Figure 21.1(a)] (4). Multiple cysts may be observed in the same patient [Figure 21.2(a)]. A variant is represented by a canalicular and/or cord-like lesion, also known as "median raphe canal" [Figure 21.3(a)] (5). Most cases are asymptomatic during childhood and become symptomatic during adolescence or adulthood especially following traumas and bacterial infections. In these cases, pain and dysuria may be referred (1, 3).

DOI: 10.1201/9781003007166-21

DIFFERENTIAL DIAGNOSIS

The differential diagnosis of MRC mainly includes epidermal cyst, dermoid cyst, steatocystoma, eccrine cystadenoma, molluscum contagiosum, genital warts, and urethral diverticulum.

DIAGNOSIS

The diagnosis is often incidental. It should be suspected when a patient presents with a cystic or nodular lesion on the ventral side of the genitalia (3). The history and the clinical aspect are generally suggestive, although histopathological examination and immunohistochemistry are sometimes necessary.

DERMOSCOPY

Dermoscopy may help in the diagnosis of MRC, especially in case of small lesions, by showing the presence of a homogeneous, whitish, or yellowish pattern [Figures 21.1(b), 21.2(b), and 21.3(b)] (6, 7). Dermoscopy may also reveal a clinically undetected connection between multiple cysts by showing a translucent tract [Figure 21.3(b)]; in this case, the final diagnosis of median raphe canal may address to a more appropriate therapeutic approach (6, 7).

HISTOPATHOLOGICAL CORRELATION

Different histopathological variants of MRC have been described. The most common type of lining is the urethral type which has stratified layers of uniform small cells overlaid by columnar epithelium (Figure 21.4) (8, 9). The cyst is not connected with either the epidermis or urethra, and the homogeneous, white/yellowish pattern observed at dermoscopy corresponds to its clear mucinous content (8).

REFERENCES

1. Syed MMA, Amatya B, Sitaula S. Median raphe cyst of the penis: a case report and review of the literature. J Med Case Rep 2019;13(1):214.
2. Amaranathan A, Sinhasan SP, Dasiah SD. Median raphe cysts of the prepucial skin, with triple histological linings: a case report and review of the literature. J Clin Diagn Res 2013;7(7):1466–8.
3. Sharma A, Agrawal S, Vishwanath T, et al. Parameatal median raphe cyst: a case report of a midline developmental defect of true urogenital origin. Indian Dermatol Online J 2020;11(2):216–8.
4. Nishida H, Kashima K, Daa T, et al. Pigmented median raphe cyst of the penis. J Cutan Pathol 2012;39:808–10.
5. Patoulias D, Kalogirou M, Chatzopoulos K, Patoulias I. Canaliform median raphe cysts (MRCs) lined by squamous epithelium in a 5-year-old male patient; report of a rare case and comprehensive review of the literature. Folia Med Cracov 2017;57(4):55–62.
6. Lacarrubba F, Tedeschi A, Francesconi L, Micali G. Canal versus cysts of the penile median raphe: advancing diagnostic methods using videodermatoscopy. Pediatr Dermatol 2010;27:667–9.
7. Micali G, Lacarrubba F. Augmented diagnostic capability using videodermatoscopy on selected infectious and non-infectious penile growths. Int J Dermatol 2011;50:1501–5.
8. Shao IH, Chen TD, Shao HT, Chen HW. Male median raphe cysts: serial retrospective analysis and histopathological classification. Diagn Pathol 2012;7:121.
9. Alphones S, Phansalkar M, Manoharan P. Median raphe cyst of the penis: a startling diagnosis for the unaccustomed clinician. Urol Ann 2019;11(3):314–6.

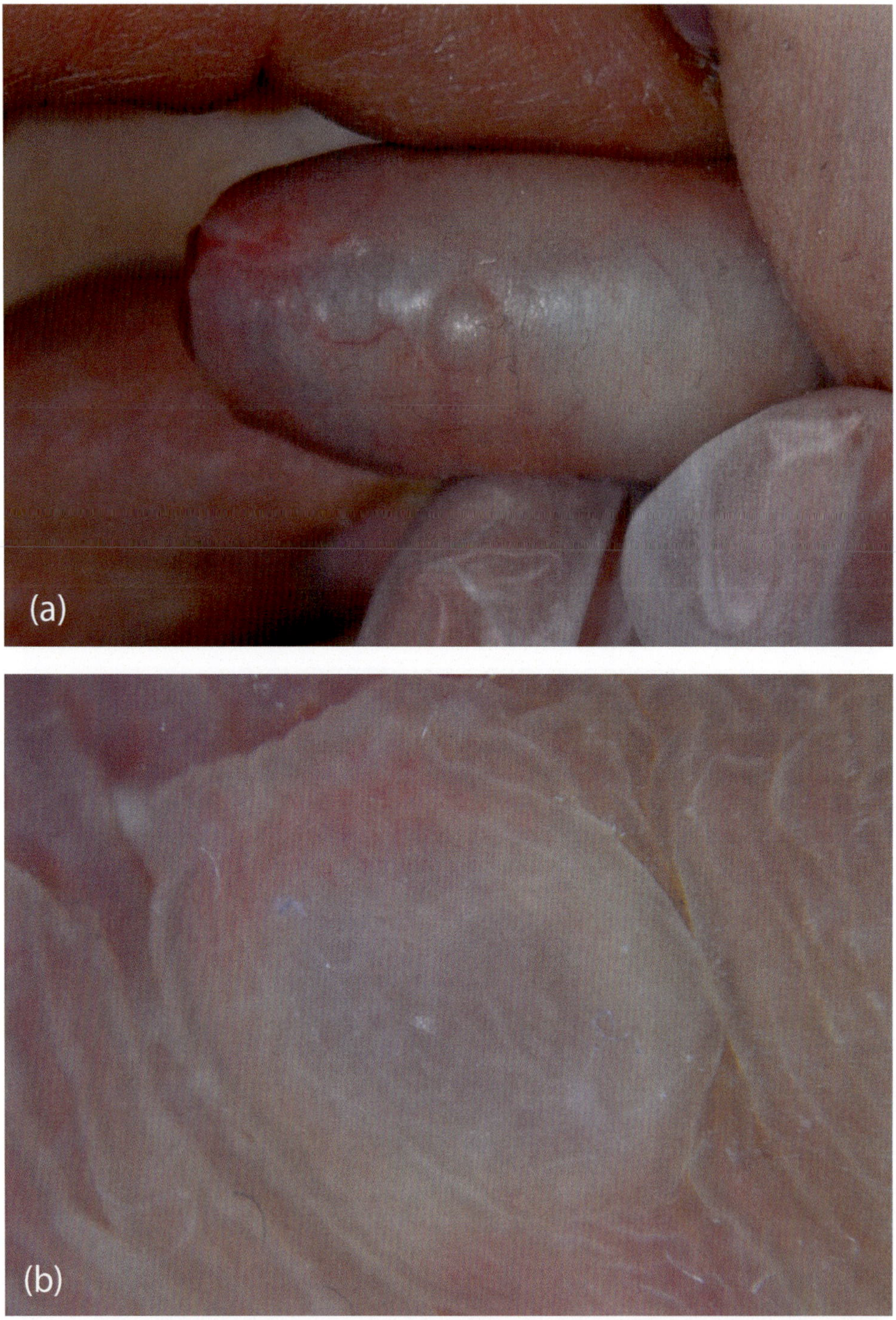

Figure 21.1 (a) Median raphe cyst. Translucent, tender nodule on the ventral side of the penis in an 11-year-old boy. (b) Dermoscopy (×10) of the nodule showing a homogeneous, whitish color.

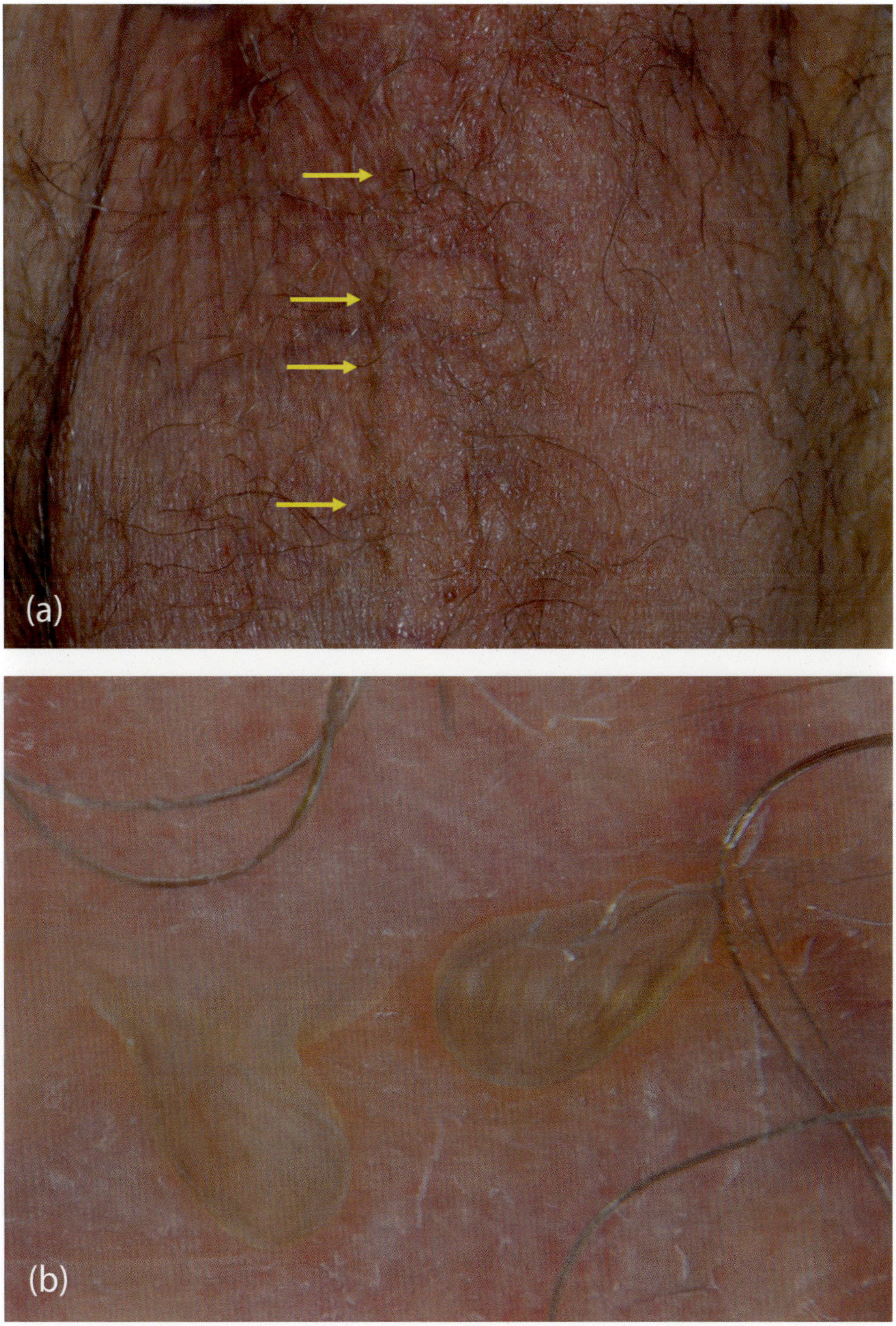

Figure 21.2 (a) Median raphe cysts. Multiple, minimal, yellowish papules linearly arranged along the median line of the scrotum in a 45-year-old man. (b) Dermoscopy (×10) of two lesions showing a homogeneous, yellowish pattern.

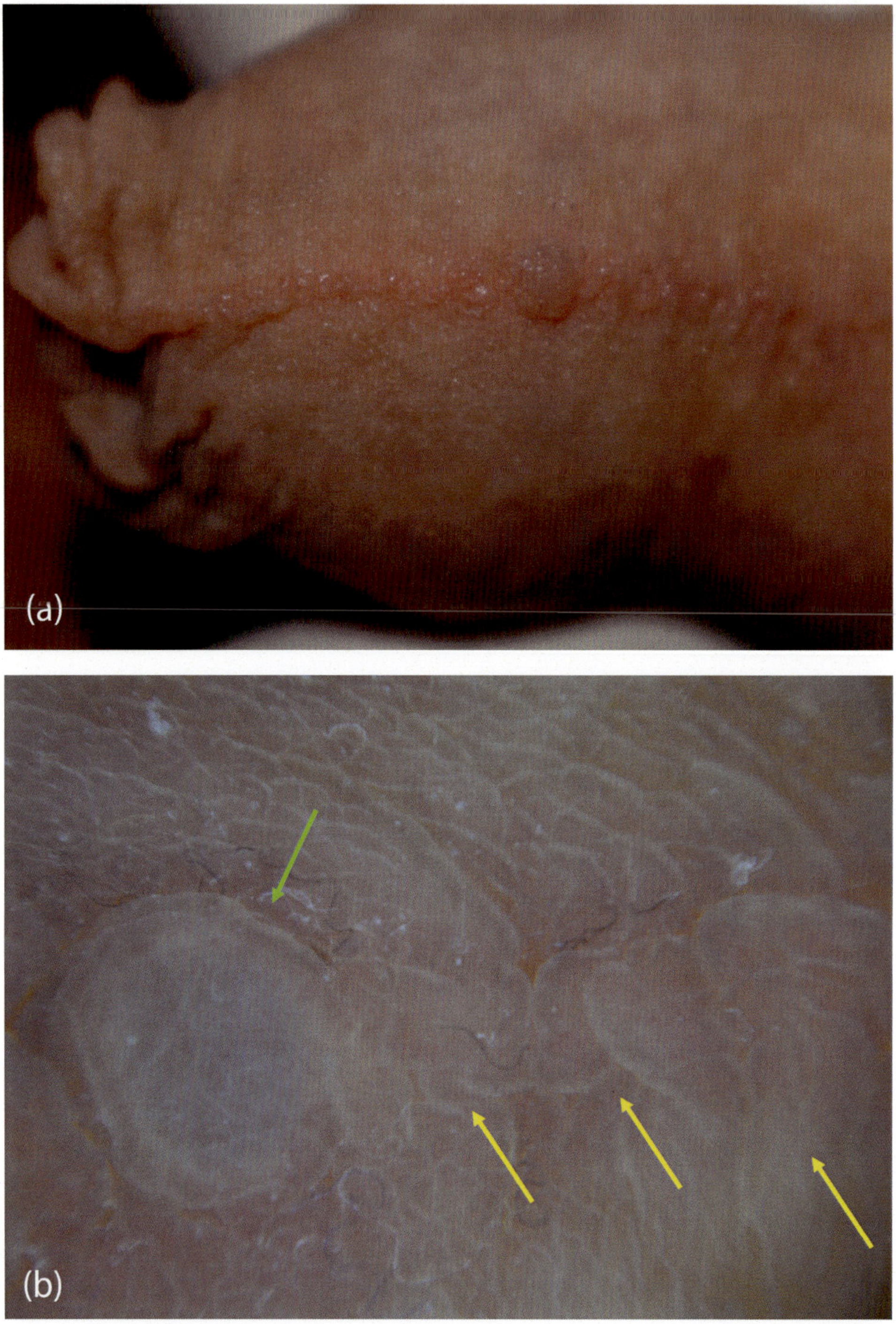

Figure 21.3 (a) Median raphe cyst. Translucent, flesh-colored papule on the ventral side of the penis in a 22-year-old man. (b) Dermoscopy (×10) of the papule showing a homogeneous, whitish color (green arrow). A translucent tract is also visible (yellow arrows) addressing the final diagnosis of the median raphe canal.

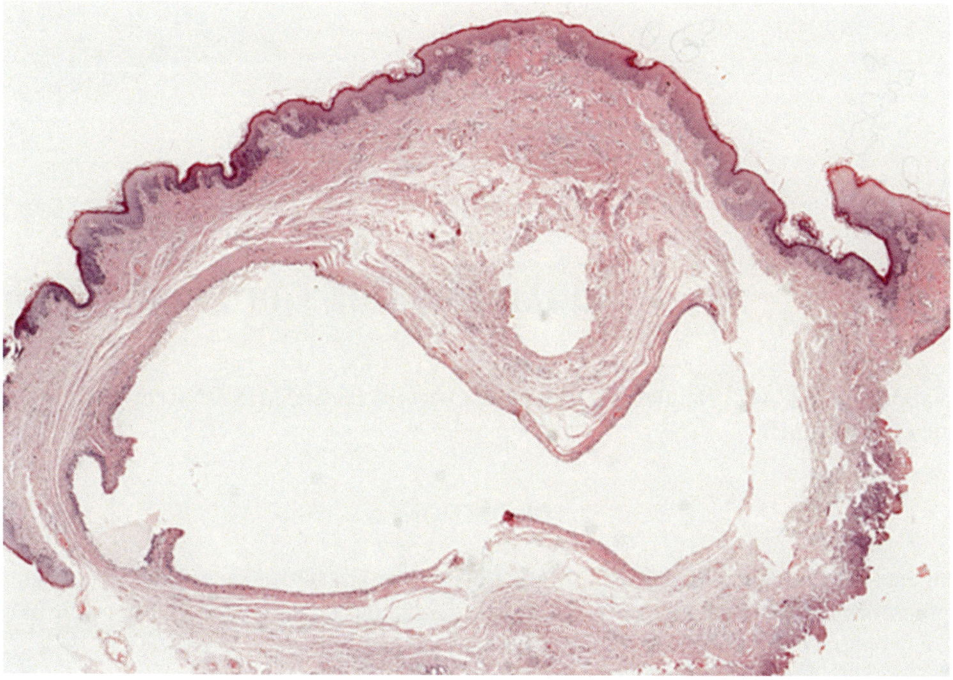

Figure 21.4 Histopathology of median raphe cyst showing pseudostratified columnar epithelium lining the cyst (H&E, ×50).

CHAPTER 22

Squamous Cell Carcinoma *In Situ*

Alessandro Borghi MD, Natale Schettini MD, Lucrezia Pacetti MD, Roberta Gafà MD, and Monica Corazza MD

DEFINITION

Squamous cell carcinoma *in situ* (SCC*is*) is a high-grade intraepithelial squamous neoplasm that can progress into an invasive cancer. When it affects genitalia, the terms of vulvar or penile intraepithelial neoplasia (VIN and PeIN, respectively) are used.

EPIDEMIOLOGY

VIN is divided into two forms: a high grade squamous intraepithelial lesion (HSIL), formerly known as usual-type vulvar intraepithelial neoplasia (uVIN), typical of younger women (mean age 63.3 years) (1) and with a lower trend in progression to infiltrating cancer (9–16% of cases) (2), and a differentiated-type (dVIN), more common in older women (mean age 70.2 years) (1) and with a higher invasive potential (30% of cases) (2). VIN presents an incidence of five cases per 100,000 women/year (3). Incidence of PeIN appears to be 0.47 cases for 100,000 men/year (4) with a risk of progression depending on clinical presentation.

ETIOLOGY

HSIL is related to the oncogenic effects of persistent human papillomavirus (HPV) infection. On the contrary, dVIN develops in a context of chronic inflammation, mostly lichen sclerosus (1). Even PeIN can be divided into HPV-dependent and -independent forms with the same pathogenetic pathways of VIN (5).

CLINICAL FEATURES

VIN – Clinical aspects of VIN are variable [Figures 22.1(a), 22.2(a), and 22.3(a)]. HSIL presents as multifocal or isolated papules or plaques around the introitus and on the labia minora. Lesions are typically whitish or erythematous in color and sharply demarcated. Verrucous or polypoid as well as pigmented variants are possible (6). In case of dVIN, poorly defined isolated and hyperkeratotic plaques with rough, irregular surfaces are described (1, 7).

PeIN – It is typically divided into three clinical entities defined as Bowenoid papulosis (BP), Bowen's disease (BD) and erythroplasia of Queyrat (EQ). BP is characterized by multiple, small, red

DOI: 10.1201/9781003007166-22

or gray-brown papules generally involving the penis and the perianal area. It may be also observed in females on the vulva [Figure 22.4(a)]. The highest incidence of BP occurs in younger subjects (20–40 years) with a lesser risk for progression (2.6%) than the other entities. BD presents as a well-demarcated patch or plaque with erythematous and sometimes pigmented surface [Figure 22.5(a)] of the keratinized penis. It generally affects patients older than 60 years and progresses into invasive cancer in 10% of cases. EQ occurs on glans or foreskin with the appearance of an erythematous plaque with a sharp demarcation and crusted or scaled aspects. The mean age of patients is 70 years. EQ shows the greatest invasive potential (10–33%) (6).

DIFFERENTIAL DIAGNOSIS

The differential diagnosis of SCC*is* includes various benign conditions such as seborrheic keratosis, inflammatory disorders like lichen simplex chronicus, lichen sclerosus, lichen planus and psoriasis, infectious balanitis and vulvitis, and genital warts. Also, malignant disorders such as melanoma, invasive SCC, basal cell carcinoma and extramammary Paget disease can mimic SCC*is*.

DIAGNOSIS

The clinical and dermoscopic suspicion of SCC*is* must be confirmed by a biopsy with histopathological examination (see below) (7).

DERMOSCOPY

Dermoscopy of intraepithelial neoplasia of genitalia may reveal lesions with asymmetry of various parameters, such as shape, structure, and/or color.

VIN – HSIL usually presents as smooth or papillomatous or cerebriform, pink to bright red plaques, with dotted and glomerular vessels (8). White dots or whitish areas as well as gray-blue/brownish elements may be seen [Figures 22.1(b), 22.2(b), and 22.3(b)]. The latter appear as either peripheral, linearly distributed dots or focal structureless areas. Pigmented variants show prominent irregularly distributed gray to brownish areas or dots. Dermoscopy of dVIN reveals serpentine and curvy vessels in the context of pink to red or whitish structureless areas. A predominance of white color appears to be a sign of progression to invasive neoplasia (10). Adjacent dermoscopic features of underlying dermatoses, mostly lichen sclerosus, may be seen (11).

PeIN – Dermoscopy typically shows structureless pink, skin-colored or white areas with polymorphic vascular pattern, most commonly dotted or glomerular (12). These vessels usually show a more diffuse and scattered arrangement than VIN (13). Linearly distributed, brown-gray dots are reported in BP [Figure 22.4(b)] and BD. Dermoscopic features of BP also include keratotic (14) or papillomatous surface (15) whereas in BD blue-black, brownish, or whitish structureless areas and gray granules or blotches can be seen [Figure 22.5(b)] (13, 16). The vascular pattern of BD may reveal glomerular, arranged both in lines and cluster (17), or hairpin vessels (13). EQ vessels typically present glomerular morphology commonly distributed in a diffused way similar to psoriatic balanitis from which EQ differs for the heterogeneity in shape, size and mutual distance of vessels (18). Scales, erosion and scar-like areas may be further findings (12).

HISTOPATHOLOGICAL CORRELATION

Histopathologically, genital SCC*is* reveals a disruption in the normal architectural structure, characterized by a proliferation of atypical basaloid cells with partial or full involvement of the epithelium (Figure 22.6). These cells present an increase in number of mitosis and in nuclear-to-cytoplasmatic ratio with nuclei that appear hyperchromatic and pleomorphic. In HPV-related forms, koilocytes can be observed. Parakeratosis and acanthosis are further features (1, 7). The pink, skin-colored or white areas with no well-defined structures seen at dermoscopy correspond histopathologically to chronic inflammation of lamina propria and fibrosis that may determine also scar-like areas. White dots and whitish area correspond to adnexal opening (19) and focal parakeratosis, respectively. The typical vascular patterns with glomerular or dotted vessels reflect the angiogenesis in lamina propria with an increase in number of capillaries (12). Gray-blue and brownish pigmentations are the consequence of the presence of melanin in atypical epidermal keratinocytes, pigment incontinence and dermal melanophages, as reported in cutaneous SCC (20).

REFERENCES

1. Preti M, Scurry J, Marchitelli CE, Micheletti L. Vulvar intraepithelial neoplasia. Best Pract Res Clin Obstet Gynaecol 2014;28:1051–62.
2. Hinten F, Molijn A, Eckhardt L, et al. Vulvar cancer: two pathways with different localization and prognosis. Gynecol Oncol 2018;149:310–7.
3. Bodelon C, Madeleine MM, Voigt LF, Weiss NS. Is the incidence of invasive vulvar cancer increasing in the United States? Cancer Causes Control 2009;20:1779–82.
4. Hoekstra RJ, Trip EJ, ten Kate FJW, et al. Penile intraepithelial neoplasia: nomenclature, incidence and progression to malignancy in the Netherlands. Int J Urol 2019;26:353–7.
5. Emmanuel A, Nettleton J, Watkin N, Berney DM. The molecular pathogenesis of penile carcinoma—current developments and understanding. Virchows Arch 2019;475:397–405.
6. Kutlubay Z, Engin B, Zara T, Tüzün Y. Anogenital malignancies and premalignancies: facts and controversies. Clin Dermatol 2013;31:362–73.
7. Del Pino M, Rodriguez-Carunchio L, Ordi J. Pathways of vulvar intraepithelial neoplasia and squamous cell carcinoma. Histopathology 2013;62:161–75.
8. Barisani A, Dika E, Fanti PA, et al. Dermoscopic findings of vulvar intraepithelial neoplasia: a series of four cases. Br J Dermatol 2017;176:227–30.
9. Ronger-Savle S, Julien V, Duru G, et al. Features of pigmented vulval lesions on dermoscopy. Br J Dermatol 2011;164:54–61.
10. Vaccari S, Barisani A, Preti EP, et al. Vulvar intraepithelial neoplasia and vulvar squamous cell carcinoma: differential dermoscopic features in a case series, and a progression model. Clin Exp Dermatol 2018;43:469–71.
11. Borghi A, Virgili A, Corazza M. Dermoscopy of inflammatory genital diseases: practical insights. Dermatol Clin 2018;36:451–61.
12. Chan SL, Watchorn RE, Panagou E, et al. Dermatoscopic findings of penile intraepithelial neoplasia: Bowenoid papulosis, Bowen disease and erythroplasia of queyrat. Australas J Dermatol 2019;60:e201–7.
13. Friedman BJ, Kohen LL. A case of pigmented penile intraepithelial neoplasia: dermoscopic and clinicohistopathologic analysis. J Am Acad Dermatol 2015;72:S71–S72.
14. Dong H, Shu D, Campbell TM, et al. Dermatoscopy of genital warts. J Am Acad Dermatol 2011; 64:859–64.
15. Marcucci C, Sabban EC, Friedman P, et al. Dermoscopic findings in bowenoid papulosis: report of two cases. Dermatol Pract Concept 2014;4:61–3.
16. Ishioka P, Yamada S, Michalany NS, Hirata SH. Dermatoscopia da doenca de Bowen: Variante pigmentada no penis. An Bras Dermatol 2012;87:482–4.
17. Giuffrida R, Conforti C, Resende FSS, et al. Clinical and dermoscopic features of genital pigmented Bowen disease. Clin Exp Dermatol 2018;43:813–6.
18. Errichetti E, Lallas A, Di Stefani A, et al. Accuracy of dermoscopy in distinguishing erythroplasia of Queyrat from common forms of chronic balanitis: results from a multicentric observational study. J Eur Acad Dermatol Venereol 2019;33:966–72.
19. Maione V, Errichetti E, Dehen L, et al. Usual-type vulvar intraepithelial neoplasia: report of a case and its dermoscopic features. Int J Dermatol 2016;55:e621–3.
20. Cameron A, Rosendahl C, Tschandl P, et al. Dermatoscopy of pigmented Bowen's disease. J Am Acad Dermatol 2010;62:597–604.

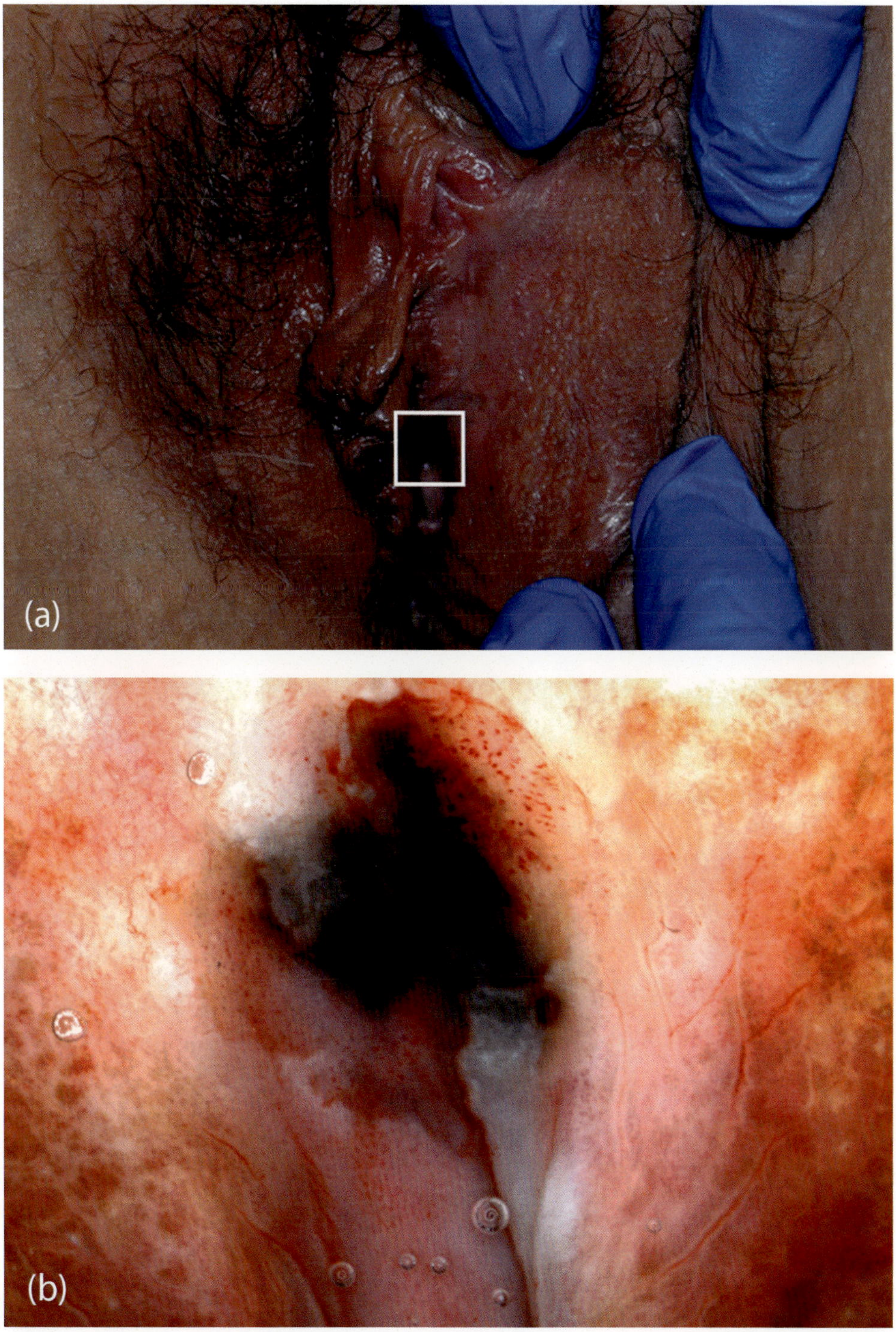

Figure 22.1 (a) Vulvar intraepithelial neoplasia of the vulvar vestibule. The square indicates the area where dermoscopy was performed. (b) Dermoscopy (×10) showing papillomatous structure varying in color from whitish to pink-grayish, with abundant dotted and linear vessels irregularly distributed. Structureless gray-blue/brownish areas are visible in the upper portion of the lesion.

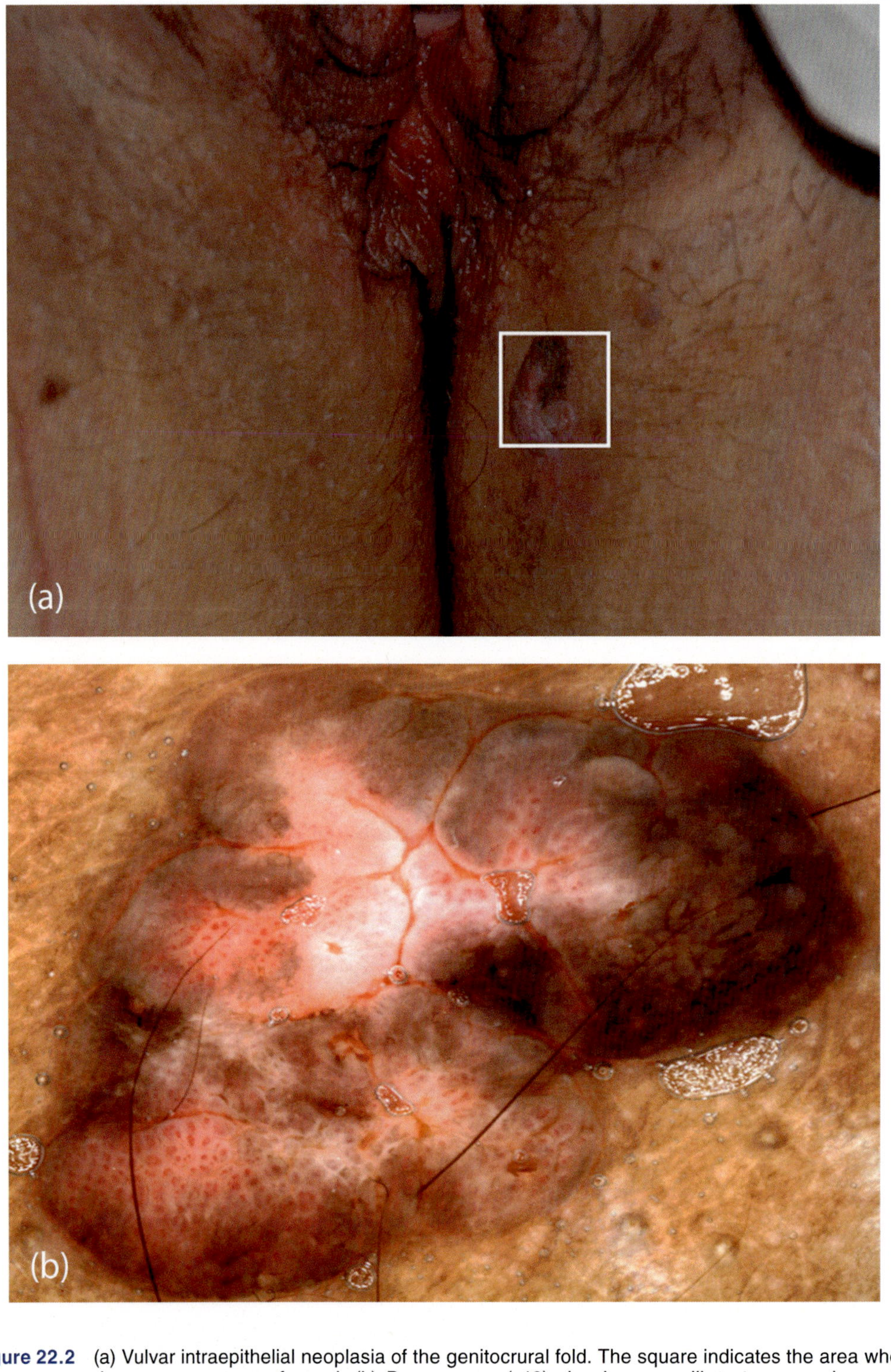

Figure 22.2 (a) Vulvar intraepithelial neoplasia of the genitocrural fold. The square indicates the area where dermoscopy was performed. (b) Dermoscopy (×10) showing a papillomatous neoplasm with cerebriform surface, pink to whitish in the center and brownish towards the periphery; Numerous glomerular vessels are observable over the lesion.

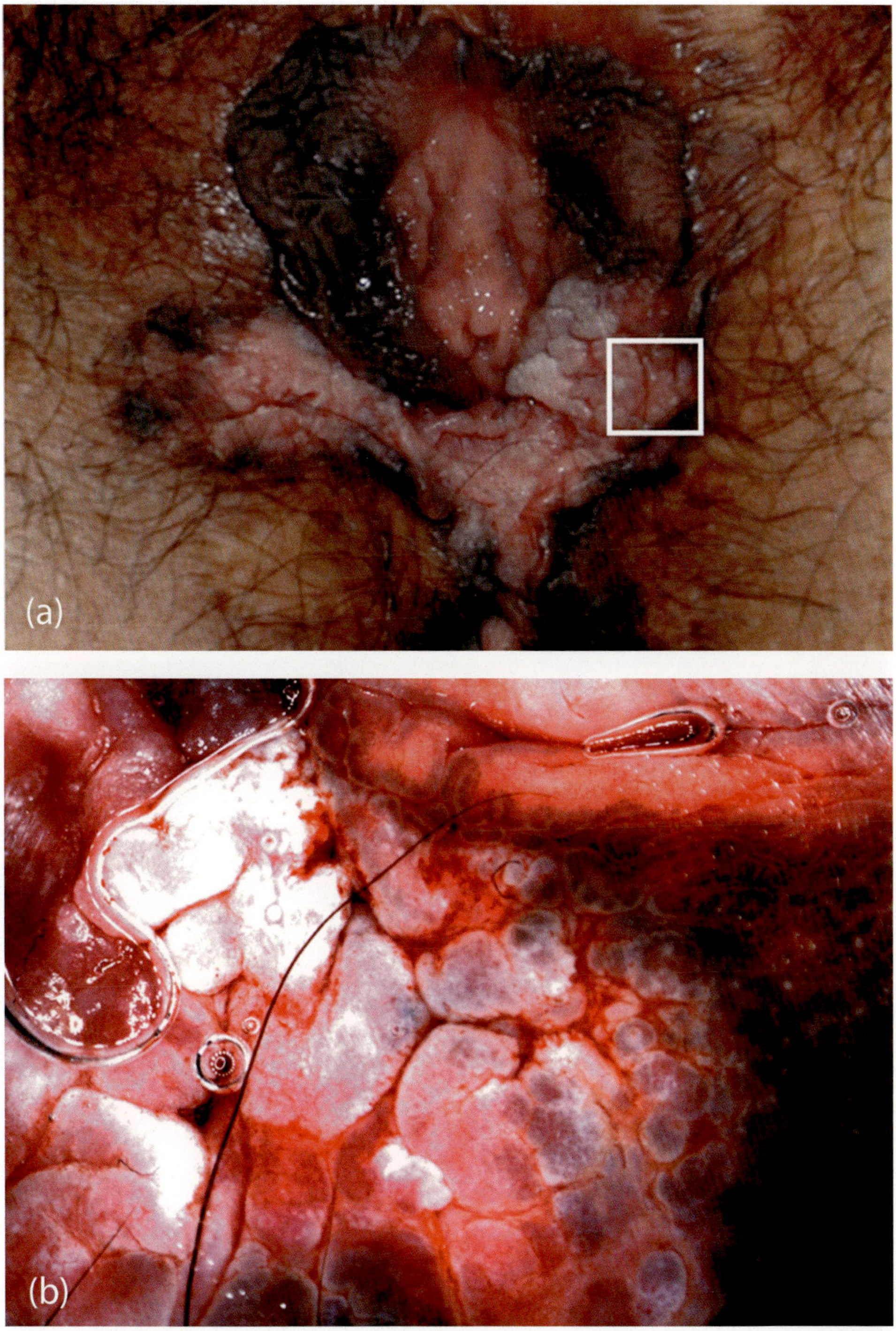

Figure 22.3 (a) Vulvar intraepithelial neoplasia involving the labia minora and the perineum. The square indicates the area where dermoscopy was performed. (b) Dermoscopy (×20) showing a papillomatous surface, with fissures and ridges, varying in color from bright red to pink-whitish, with brownish, edge pigmentation. A thick vascularization, mainly dotted in shape, is distributed over the lesion surface.

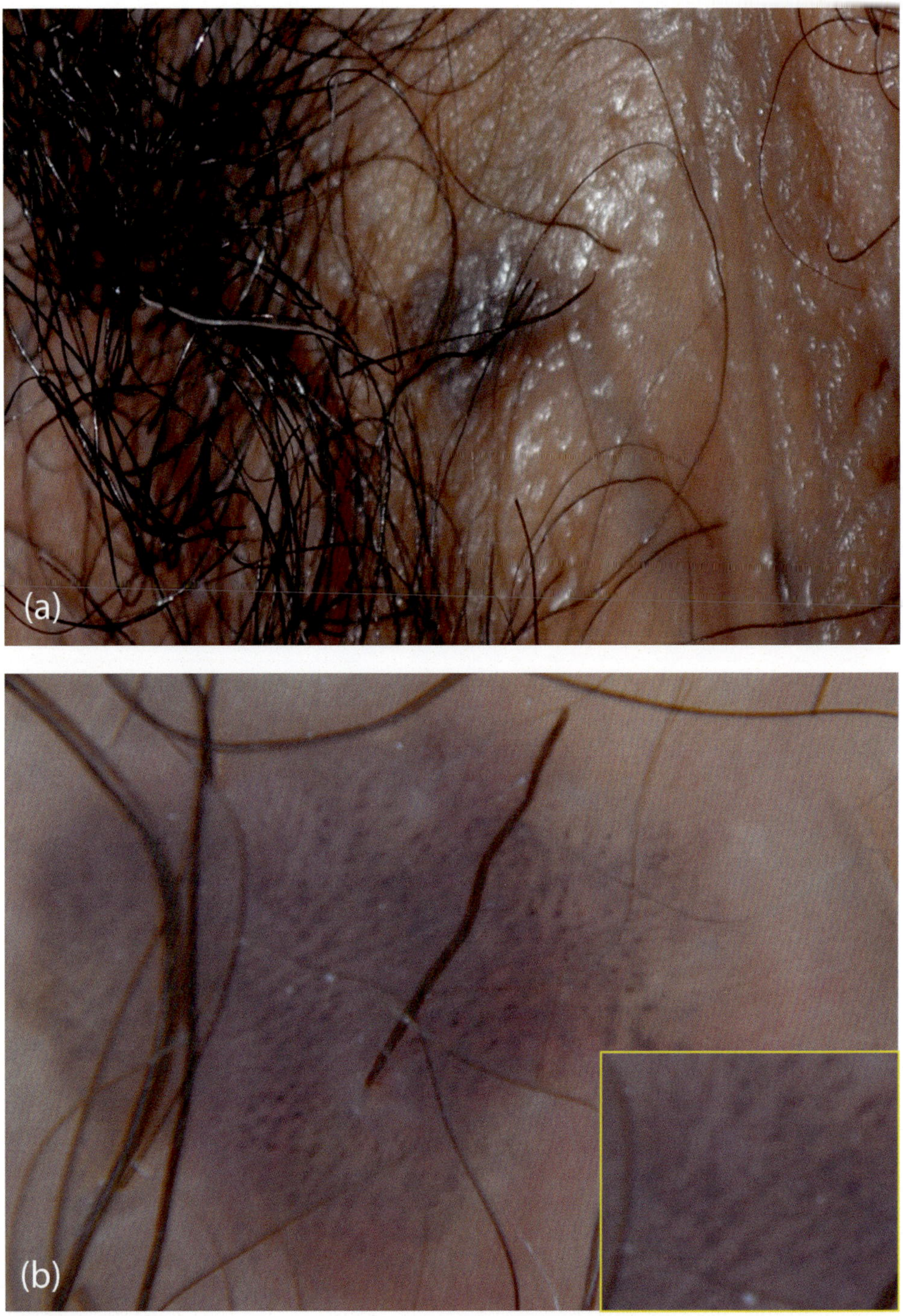

Figure 22.4 (a) Bowenoid papulosis of the vulva. Brownish papule of the labium major. (b) Dermoscopy (×10) showing linearly distributed, brown-gray dots (insert: a detail).

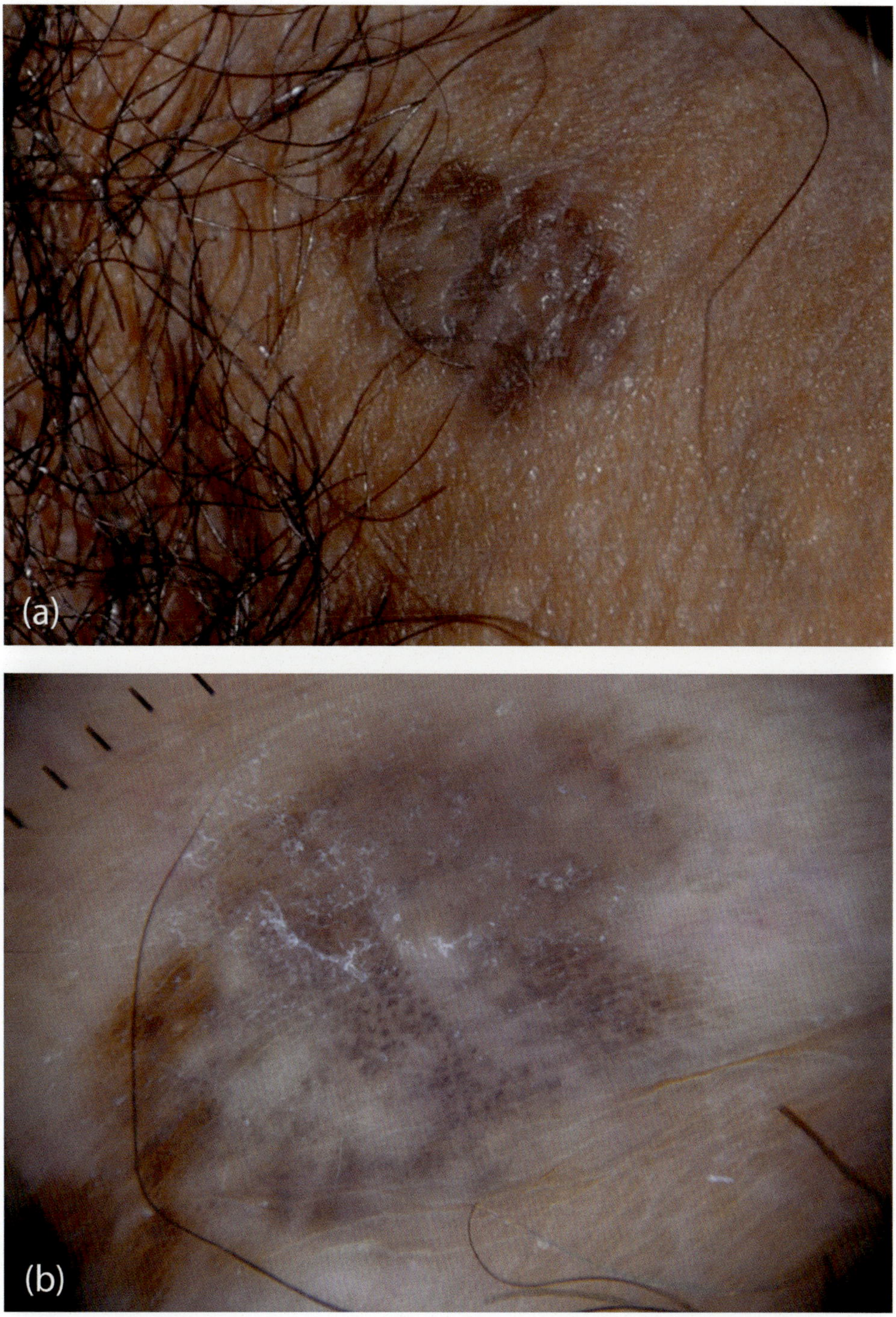

Figure 22.5 (a) Pigmented Bowen's disease. Brownish macule of the penis. (b) Dermoscopy (×10) showing irregular brownish pigmentation, structureless whitish areas, and brown-gray dots.

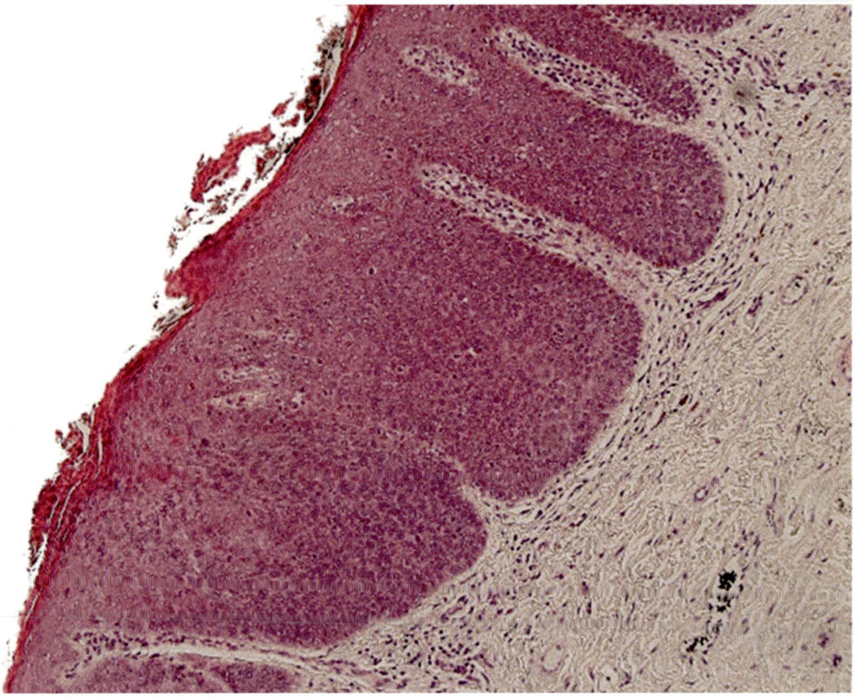

Figure 22.6 Histopathology of vulvar intraepithelial neoplasia showing full thickness atypia with hypercromasia and crowding; frequent mitoses are visible in all layers (H&E, ×100).

CHAPTER 23

Invasive Squamous Cell Carcinoma

Monica Corazza MD, Lucrezia Pacetti MD, Natale Schettini MD, Roberta Gafà MD, and Alessandro Borghi MD

DEFINITION

Invasive squamous cell carcinoma (SCC) is a high-grade neoplasia originating from cutaneous squamous cells, often following a progressive model from healthy skin cells to progressively more malignant entities.

EPIDEMIOLOGY

SCC is the most common malignant tumor of both the vulva (83%) (1) and penis (95%) (2), with an incidence of 1.2 × 100,000 in women and in 0.1–0.9 × 100,000 in men per year in Western Europe (3, 4). The overall 5-year survival rate for genital SCC is 71% in women and 67% in men.

ETIOLOGY

Vulvar SCC can arise from one of following predisposing conditions: i) human papillomavirus (HPV) infection that causes an intraepithelial cancer (high grade squamous intraepithelial lesion or HSIL, formerly known as usual-type vulvar intraepithelial neoplasia, uVIN); this is a precursor of invasive cancer mostly in younger women (between 35 and 65 years of age); ii) a non-neoplastic chronic inflammatory dermatosis, which can cause differentiated-type vulvar intraepithelial neoplasia (dVIN); dVIN can lead to SCC in older subjects (between 55 and 85 years) (5).

Penile SCC may evolve from penile intraepithelial neoplasia (PeIN) or arise *de novo* and has been associated with high-risk HPV infections. SCC of the penis occurs almost exclusively in uncircumcised men, most commonly between the ages of 50 and 70 years (6).

CLINICAL FEATURES

SCC usually presents as an isolated lesion, sometimes associated with pruritus. The lesion can manifest as an infiltrated plaque or an exophytic mass, which may show ulceration, or be either leukoplakic, fleshy, or warty, with or without surrounding erythema [Figures 23.1(a), 23.2(a), 23.3(a)]. More rarely, it can be associated with bleeding, discharge, foul odour, and pain, which may be clinical markers of disease progression (5, 6).

DOI: 10.1201/9781003007166-23

DIFFERENTIAL DIAGNOSIS

Genital SCC can be put in differential diagnosis with a plethora of different disorders, both inflammatory and neoplastic, such as SCC *in situ*, basal cell carcinoma, amelanotic melanoma, extramammary Paget's disease and lichen sclerosus (LS).

DIAGNOSIS

Although SCC is typically unifocal, a thorough clinical examination is indicated to rule out the presence of multiple foci of disease. A biopsy with histopathological exam is essential for the conclusive diagnosis (see below) (7).

DERMOSCOPY

Dermoscopically, SCC shows no pathognomonic features, and its identification is based mainly on the presence of altered and chaotic patterns, predominance of white color (8), and polymorphous vessels with irregular distribution. Ulceration and dermoscopic signs of altered keratinization, albeit less evident than in cutaneous SCC, may be further features. More in detail, asymmetry in both structures and color is a distinctive dermoscopic characteristic of SCC (9). White structures, varying from roundish lobules to amorphous areas, seem to have the highest specificity among all dermoscopic criteria for distinguishing SCC from other differential diagnoses [Figure 23.1(b)]. Scales may arise from a hyperkeratotic, whitish background [Figure 23.2(b)]. The increasing amount of white color within a lesion was found to be correlated with a progression from SCC *in situ*, to microinvasive and later invasive SCC (8). Red color, corresponding to erosive or ulcerated surfaces, and peripheral brown structureless areas may also be observed [Figure 23.3(b)].

Linear-irregular vessels, mainly located centrally within the lesion, and hairpin vessels, more peripherally, are quite typical in the described cases of invasive genital SCC and allow to differentiate it from other entities (8). Curvy and short-serpentine vessels are more typical of intraepithelial SCC (8), although this is not a rule for some clinical variants, such as Bowen's disease and erythroplasia of Queyrat (10). Fine, reddish, well-focused arborizing vessels, together with blue-gray ovoid globules, homogeneous whitish shiny areas and pinkish background, are dermoscopic features of genital basal cell carcinoma (10). Amelanotic melanoma show polymorphic vascular patterns associated with a pinkish background hue. The dermoscopic presence of a whitish background as well as the lack of both a negative network and peripheral residual areas of melanocytic pigmentation can point to a diagnosis of SCC (11).

Extramammary Paget's disease shares clinical and dermoscopic features with SCC too. However, the presence of primarily dotted and glomeruloid vessels, together with milky red areas, pigmentary structures and shiny white lines, leads towards a diagnosis of Paget's disease instead of SCC (10).

Lastly, SCC can also be put in differential diagnosis with LS, from which it can arise. Also, these two conditions share dermoscopic features, but a decrease in vessel concentration, gray-brown dots arranged in a peppering pattern, and comedo-like openings are strong indicators for LS (10, 12).

HISTOPATHOLOGICAL CORRELATION

Histopathologically, SCC can be grouped into one of three main subtypes: warty, basaloid, and keratinizing. The keratinizing type (Figure 23.4) is predominant (65–80%) and mainly occurs in postmenopausal women. The basaloid and warty types (20–35%) occur more often in premenopausal or perimenopausal women and are more commonly associated with HPV infection and history of HSIL or PeIN (5). The extent and the arrangement of the most common dermoscopic features observed in invasive SCC, such as white areas, elongated and irregular vessels and ulceration, depend on both the degree of tumor vertical growth and differentiation (8, 13). Shape and distribution of the whitish structures tend to be somewhat homogeneous in well-differentiated SCC (14). On the other hand, poorly differentiated SCCs show altered and chaotic dermoscopic architecture; ulceration and highly polymorphous elongated vessels, with great variability in both shape and diameter, are further dermoscopic signs of poor cyto-architectural differentiation (8, 14). White areas and structures broadly correlate with the presence of keratin at histopathology (Figure 23.4) (15). Elongated vessels at dermoscopy may indicate the presence of capillary loops that extend with tumor growth (16).

REFERENCES

1. Hoang LN, Park KJ, Soslow RA, Murali R. Squamous precursor lesions of the vulva: current classification and diagnostic challenges. Pathology 2016;48:291–302.
2. Hakenberg OW, Dräger DL, Erbersdobler A, et al. The diagnosis and treatment of penile cancer. Dtsch Arztebl Int 2018;115:646–652.
3. Iacoponi S, Zapardiel I; VULCAN Study Collaborative Group. European nationality influence in the management of squamous cell vulvar cancer. Gynecol Obstet Invest 2017; 82:349–354.
4. Novara G, Galfano A, De Marco V, et al. Prognostic factors in squamous cell carcinoma of the penis. Nat Clin Pract Urol 2007;4:140–146.
5. Alkatout I, Schubert M, Garbrecht N, et al. Vulvar cancer: epidemiology, clinical presentation, and management options. Int J Womens Health 2015;20:305–313.
6. Marchionne E, Perez C, Hui A, Khachemoune A. Penile squamous cell carcinoma: a review of the literature and case report treated with Mohs micrographic surgery. An Bras Dermatol 2017;92:95–99.
7. Buchanan T, Mutch D. Squamous cell carcinoma of the vulva: a review of present management and future considerations. Expert Rev Anticancer Ther 2019;19:43–50.
8. Vaccari S, Barisani A, Preti EP, et al. Vulvar intraepithelial neoplasia and vulvar squamous cell carcinoma: differential dermoscopic features in a case series, and a progression model. Clin Exp Dermatol 2018;43:469–471.
9. Oakley A. Dermatoscopic features of vulval lesions in 97 women. Australas J Dermatol 2016;57:48–53.
10. Kamat D, Vinay K. Dermatoscopy of nonvenereal genital dermatoses: a brief review. Indian J Sex Transm Dis AIDS 2019;40:13–19.
11. Russo T, Piccolo V, Lallas A, et al. Dermoscopy of malignant skin tumours: what's New? Dermatology 2017;233:64–73.
12. Borghi A, Virgili A, Corazza M. Dermoscopy of inflammatory genital diseases: practical insights. Dermatol Clin 2018;36:451–461.
13. Zalaudek I, Giacomel J, Schmid K, et al. Dermatoscopy of facial actinic keratosis, intraepidermal carcinoma, and invasive squamous cell carcinoma: a progression model. J Am Acad Dermatol 2012;66:589–97.
14. Vaccari S, Barisani A, Tosti G, et al. Vulval squamous cell carcinoma: a clinicodermoscopic correlation. Clin Exp Dermatol 2019;44:939–941.
15. Wolner ZJ, BA, Yelamos O, Liopyris K, et al. Enhancing skin cancer diagnosis with dermoscopy. Dermatol Clin 2017;35:417–437.
16. Pyne J, Sapkota D, Wong JC. Squamous cell carcinoma: variation in dermatoscopic vascular features between well and non-well differentiated tumours. Dermatol Pract Concept 2012;2:204–205.

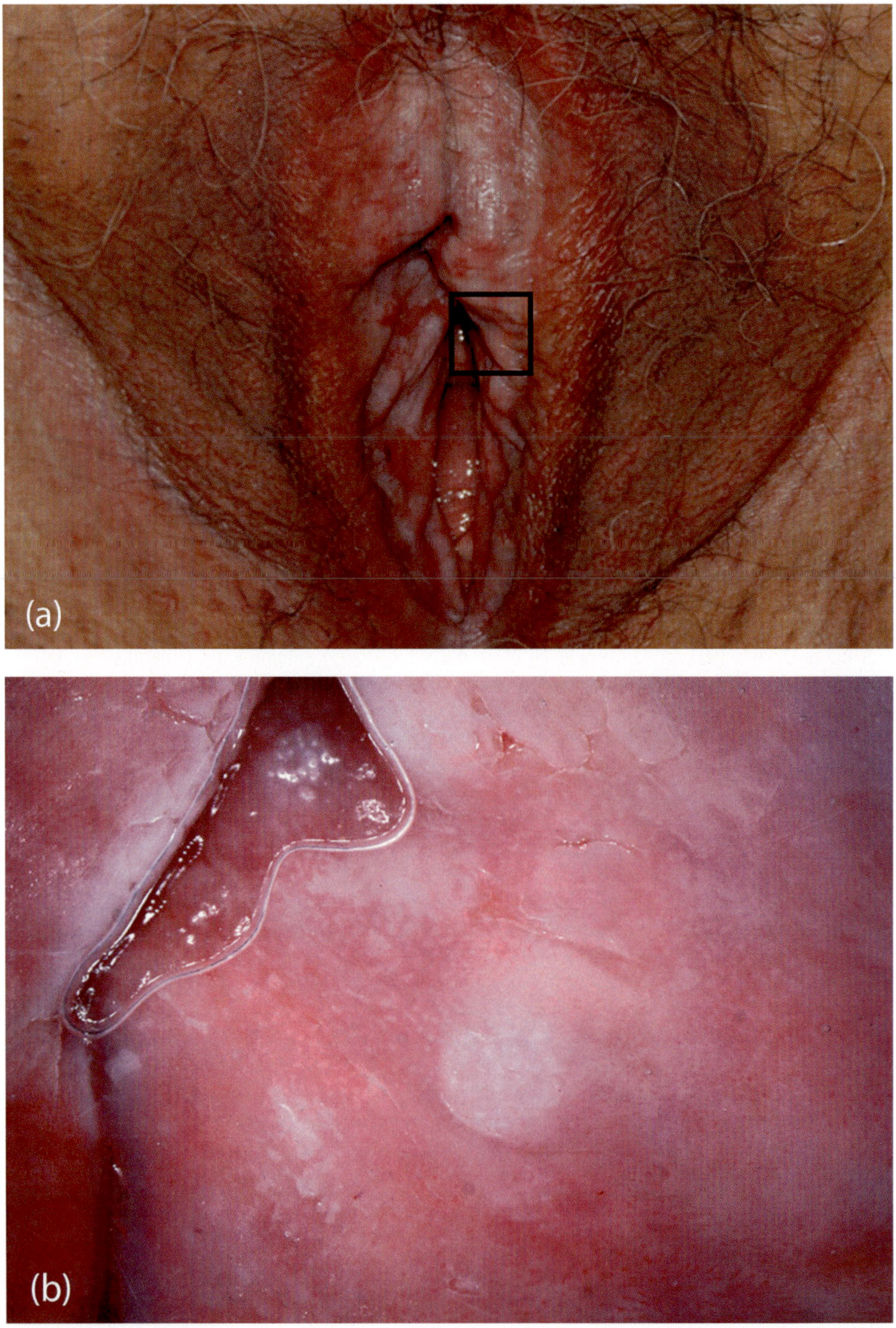

Figure 23.1 (a) Invasive squamous cell carcinoma extensively affecting the vulva. The square indicates the area where dermoscopy was performed. (b) Dermoscopy (×10) showing a whitish, papillomatous surface with dotted, glomerular and linear vessels irregularly arranged in loose clusters over the lesion.

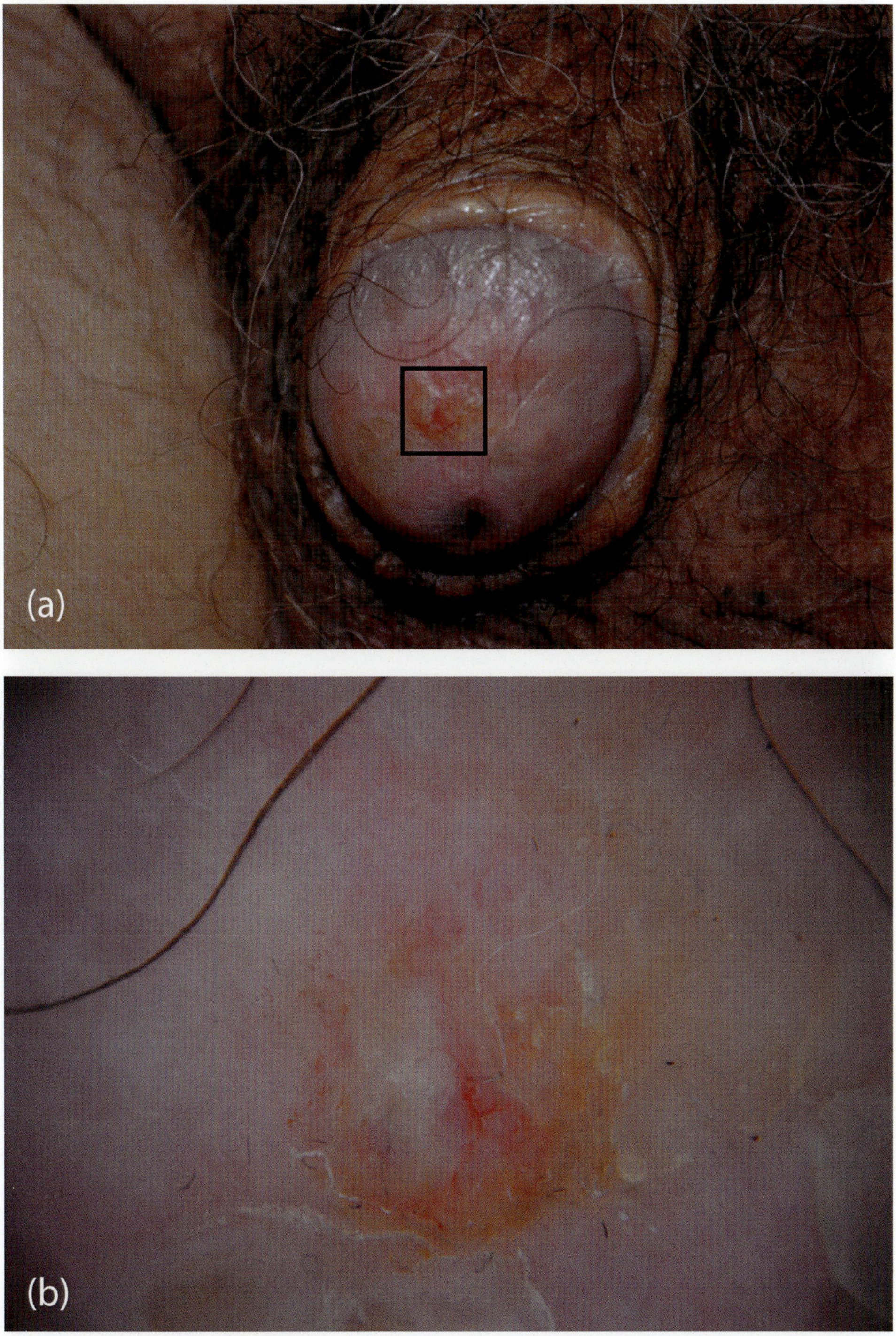

Figure 23.2 (a) Invasive squamous cell carcinoma involving the glans penis, consisting of a polycyclic squamous plaque with an erosive area. The square indicates the area where dermoscopy was performed. (b) Dermoscopy (×10) showing a white background topped with yellowish-white scaly lamellae. An erosive area of roughly triangular shape appears pinkish in color. Irregularly distributed linear vessels are visible on the surfaces not covered with scales.

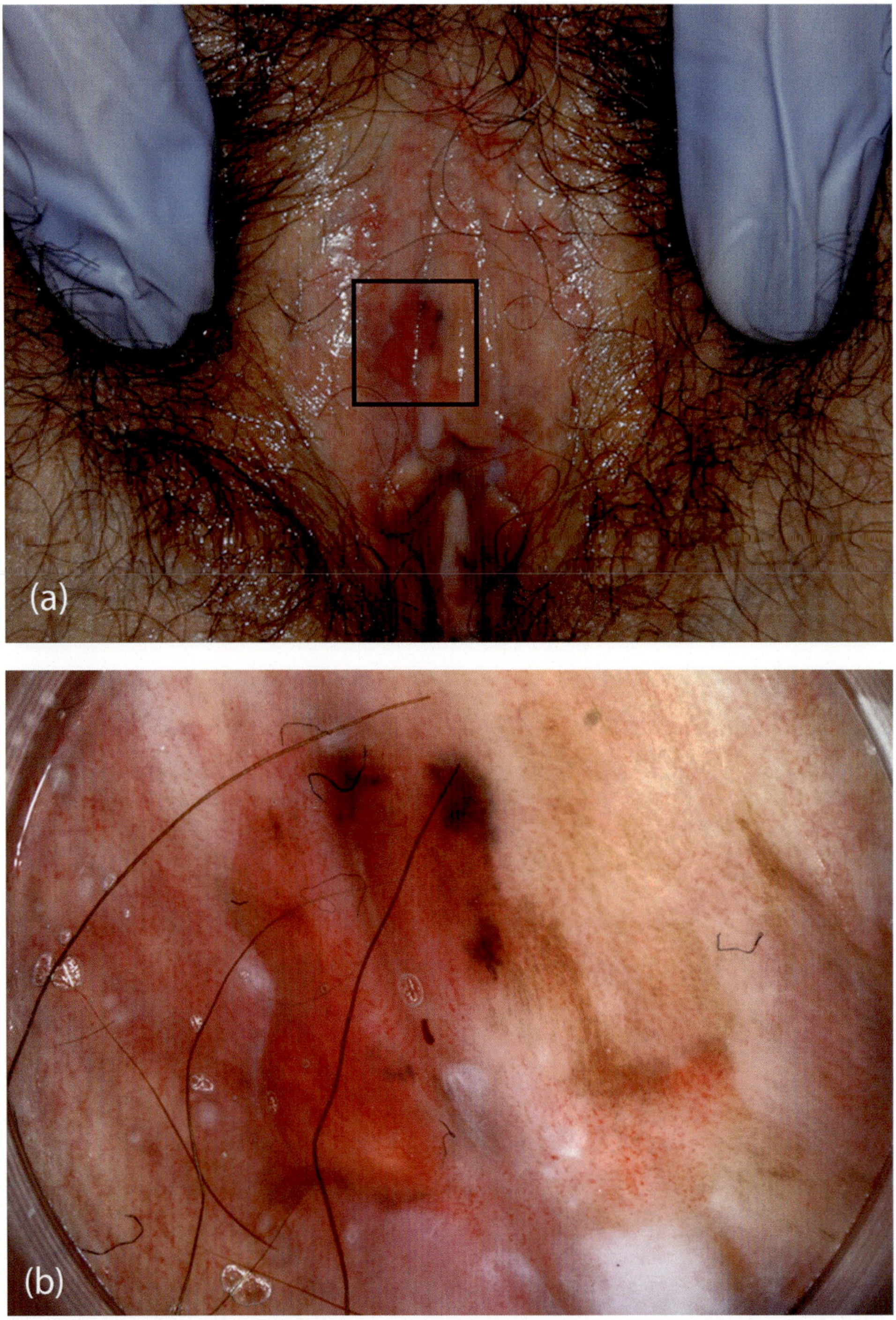

Figure 23.3 (a) Invasive squamous cell carcinoma of clitoral hood, clinically characterized by erosion. The square indicates the area where dermoscopy was performed. (b) Dermoscopy (×7) showing a whitish background surrounding the erosive area which appears red to pinkish in color, with a rich vascularization composed of polymorphous vessels, curvy, linear–irregular and hairpin in shape. Gray to brown blotches are present at the edge of the erosion.

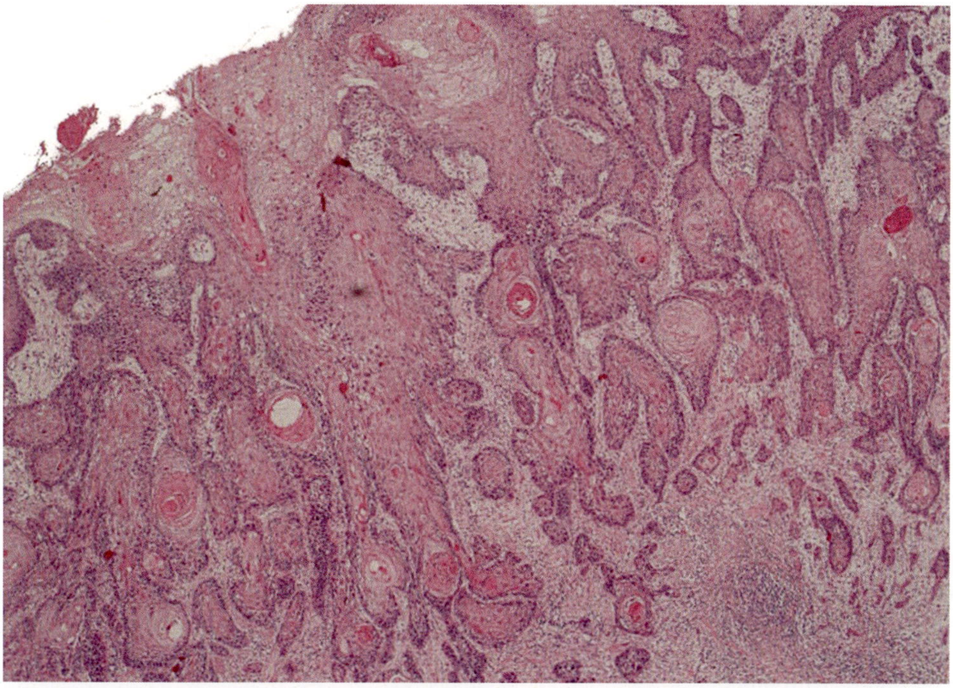

Figure 23.4 Histopathology of the case shown in Figure 23.1. Squamous cell carcinoma with squamous pearls and irregular nests of atypical squamous cells infiltrating the stroma (H&E, ×40).

CHAPTER 24

Extramammary Paget's Disease

Flavio Giulio Liso MD, Pietro Rubegni MD, Jean-Luc Perrot MD, and Elisa Cinotti MD

DEFINITION

Extramammary Paget's disease (EMPD) is a rare cutaneous malignancy that affects the rich in apocrine sweat glands areas. Although perineal, perianal, scrotal, penile, and axillae skin may be affected, the vulva represents the most common localization. It is an intraepithelial adenocarcinoma that may originate from the intraepidermal portion of apocrine sweat glands or primitive basal cells with the ability to differentiate towards glandular elements (1, 2). Less frequently, it can also arise from a visceral tumor that invades the skin (3, 4). EMPD can infiltrate the dermis and form metastases.

EPIDEMIOLOGY

EMPD typically affects the anogenital area in the elderly. Due to its rarity, the precise incidence is unknown and has been reported to range from 0.1 to 2.4 patients per million person-years (4). Although a male predominance exists in Asia, it occurs more frequently in Caucasian women. It commonly affects patients over 65 years of age (4). Familial occurrence is exceedingly rare (5).

ETIOLOGY

Primary EMPD is not associated with other tumors and appears to be of apocrine origin. Secondary EMPD represents an extension of an underlying adnexal adenocarcinoma or an underlying visceral malignancy (but often without anatomical or histological continuity), most commonly urothelial, cervical, ovarian, or endometrial for vulvar forms, anorectal for perianal and perineal forms, and prostatic or urothelial for forms of the male genital organs (2).

CLINICAL FEATURES

The genital and perianal regions are the most frequently affected sites. Cases of "ectopic EMPD" have been described and are localized in particular on the cheek, abdomen and external ear (5).

EMPD lesions present as a well-demarcated slow growing erythematous or brown patch or plaque [Figures 24.1(a) and 24.2(a)]. Scattered hyperkeratotic areas of white scales and erosion can give a "strawberries and cream" appearance (6). Eczematous areas may be present. Erythema of the covered underpants area has been described as a sign of advanced stage EMPD

 DOI: 10.1201/9781003007166-24

with lymphatic infiltration (7). The lesions may become erosive or ulcerated with nodule formation and bleeding at a later stage. Hypo- and hyperpigmentation can occur. Although EMPD generally arises as a single lesion, simultaneous multiple lesions involving the anogenital and axillary regions have been described. The distribution of the disease has a characteristically asymmetric development. Subjective symptoms can be present and include itching, burning, and pain (4).

DIFFERENTIAL DIAGNOSIS

This clinical entity is frequently misdiagnosed, since EMPD may mimic skin infectious, benign inflammatory skin diseases and malignant conditions. When symptoms or lesions persist and empiric therapy fails, clinicians should be alerted to consider an alternative diagnosis. The most frequent differential diagnoses are eczema (allergic or irritant contact dermatitis), fungal infection, psoriasis, seborrheic dermatitis, lichen sclerosus, Bowen's disease, squamous cell carcinoma, basal cell carcinoma, melanoma (especially for pigmented EMPD), mycosis fungoides, histiocytosis, hidradenitis suppurativa, or Crohn's disease (8).

DIAGNOSIS

The correct diagnosis is usually delayed by an average of 2 years (2). Early diagnosis of EMPD is desirable for a favorable prognosis because a delayed diagnosis can result in a more extensive lesion, dermal invasion or distant metastasis. Although there are few data on the diagnostic accuracy of non-invasive dermatologic imaging techniques for EMPD lesions, it seems that dermoscopy and reflectance confocal microscopy (9, 10) can add relevant information that, integrated with clinical examination, may assist this challenging diagnosis and help to define surgical margins (11). The definitive diagnosis of EMPD is based on histopathological examination (see below) (11).

DERMOSCOPY

Owing to its rarity, dermoscopic features of EMPD are not yet well established. Dermoscopic characteristics can be similar to those of several conditions including eczematous dermatitis, fungal infection, Bowen's disease, and basal cell carcinoma (12). Pigmented forms can mimic melanoma (13). For educational purposes, two EMPD dermoscopic entities can be distinguished: non-pigmented and pigmented EMPD. In non-pigmented lesions, vascular structures, like dotted, glomerular and linear vessels, milky red areas, shiny white lines, white clods or white structureless areas resembling stratus clouds are more common [Figures 24.1(b)–(d) and 24.2(b)] (14, 15). Surface scales and erosions may also be detected. Polymorphous vessels and ulceration are more frequently observed in invasive lesions (10). In pigmented forms, gray/brown dots and globules and gray/brown structureless areas have been reported (15). In a case of scrotal EMPD, a white negative pigment network consisting of a linear arrangement of globules on a white background has been described.

Red dots and yellow scales could aid in differentiating eczema from EMPD. In fungal infection, scales are more peripheral and vessels are fewer. Milky red area, polymorphous vessels, shiny white lines, pigmentation and ulceration are also found in melanoma (11). However, melanoma has a faster extension.

HISTOPATHOLOGICAL CORRELATION

Typical histopathological findings of EMPD include isolated or aggregated in nests, roundish cells with ample pale cytoplasm and large pleomorphic nuclei, sometimes with a prominent nucleolus (Paget cells) in the epidermis that can be stained by Periodic acid–Schiff (PAS) (Figure 24.3) (11). Immunohistochemistry usually shows positivity for eccrine and apocrine markers, such as CK7, and thus helps in the histological differentiation from other diseases such as Bowen's disease, mycosis fungoides, malignant melanoma, and sebaceous carcinoma (4).

Vascular proliferation and dilatation in the papillary dermis correlate with dermoscopic dotted and glomerular vessels and milky red areas. Polymorphous vessels at dermoscopy are associated with invasive EMPD. Dermal melanophages may also be detected and can be seen as gray dots. Bowen's disease and EMPD share dotted and/or glomerular vessels at dermoscopy because both diseases are intraepidermal malignancies with dilated capillaries at the top of dermal papillae. Nevertheless, the patchy distribution of the vessels and the presence of scales and erosions can help to identify Bowen's disease (10). Surface scales in EMPD are related to possible hyperkeratosis of the epidermis.

REFERENCES

1. Miracco C, Francini E, Torre P, et al. Extramammary invasive Paget's disease and apocrine angiomatous hamartoma: an unusual association. Eur J Dermatol 2018;28(6):853–5.
2. McDaniel B, Brown F, Crane JS Extramammary Paget Disease. In: StatPearls [Internet]. Treasure Island, FL: StatPearls Publishing; 2021.
3. Bayan CY, Khanna T, Rotemberg V, et al. A review of non-invasive imaging in extramammary Paget's disease. J Eur Acad Dermatol Venereol 2018;32(11):1862–73.
4. Ito T, Kaku-Ito Y, Furue M. The diagnosis and management of extramammary Paget's disease. Expert Rev Anticancer Ther 2018;18(6):543–53.
5. Simonds RM, Segal RJ, Sharma A. Extramammary Paget's disease: a review of the literature. Int J Dermatol 2019;58(8):871–9.
6. Scarbrough CA, Vrable A, Carr DR. Definition, association with malignancy, biologic behavior, and treatment of ectopic extramammary Paget's disease: a review of the literature. J Clin Aesthet Dermatol 2019;12(8):40–4.
7. Murata Y, Kumano K, Tani M. Underpants-pattern erythema: a previously unrecognized cutaneous manifestation of extramammary Paget's disease of the genitalia with advanced metastatic spread. J Am Acad Dermatol 1999;40(6 Pt 1):949–56.
8. Cinotti E, Galluccio D, Tognetti L, et al. Nipple and areola lesions: review of dermoscopy and reflectance confocal microscopy features. J Eur Acad Dermatol Venereol 2019;33(10):183746.
9. Cinotti E, Galluccio D, Ardigò M, et al. Nipple and areola lesions: dermoscopy and reflectance confocal microscopy features. J Am Acad Dermatol 2019;81(2):610–3.
10. Terrier JE, Tiffet O, Raynaud N, Cinotti E. In vivo reflectance confocal microscopy combined with the "spaghetti" technique: a new procedure for defining surgical margins of genital Paget disease. Dermatol Surg 2015;41(7):862–4.
11. Wagner G, Sachse MM. Extramammary Paget disease – clinical appearance, pathogenesis, management. J Dtsch Dermatol Ges 2011;9(6):448–54.
12. Barisani A, Dika E, Fanti PA, Patrizi A, Vaccari S. Erythematous plaques of the vulvo-perineal region: diagnostic role of dermatoscopy. J Dtsch Dermatol Ges 2017;15(8):856–9.
13. Bolognia J, Schaffer J, Cerroni L (Eds). Dermatology (4th edition), Elsevier, 2017.
14. Mun JH, Park SM, Kim GW, et al. Clinical and dermoscopic characteristics of extramammary Paget disease: a study of 35 cases. Br J Dermatol 2016;174(5):1104–7.
15. Coras-Stepanek B, von Portatius A, Dyall-Smith D, Stolz W. Dermatoscopy of pigmented extramammary Paget disease simulating melanoma. J Am Acad Dermatol 2012;67(4):e144–6.
16. Payapvipapong K, Nakakes A, Tanaka M. Lava lake structure and cloud-like structureless area: new clues for diagnosing extramammary Paget disease. J Eur Acad Dermatol Venereol 2017;31(10):e459-e461.

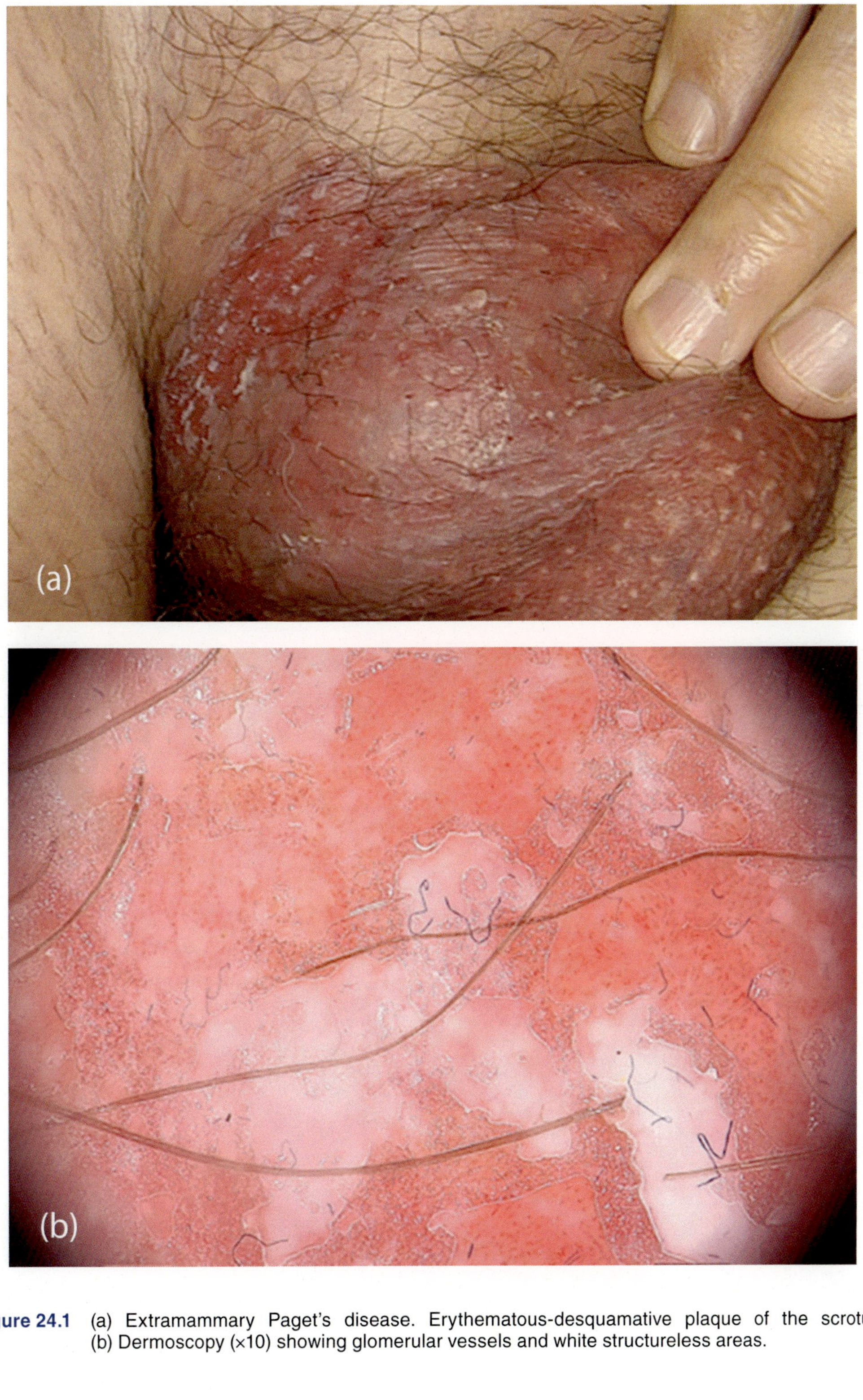

Figure 24.1 (a) Extramammary Paget's disease. Erythematous-desquamative plaque of the scrotum. (b) Dermoscopy (×10) showing glomerular vessels and white structureless areas.

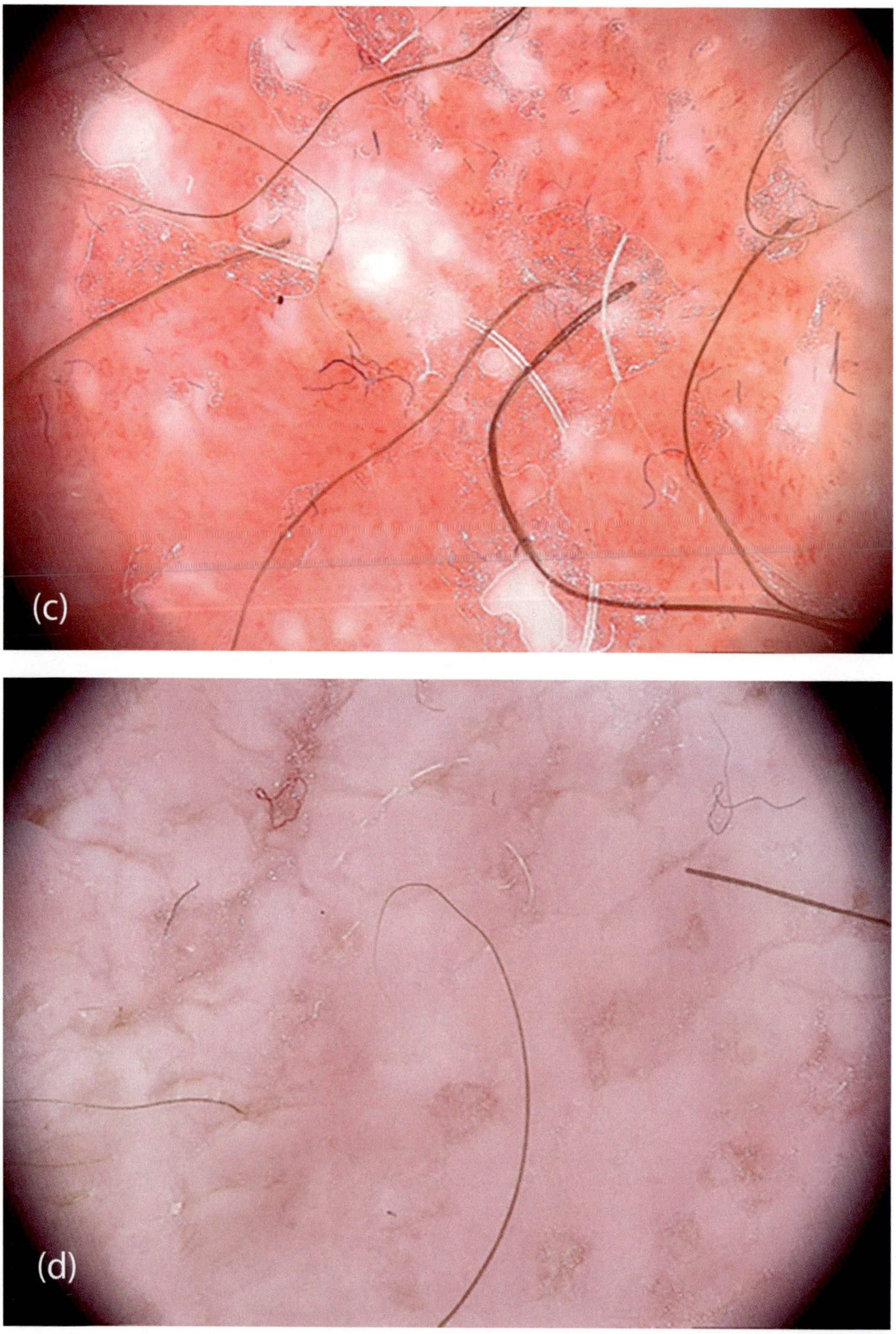

Figure 24.1 (c) Dermoscopy (×10) showing glomerular, linear, and corkscrew irregular vessels, white structureless areas and small milky red areas. (d) Dermoscopy (×10) showing whitish/pinkish structureless areas.

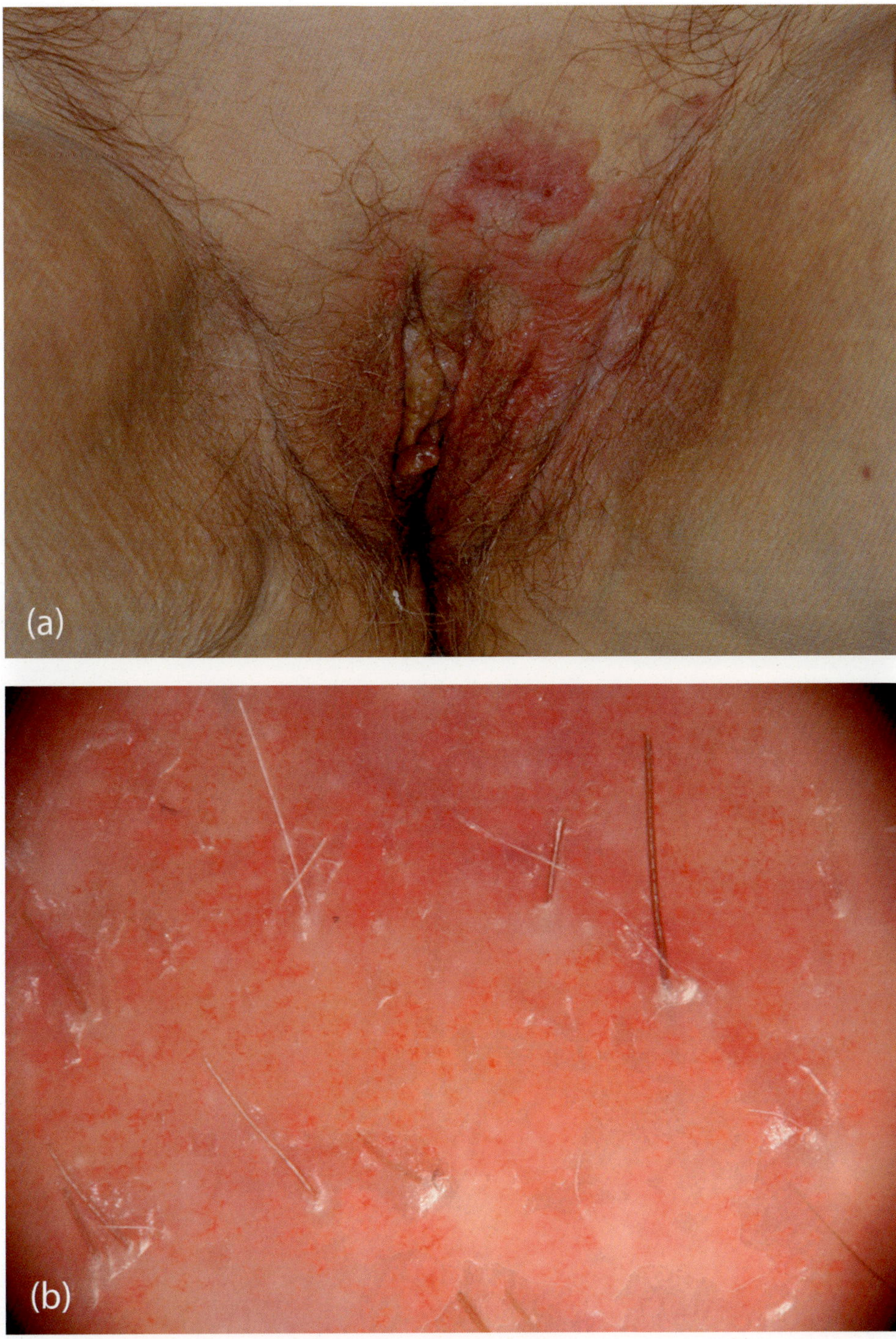

Figure 24.2 (a) Extramammary Paget's disease. Irregular, erythematous plaque involving the vulva and the perivulvar area. (b) Dermoscopy (×10) showing irregular vessels and milky red areas.

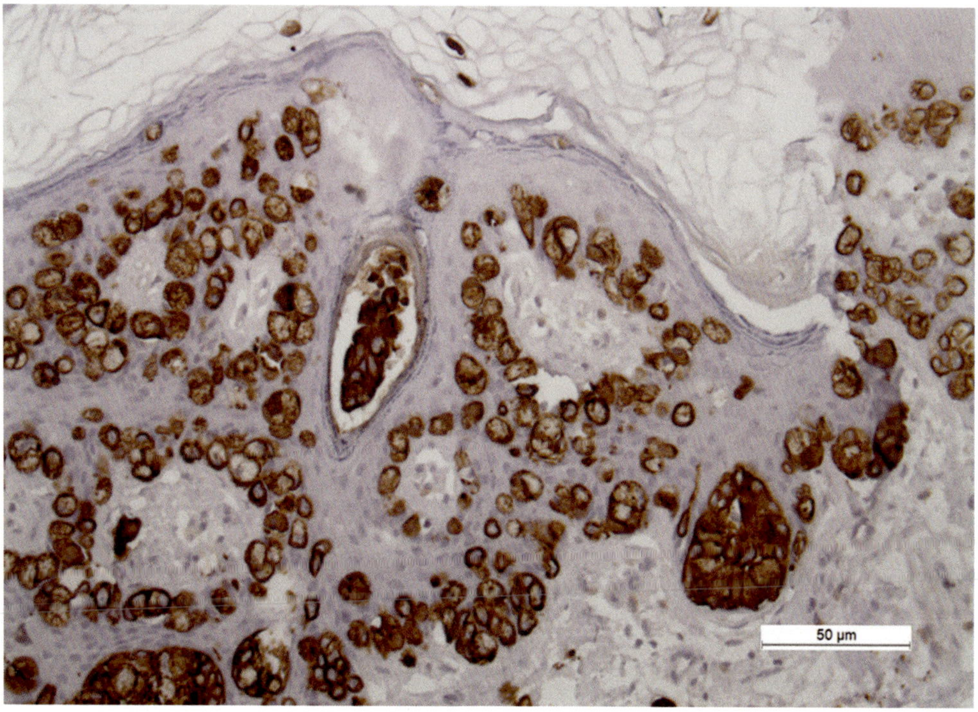

Figure 24.3 Histopathology of extramammary Paget's disease showing large roundish cells in the epidermis corresponding to Paget's cells (CK7, ×20).

CHAPTER 25

Melanoma

Elisa Cinotti MD, Flavio Giulio Liso MD, Pietro Rubegni MD, and Jean-Luc Perrot MD

DEFINITION

Genital melanoma is a malignant tumor that originates from the melanocytes of the mucous membranes (1) and the hairy skin of the genital area. In the latter case, it is mostly described together with mucosal melanoma due to its sun shielded location and continuity with mucosa which covers most of the genital area (2). Genital melanoma is a rare and aggressive tumor with an unfavorable prognosis.

EPIDEMIOLOGY

A small share of melanomas occurs in the genital area. Primary genital melanoma includes less than 1% of the total melanomas and 3% of melanomas in women (3). The median age at diagnosis is around 60 years (4). Most of the cases are in older women and involve the vulva and vagina. The female genital tract accounts for 18% of all mucosal melanomas (2) and vulvar melanoma is the second most common malignancy of the vulva, after squamous cell carcinoma. The 5-year survival rate is very low (<25%) (5). Rarely, genital melanoma can occur in men, mainly in the glans penis (1, 6).

ETIOLOGY

The etiology of genital melanoma remains unclear. Due to its anatomic site of origin, ultraviolet light exposure, known risk factor for cutaneous melanomas, cannot be implicated in the occurrence of genital melanoma. Possible risk factors are chronic inflammatory diseases and exposure to irritants. No association with viral infections has been drawn (2, 7). Moreover, mucosal melanomas have different mutation profiles than cutaneous melanomas: BRAF mutations are infrequent and unlike cutaneous melanoma, there is an increased rate of c-KIT overexpression. This comparatively higher proportion of c-KIT mutations and lower proportion of BRAF mutations suggests that mucosal melanoma has different biology than cutaneous melanoma (3).

DOI: 10.1201/9781003007166-25

CLINICAL FEATURES

Clinically, genital melanoma is often a solitary, brown to black macule. However, it is estimated that about a fifth of mucosal melanomas are amelanotic, which makes the diagnosis even more difficult (2). In the initial phase of growth, genital melanomas are indolent, asymptomatic, and most people do not undergo medical attention until swelling, ulceration, and bleeding occur. Long-lasting lesions are asymmetric, large, and irregular in outline patches or plaques/nodular lesions, with a wide range of colors, including white, red, and blue [Figures 25.1(a), 25.2(a), and 25.3(a)]. The lesions can also be ulcerated [Figures 25.1(a), 25.2(a), and 25.3(a)], polypoid and papillomatous (3, 6). Occasionally, satellite lesions surround the initial tumor (1, 3, 8).

DIFFERENTIAL DIAGNOSIS

Melanomas should be differentiated from other pigmented lesions, including nevi and melanoses (9). Genital nevi tend to present clinically as evenly pigmented papules or macules with regular borders. Their colors range from red to dark brown-black and they typically measure less than 1 cm. Genital melanosis is characterized by single or multiple, irregularly pigmented, tan to black macules or patches with uneven borders.

DIAGNOSIS

Early diagnosis is the mainstay to improve the prognosis of this tumor. Dermoscopy and reflectance confocal microscopy are widely used non-invasive imaging techniques to help the clinical diagnosis of skin melanoma (10), but their diagnostic performance for mucosal melanoma is not well established. These techniques are applicable only to the skin and external mucosa of the genitalia that are the most frequently affected sites. The examination and evaluation of mucosal lesions with these techniques could be more problematic than in other body sites. First, especially in female patients, the lesion may be on a location difficult to examine and patients may be embarrassed; second, the dermoscopic findings could be affected by the mucosa stretching during the examination; and third, the contact probes should be protected or disinfected to prevent infection (11, 12).

DERMOSCOPY

There are few data on dermoscopy of genital melanoma and they are mainly driven from small studies and case reports (13–16). Multicomponent and structureless are the most frequently reported dermoscopic patterns [Figures 25.1(b) and (c), 25.2(b) and (c), and 25.3(b)] (12, 14, 17). Multicomponent pattern is defined, according to Ronger-Savle et al., as the presence in the same lesion of multiple patterns, like the homogeneous, reticular, and the globular ones combined asymmetrically (14). According to Blum et al., structureless pattern could be defined as the absence of any discernible structure (dots, globules or clods, circles, or lines) (16). One of the main dermoscopic features of genital melanoma is the presence of multiple colors, being blue, gray, and white the most frequent (16). Moreover, dermoscopic features that support the diagnosis of cutaneous melanoma, such as blue-whitish veil, regression structures, irregular streaks, and irregular globules were also found.

Vessels are often visible and are irregular or form milky-red areas [Figures 25.1(b) and (c), 25.2(b) and (c), and 25.3(b)] (18).

Ronger-Savle et al. proposed an algorithm for vulvar pigmented lesions derived from multiple correspondence analysis. They gave one or two points for each variable statistically associated with melanoma (multicomponent pattern, blue-whitish veil, irregular vessels, three or more colors, palpable lesion, unilateral and unifocal lesion, polycircular pattern, white veil, and irregular globules) and a total score four was defined as a threshold for the diagnosis of melanoma. Sensitivity and specificity were respectively 100% and 94% (14). Blum et al. established two diagnostic models for the diagnosis of mucosal melanoma by dermoscopy. According to the first model, the presence of blue, gray, or white color plus the presence of a structureless zone (even if only parts of the lesion were structureless) was regarded as suspicious. Regarding the diagnosis of melanoma, this model had a sensitivity of 100% and a specificity of 82.2%. In the second model, they used only colors: every lesion that contained blue, gray, or white color was regarded as suspicious, irrespective of the pattern. The sensitivity for melanoma of this model was 100%, the specificity 64.3% (16).

HISTOPATHOLOGICAL CORRELATION

Histopathologically, many genital melanomas are of the mucosal lentiginous subtype, but they can also be of the superficial spreading or nodular subtypes, especially on keratinized surfaces (Figures 25.4 and 25.5) (19). The presence of structureless brown areas and the presence of gray may be indicative of an early stage. On the contrary, multicomponent patterns and additional colors, especially blue or white, seem to be more indicative of late stages because they are correlated with more irregular cell proliferation (multicomponent pattern), a deep proliferation of pigmented cells (blue) or loss of differentiation of the melanocytes and fibrosis (loss of pigmentation, white areas) (20).

REFERENCES

1. Tacastacas JD, Bray J, Cohen YK, et al. Update on primary mucosal melanoma. J Am Acad Dermatol 2014;71(2):366–75.
2. Mihajlovic M, Vlajkovic S, Jovanovic P, Stefanovic V. Primary mucosal melanomas: a comprehensive review. Int J Clin Exp Pathol 2012;5(8):739–53.
3. Shokrani M. Evaluation of 6 patients with genital melanoma from onset of symptoms to death: evaluate the factors affecting the prognosis of the disease. Med Arch 2015;69(5):293–7.
4. Cinotti E, Chevallier J, Labeille B, et al. Mucosal melanoma: clinical, histological and c-kit gene mutational profile of 86 French cases. J Eur Acad Dermatol Venereol 2017;31(11):1834–40.
5. Hahn HM, Lee KG, Choi W, et al. An updated review of mucosal melanoma: survival meta-analysis. Mol Clin Oncol 2019;11(2):116–126.
6. Özkur E, Altunay İK. Primary scrotal melanoma: it is time to destigmatize genital lesions. An Bras Dermatol 2019;94(6):721–23.
7. Yde SS, Sjoegren P, Heje M, Stolle LB. Mucosal melanoma: a literature review. Curr Oncol Rep 2018;20(3):28.
8. Cinotti E, Couzan C, Perrot JL, et al. In vivo confocal microscopic substrate of grey colour in melanosis. J Eur Acad Dermatol Venereol 2015;29(12):2458–62.
9. Murzaku EC, Penn LA, Hale CS, et al. Vulvar nevi, melanosis, and melanoma: an epidemiologic, clinical, and histopathologic review. J Am Acad Dermatol 2014;71(6):1241–9.
10. Argenziano G, Soyer HP, Chimenti S, et al. Dermoscopy of pigmented skin lesions: results of a consensus meeting via the internet. J Am Acad Dermatol 2003;48(5):679–93.
11. Hofmann-Wellenhof R. Special criteria for special locations 2: scalp, mucosal, and milk line. Dermatol Clin 2013;31(4):625–36, ix.

12. Cinotti E, Campoli M, Pataia G, et al. How transparent film applied on dermatologic imaging devices in order to prevent infections affects image quality? Skin Res Technol 2019;25(2):229–33.
13. Lin J, Koga H, Takata M, Saida T. Dermoscopy of pigmented lesions on mucocutaneous junction and mucous membrane. Br J Dermatol 2009;161(6):1255–61.
14. Ferrari A, Zalaudek I, Argenziano G, et al. Dermoscopy of pigmented lesions of the vulva: a retrospective morphological study. Dermatology 2011;222(2):157–66.
15. Ronger-Savle S, Julien V, Duru G, Raudrant D, et al. Features of pigmented vulval lesions on dermoscopy. Br J Dermatol 2011;164(1):54–61.
16. Oakley A. Dermatoscopic features of vulval lesions in 97 women. Australas J Dermatol 2016;57(1):48–53.
17. Blum A, Simionescu O, Argenziano G, et al. Dermoscopy of pigmented lesions of the mucosa and the mucocutaneous junction: results of a multicenter study by the International dermoscopy society (IDS). Arch Dermatol 2011;147(10):1181–7.
18. Rogers T, Pulitzer M, Marino ML, et al. Early diagnosis of genital mucosal melanoma: how good are our dermoscopic criteria? Dermatol Pract Concept 2016;6(4):43–46.
19. Nucci MR, Parra-Herran C (Eds). Gynecologic Pathology (Vulvar Neoplasia) Elsevier, Churchill Livingston, 2009, pp. 31–75.
20. Papageorgiou C, Ioannides D, Apalla Z, et al. Dermoscopy of difficult-to-diagnose melanomas. Serbian J Dermatol Venereol 2016;8(3):121–27.

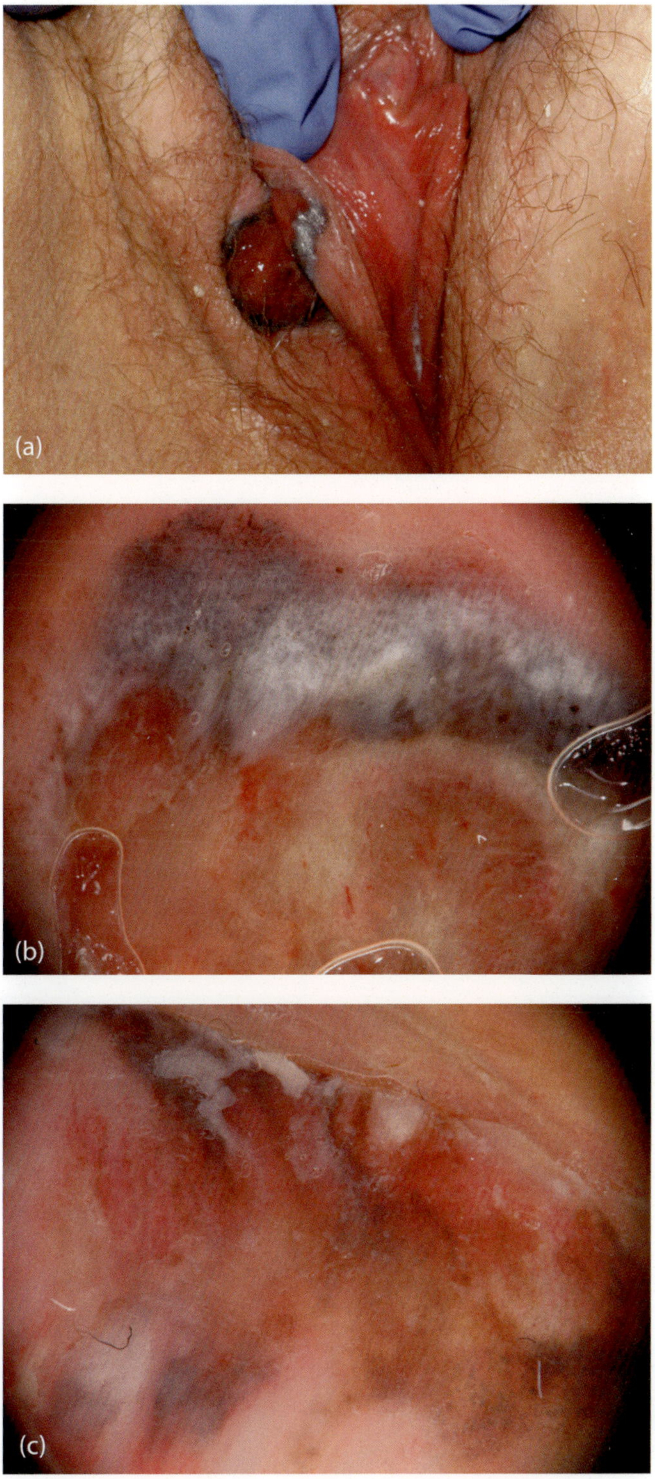

Figure 25.1 (a) Melanoma of the vulva. Reddish nodule with peripheral pigmentation. (b) Dermoscopy (×10) showing structureless white and pinkish areas, irregular vessels, and irregular brown globules and dots. (c) Dermoscopy (×10) showing structureless white, pinkish and gray areas, irregular vessels, milky red areas, blue-white veil, irregular brown and gray globules and dots.

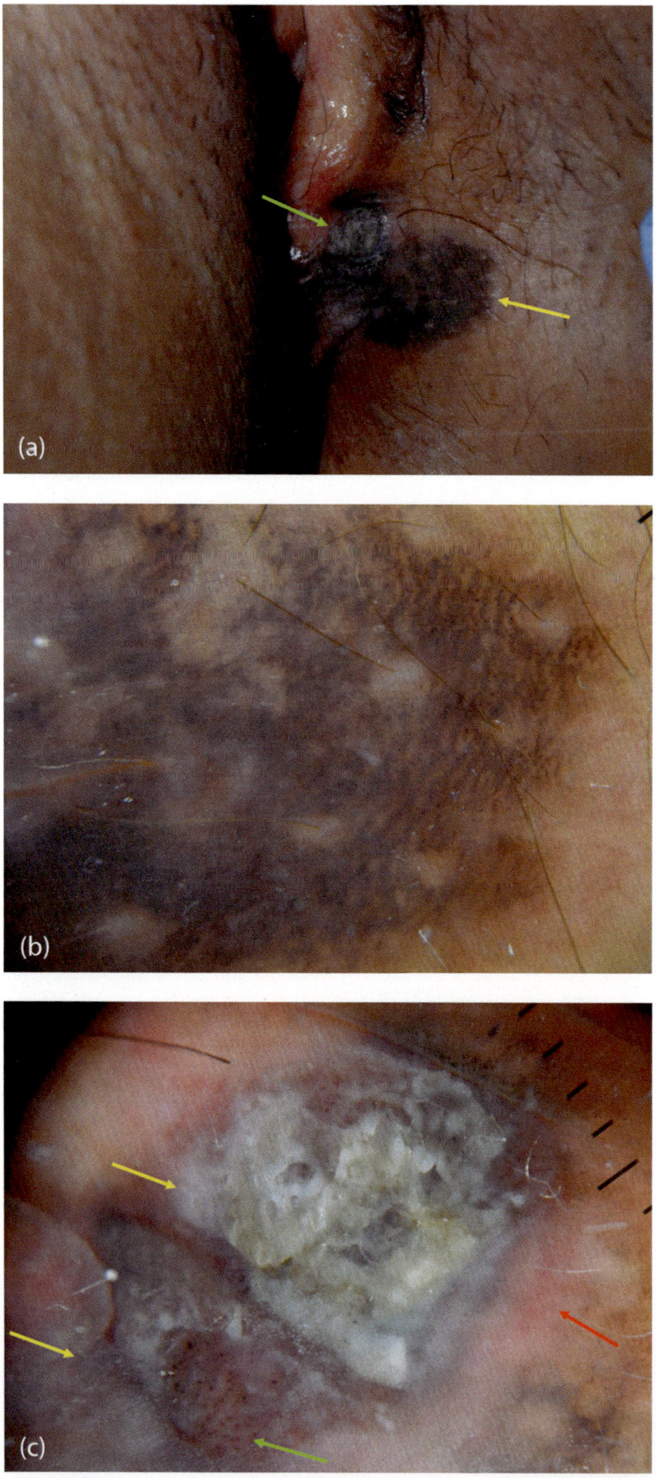

Figure 25.2 (a) Melanoma of the vulva. Brownish lesion showing both a nodular (green arrow) and a macular (yellow arrow) component. (b) Dermoscopy (×10) of the macular area showing an atypical reticular pattern. (c) Dermoscopy (×10) of the nodular component showing structureless whitish and grayish areas (yellow arrows), milky red areas (red arrow), and ulceration (green arrow).

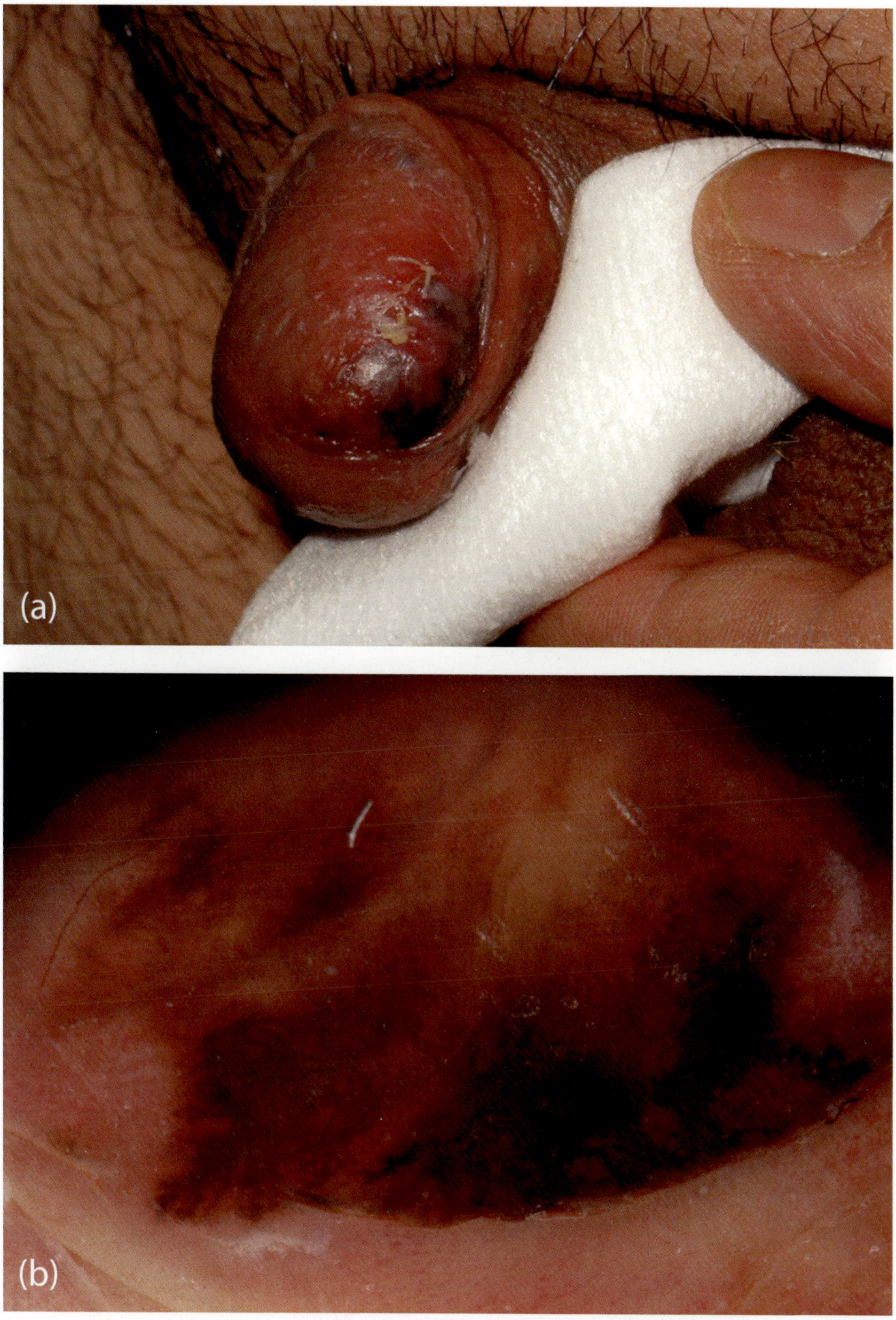

Figure 25.3 (a) Melanoma of the penis. Multicolored macule of the glans. (b) Dermoscopy (×10) showing structureless brown areas, irregular lines (irregular network-like pattern) and irregular peripheral streaks.

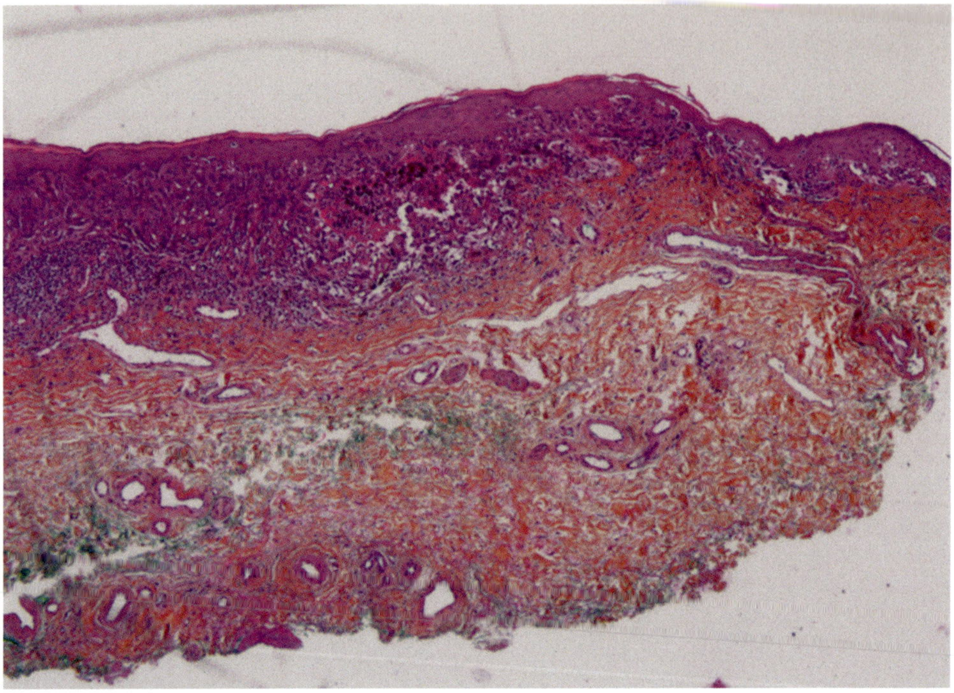

Figure 25.4 Histopathology of the melanoma of Figure 25.1 showing an atypical melanocyte proliferation (H&E, ×50).

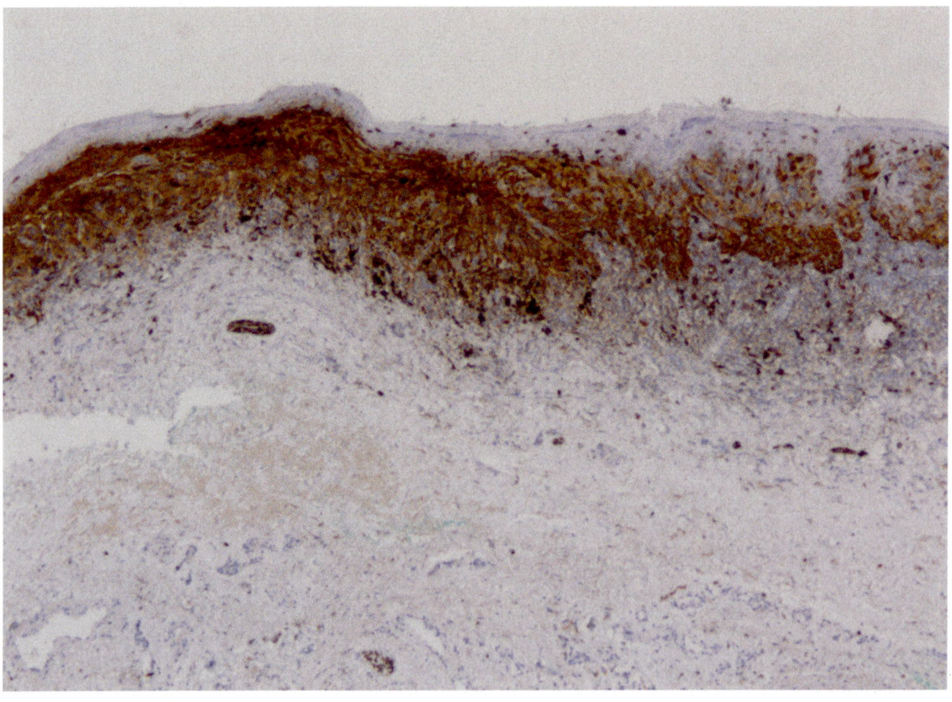

Figure 25.5 Histopathology of the melanoma of Figure 25.1 showing an atypical melanocyte proliferation (PS100, ×50).